GW00578206

Pharmacokinetics

DRUGS AND THE PHARMACEUTICAL SCIENCES

A Series of Textbooks and Monographs

Edited by
James Swarbrick
School of Pharmacy
University of North Carolina
Chapel Hill, North Carolina

Other Volumes in Preparation

Pharmacokinetics

SECOND EDITION, REVISED AND EXPANDED

Milo Gibaldi
University of Washington
School of Pharmacy
Seattle, Washington

Donald Perrier
School of Pharmacy
University of Arizona
Tucson, Arizona

MARCEL DEKKER, INC.   New York and Basel

Library of Congress Cataloging in Publication Data

Gibaldi, Milo.
    Pharmacokinetics.

    (Drugs and the pharmaceutical sciences; v. 15)
    Includes bibliographical references and indexes.
    1. Pharmacokinetics. I. Perrier, Donald.
II. Title. III. Series. [DNLM: 1. Drugs—Metabolism.
2. Kinetics. W1 DR893B v.14 / QV 38 G437p]
RM301.5.G5 1982   615'.7   82-4608
ISBN 0-8247-1042-8

MARCEL DEKKER, INC.
270 Madison Avenue, New York, New York 10016

Current printing (last digit):
10   9   8   7   6   5

PRINTED IN THE UNITED STATES OF AMERICA

Preface

Pharmacokinetics is the study of the time course of drug absorption, distribution, metabolism, and excretion. It also concerns the relationship of these processes to the intensity and time course of pharmacologic (therapeutic and toxicologic) effects of drugs and chemicals. Pharmacokinetics is a quantitative study that requires a preexisting competence in mathematics at least through calculus. It is also a biologic study and can be very useful to the biomedical scientist.

At a fundamental level, pharmacokinetics is a tool to optimize the design of biological experiments with drugs and chemicals. All biologists would benefit from some knowledge of pharmacokinetics whenever they engage in data analysis. It has become increasingly important in the design and development of new drugs and in the reassessment of old drugs. Clinical applications of pharmacokinetics have resulted in improvements in drug utilization and direct benefits to patients.

There is consensus that the origin of pharmacokinetics can be traced to two papers entitled "Kinetics of distribution of substances administered to the body" written by Torsten Teorell and published in the *International Archives of Pharmacodynamics* in 1937. Since this unheralded beginning, the study of pharmacokinetics has matured rapidly; undoubtedly growth has been stimulated by major breakthroughs in analytical chemistry, which permit us to quantitatively detect minute concentrations of drugs and chemicals in exceedingly small volumes of biological fluids, in data processing, and by the brilliant insights of many scientists. Dost, Kruger-Theimer, Nelson, Wagner, Riegelman, and Levy are among those scientists and must be reserved a special place in the history of the development of pharmacokinetics.

Our goals in preparing this revision were similar to those that prompted us to undertake the initial effort. The need for revision was amply clear to us each time we looked at our files, bulging with research papers and commentaries on pharmacokinetic methods and applications published since 1975. The buzz words today are clearance concepts, noncompartmental models, and physiologic pharmacokinetics. Again, we strived to present the material in an explicit and detailed manner. We continue to believe that *Pharmacokinetics* can be used in formal courses, for self-study, or for reference purposes.

We thank our colleagues for their work and publications, our staffs for their labors and support, and our families for their love and understanding.

Milo Gibaldi
Donald Perrier

Contents

Contents

1
One-Compartment Model

The most commonly employed approach to the pharmacokinetic characterization of a drug is to represent the body as a system of compartments, even though these compartments usually have no physiologic or anatomic reality, and to assume that the rate of transfer between compartments and the rate of drug elimination from compartments follow first-order or linear kinetics. The one-compartment model, the simplest model, depicts the body as a single, kinetically homogeneous unit. This model is particularly useful for the pharmacokinetic analysis of drugs that distribute relatively rapidly throughout the body. Almost invariably, the plasma or serum is the anatomical reference compartment for the one-compartment model, but we do not assume that the drug concentration in plasma is equal to the concentration of drug in other body fluids or in tissues, for this is rarely the case. Rather, we assume that the rate of change of drug concentration in plasma reflects quantitatively the change in drug concentrations throughout the body. In other words, if we see a 20% decrease in drug concentration in plasma over a certain period of time, we assume that the drug concentrations in kidney, liver, cerebrospinal fluid, and all other fluids and tissues also decrease by 20% during this time.

Drug elimination from the body can and often does occur by several pathways, including urinary and biliary excretion, excretion in expired air, and biotransformation in the liver or other fluids or tissues. Glomerular filtration in the kidneys is clearly a diffusional process, the rate of which can be characterized by first-order kinetics, but tubular secretion in the kidneys, biliary secretion, and biotransformation usually involves enzymatic (active) processes that are capacity limited. However, as demonstrated in subsequent sections of the text dealing with capacity-limited and nonlinear processes (Chap. 7), at low concentrations of drug (i.e., concentrations typically associated with therapeutic doses) the rate of these enzymatic processes can be approximated very well by first-order kinetics. Hence we find

1

that the elimination of most drugs in humans and animals following therapeutic or nontoxic doses can be characterized as an apparent first-order process (i.e., the rate of elimination of drug from the body at any time is proportional to the amount of drug in the body at that time). The proportionality constant relating the rate and amount is the first-order elimination rate constant. Its units are reciprocal time (i.e., min^{-1} or h^{-1}). The first-order elimination rate constant characterizing the overall elimination of a drug from a one-compartment model is usually written as K and usually represents the sum of two or more rate constants characterizing individual elimination processes:

$$K = k_e + k_m + k'_m + k_b + \cdots \tag{1.1}$$

where k_e and k_b are apparent first-order elimination rate constants for renal and biliary excretion, respectively, and k_m and k'_m are apparent first-order rate constants for two different biotransformation (metabolism) processes. These constants are usually referred to as apparent first-order rate constants to convey the fact that the kinetics only approximate first-order.

INTRAVENOUS INJECTION

Drug Concentrations in the Plasma

Following rapid intravenous injection of a drug that distributes in the body according to a one-compartment model and is eliminated by apparent first-order kinetics, the rate of loss of drug from the body is given by

$$\frac{dX}{dt} = -KX \tag{1.2}$$

where X is the amount of drug in the body at time t after injection. K, as defined above, is the apparent first-order elimination rate constant for the drug. The negative sign indicates that drug is being lost from the body.

To describe the time course of the amount of drug in the body after injection, Eq. (1.2) must be integrated. The method of Laplace transforms in Appendix A will be employed. The transform of (1.2) is

$$s\overline{X} - X_0 = -K\overline{X} \tag{1.3}$$

where X_0 is the amount injected (i.e., the dose) and s is the Laplace operator. Rearrangement of (1.3) yields

$$\overline{X} = \frac{X_0}{s + K} \tag{1.4}$$

which when solved using a table of Laplace transforms (Appendix A) gives

$$X = X_0 e^{-Kt} \qquad (1.5)$$

where e represents the base of the natural logarithm. Taking the natural logarithm of both sides of (1.5) gives

$$\ln X = \ln X_0 - Kt \qquad (1.6)$$

Then, based on the relationship

$$2.303 \log a = \ln a \qquad (1.7)$$

Eq. (1.6) can be converted to common logarithms (base 10, log):

$$\log X = \log X_0 - \frac{Kt}{2.303} \qquad (1.8)$$

The body is obviously not homogeneous even if plasma concentration and urinary excretion data can be described by representing the body as a one-compartment model. Drug concentrations in the liver, kidneys, heart, muscle, fat, and other tissues usually differ from one another as well as from the concentration in the plasma. If the relative binding of a drug to components of these tissues and fluids is essentially independent of drug concentration, the ratio of drug concentrations in the various tissues and fluids is constant. Consequently, there will exist a constant relationship between drug concentration in the plasma C and the amount of drug in the body:

$$X = VC \qquad (1.9)$$

The proportionality constant V in this equation has the units of volume and is known as the apparent volume of distribution. Despite its name, this constant usually has no direct physiologic meaning and does not refer to a real volume. For example, the apparent volume of distribution of a drug in a 70 kg human can be several hundred liters.

The relationship between plasma concentration and the amount of drug in the body, as expressed by Eq. (1.9), enables the conversion of Eq. (1.8) from an amount-time to a concentration-time relationship:

$$\log C = \log C_0 - \frac{Kt}{2.303} \qquad (1.10)$$

where C_0 is the drug concentration in plasma immediately after injection. Equation (1.10) indicates that a plot of log C versus t will be linear under the conditions stated (Fig. 1.1). C_0 may be obtained by extrapolation of the log C versus t plot to time zero. This intercept, C_0, may be used in the calculation of the apparent volume of distribution. Since X_0 equals the amount of drug injected intravenously (i.e., the intravenous dose), V may be estimated from the relationship

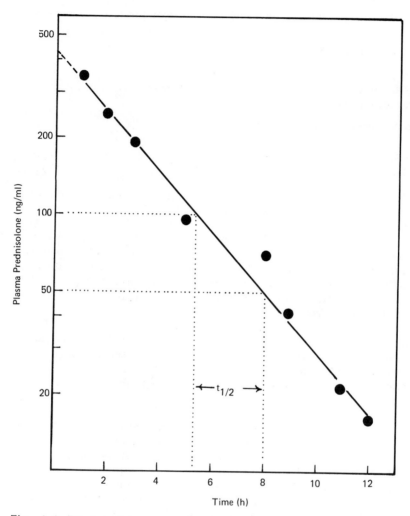

Fig. 1.1 Prednisolone concentration in plasma following an intravenous dose equivalent to 20 mg prednisone to a kidney transplant
patient. The data show monoexponential decline that can be described
by Eq. (1.10). C_0 = intravenous dose/V; slope = $-K/2.303$. (Data
from Ref. 1.)

$$V = \frac{\text{intravenous dose}}{C_0} \qquad (1.11)$$

Equation (1.11) is theoretically correct only for a one-compartment
model where instantaneous distribution of drug between plasma and

tissues takes place. Since this is rarely true, a calculation based on Eq. (1.11) will almost always overestimate the apparent volume of distribution. Sometimes the error is trivial, but often the overestimate is substantial and the calculation may be misleading. More accurate and more general methods of estimating V will be discussed subsequently.

The slope of the line resulting from a plot of log C versus time is equal to $-K/2.303$ and K may be estimated directly from this slope. It is easier, however, to estimate K from the relationship

$$K = \frac{0.693}{t_{1/2}} \qquad\qquad (1.12)$$

where $t_{1/2}$ is the biologic or elimination half-life of the drug. This parameter is readily determined from a semilogarithmic plot of plasma drug concentration (on logarithmic scale) versus time (on linear scale), as illustrated in Fig. 1.1. The time required for the drug concentration at any point on the straight line to decrease by one-half is the biologic half-life. An important characteristic of first-order processes is that the time required for a given concentration to decrease by a given percentage is independent of concentration. Equation (1.12) is easily derived by setting C equal to $C_0/2$ and t equal to $t_{1/2}$ in Eq. (1.10).

In principle, a plot of the logarithm of tissue drug concentration versus time should also be linear and give exactly the same slope as the plasma concentration-time curve. This is illustrated in Fig. 1.2.

Estimates of C_0, $t_{1/2}$, and K are often obtained from the best straight-line fit (by eye) to the log C versus time data. However, a more objective method is to convert all concentration values to logarithms, and then to determine the best-fitting line by the method of least squares, described in elementary textbooks of statistics [3]. Computer programs are available (see Appendix H) that do not require logarithmic conversions for nonlinear least-squares fitting of data.

Urinary Excretion Data

It is sometimes possible to determine the elimination kinetics of a drug from urinary excretion data. This requires that at least some of the drug be excreted unchanged. Consider a drug eliminated from the body partly by renal excretion and partly by nonrenal processes such as biotransformation and biliary excretion, as shown in Scheme 1,

Scheme 1

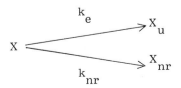

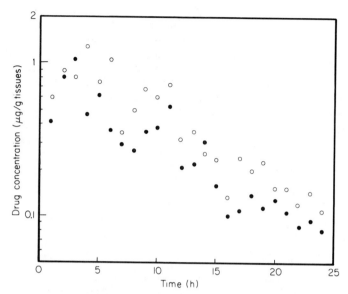

Fig. 1.2 Dipyridamole concentrations in serum (O) and heart tissue (●) after a single oral dose of the drug to guinea pigs. Drug concentrations in serum and heart decline in a parallel manner. (Data from Ref. 2.)

where X_u and X_{nr} are the cumulative amounts of drug eliminated unchanged in the urine and eliminated by all nonrenal pathways, respectively. The elimination rate constant K is the sum of the individual rate constants that characterize the parallel elimination processes. Thus

$$K = k_e + k_{nr} \tag{1.13}$$

where k_e is the apparent first-order rate constant for renal excretion and k_{nr} is the sum of all other apparent first-order rate constants for drug elimination by nonrenal pathways. Since in first-order kinetics, the rate of appearance of intact drug in the urine is proportional to the amount of drug in the body, the excretion rate of unchanged drug, dX_u/dt, can be defined as

$$\frac{dX_u}{dt} = k_e X \tag{1.14}$$

where X is the amount of drug in the body at time t.

Substitution for X according to Eq. (1.5) yields

$$\frac{dX_u}{dt} = k_e X_0 e^{-Kt} \tag{1.15}$$

Therefore,

$$\log \frac{dX_u}{dt} = \log k_e X_0 - \frac{Kt}{2.303} \tag{1.16}$$

Equation (1.16) states that a semilogarithmic plot of excretion rate of unmetabolized drug versus time is linear, with a slope of $-K/2.303$. This slope is the same as that obtained from a semilogarithmic plot of drug concentration in plasma versus time. Thus the elimination rate constant of a drug can be obtained from either plasma concentration or urinary excretion data. It must be emphasized that the slope of the log excretion rate versus time plot is related to the elimination rate constant K, not to the excretion rate constant k_e.

Urinary excretion rates are estimated by collecting all urine for a fixed period of time, determining the concentration of drug in the urine, multiplying the concentration by the volume of urine collected to determine the amount excreted, and dividing the amount excreted by the collection time. These experimentally determined excretion rates are obviously not instantaneous rates (i.e., dX_u/dt) but are average rates over a finite time period (i.e., $\Delta X_u/\Delta t$). However, we often find that the average excretion rate closely approximates the

Table 1.1 Calculation of Excretion Rate Versus Time Data for Estimating Half-Life

t (h)	X_u (mg)	Δt	ΔX_u	$\Delta X_u/\Delta t$ (mg/h)	t_m
0	0.0	1	4.0	4.0	0.5
1	4.0	1	3.8	3.8	1.5
2	7.8	1	3.5	3.5	2.5
3	11.3	3	9.1	3.0	4.5
6	20.4	6	13.5	2.2	9.0
12	33.9	12	14.7	1.2	18.0
24	48.6	12	6.4	0.53	30.0
36	55.0	12	2.8	0.23	42.0
48	57.8				

Note: The symbols are as follows: t, cumulative time after intravenous administration; X_u, cumulative amount of unmetabolized drug excreted in the urine; Δt, urine collection interval; ΔX_u, amount of drug excreted during each interval; $\Delta X_u/\Delta t$, experimentally determined excretion rate; t_m, midpoint of the collection interval.

instantaneous excretion rate at the midpoint of the urine collection period. The validity of this approximation depends on the collection period relative to the half-life of the drug. An individual collection period should not exceed one biologic half-life and, ideally, should be considerably less. These considerations are discussed in Appendix F. It is important to remember that urinary excretion rates must be plotted against the midpoints of the urine collection periods and not at the beginning or end of these periods (see Table 1.1 and Figs. 1.3 and 1.4).

Fluctuations in the rate of drug elimination are reflected to a high degree in excretion rate plots. At times the data are so scattered that an estimate of the half-life is difficult. To overcome this problem an

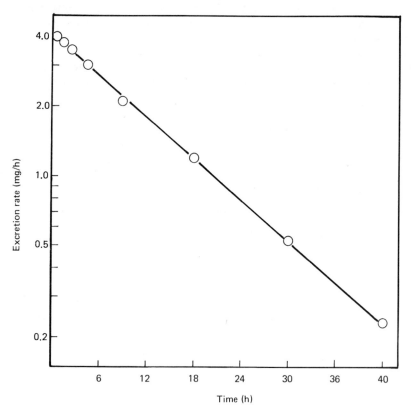

Fig. 1.3 Semilogarithmic plot of excretion rate versus time after intravenous administration of a drug. Data taken from Table 1.1. Each excretion rate is plotted at the midpoint of the urine collection interval. The data are described by Eq. (1.16). Slope = $-K/2.303$.

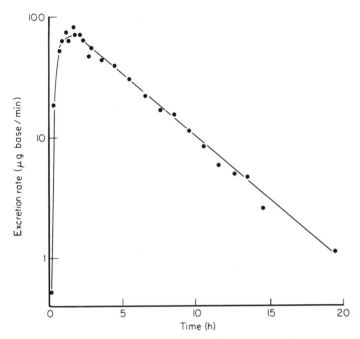

Fig. 1.4 Urinary excretion rate of norephedrine after oral administration of a single dose of the drug to a healthy adult subject. [From Ref. 4. © 1968 American Society for Pharmacology and Experimental Therapeutics, The Williams and Wilkins Company (agent).]

alternative approach, termed the sigma-minus method, is available. This method is considered less sensitive to fluctuations in drug elimination rate. The Laplace transform of Eq. (1.14) is

$$s\overline{X}_u = k_e \overline{X} \tag{1.17}$$

Substitution for $\overline{X}$ from Eq. (1.4) and rearrangement yields

$$\overline{X}_u = \frac{k_e X_0}{s(s + K)} \tag{1.18}$$

which when solved gives the following relationship between amount of drug in the urine and time:

$$X_u = \frac{k_e X_0}{K} (1 - e^{-Kt}) \tag{1.19}$$

where X_u is the cumulative amount of unchanged drug excreted to time t. The amount of unmetabolized drug ultimately eliminated in the urine, X_u^{∞}, can be determined by setting time in (1.19) equal to infinity; it is given by

$$X_u^\infty = \frac{k_e X_0}{K} \tag{1.20}$$

For a drug eliminated solely by renal excretion, $K = k_e$ and the amount ultimately excreted, X_u^∞, will be equal to the intravenous dose, X_0. In all cases the ratio of X_u^∞ to X_0 equals the ratio of k_e to K. This relationship is commonly employed to estimate k_e from urinary excretion data once the half-life of the drug is determined.

Substitution of X_u^∞ for $k_e X_0/K$ in (1.19) and rearrangement yields

$$X_u^\infty - X_u = X_u^\infty e^{-Kt} \tag{1.21}$$

which in logarithmic form is

$$\log (X_u^\infty - X_u) = \log X_u^\infty - \frac{Kt}{2.303} \tag{1.22}$$

The term $(X_u^\infty - X_u)$ is commonly called the *amount* of unchanged drug *remaining* to be *excreted*, or A.R.E. A plot of log A.R.E. versus time is linear (Fig. 1.5) with a slope equal to $-K/2.303$. Hence the elimination rate constant may be estimated from plots of log drug concentration in plasma versus time, log excretion rate versus time (the rate method), and log A.R.E. versus time (the sigma-minus method). To determine X_u^∞, total urine collection must be carried out until no unchanged drug can be detected in the urine. It is incorrect to plot log (dose $- X_u$) rather than log $(X_u^\infty - X_u)$ versus time.

When possible, total urine collection should be continued for a period of time equal to about seven half-lives of the drug to accurately estimate X_u^∞. This can be very difficult if the drug has a long half-life. The problem does not arise if the log excretion rate versus time plots are used since urine need be collected for only three or four half-lives to obtain an accurate estimate of the elimination rate constant. The rate method also obviates the need to collect all urine (i.e., urine samples may be lost or intentionally discarded to minimize the number of assays) since the determination of a single point on a rate plot simply requires the collection of two consecutive urine samples.

Renal Clearance

The kinetics of renal excretion of a drug may be characterized not only by a renal excretion rate constant k_e, but also by a renal clearance Cl_r. The concept of drug clearance is discussed in Chap. 8. At this point it suffices to state that the renal clearance of drug is equal to the volume of blood flowing through the kidneys per unit time from which all drug is extracted and excreted.

The renal clearance of a drug cannot exceed the renal blood flow. Clearance has units of flow (i.e., ml/min or liters/h). In pharmaco-

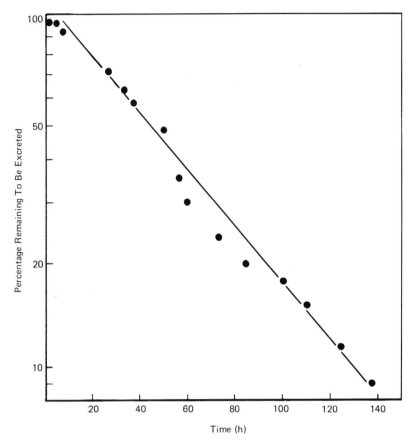

Fig. 1.5 Semilogarithmic plot of the average percentage unmetabolized drug remaining to be excreted versus time after oral administration of 250 mg of chlorpropamide to six healthy subjects. $t_{1/2} = 36$ h. (Data from Ref. 5.)

kinetic terms renal clearance is simply the ratio of urinary excretion rate to drug concentration in the blood or plasma:

$$Cl_r = \frac{dX_u/dt}{C} \qquad (1.23)$$

In practice, renal clearance is estimated by dividing the average urinary excretion rate, $\Delta X_u/\Delta t$, by the drug concentration in plasma at the time corresponding to the midpoint of the urine collection period.

Since excretion rate is the product of the urinary excretion rate constant and the amount of drug in the body [Eq. (1.14)], we can write

$$Cl_r = \frac{k_e X}{C} \tag{1.24}$$

Recognizing that X/C is simply the apparent volume of distribution [Eq. (1.9)], we can shown that renal clearance is the product of the urinary excretion rate constant and the apparent volume of distribution:

$$Cl_r = k_e V \tag{1.25}$$

All clearance terms can be expressed in terms of a rate constant and a volume.

An estimation of renal clearance by means of Eq. (1.23) may be misleading because like all rate processes in the body, renal excretion is subject to biologic variability. A more satisfactory approach is to plot urinary excretion rate versus drug concentration in plasma at the times corresponding to the midpoints of the urine collection periods (see Fig. 1.6). Since rearrangement of Eq. (1.23) yields

$$\frac{dX_u}{dt} = Cl_r C \tag{1.26}$$

the slope of an excretion rate-plasma concentration plot is equal to renal clearance.

A second method for calculating renal clearance requires simultaneous collection of plasma and urine. Integrating Eq. (1.26) from t_1 to t_2 yields

$$(X_u)_{t_1}^{t_2} = Cl_r \int_{t_1}^{t_2} C \, dt, \tag{1.27}$$

where $(X_u)_{t_1}^{t_2}$ is the amount of unmetabolized drug excreted in the urine during the time interval from t_1 to t_2 and $\int_{t_1}^{t_2} C \, dt$ is the area under the drug concentration in plasma versus time curve during the same time interval (see Fig. 1.7). Terms for area have units of concentration-time. A plot of $(X_u)_{t_1}^{t_2}$ versus $\int_{t_1}^{t_2} C \, dt$ yields a straight line with a slope equal to renal clearance.

Integration of Eq. (1.26) from time zero to time infinity, and rearrangement, gives an expression for the average renal clearance over the entire time course of drug in the body after a single dose:

$$Cl_r = \frac{X_u^{\infty}}{\int_0^{\infty} C \, dt} = \frac{X_u^{\infty}}{AUC} \tag{1.28}$$

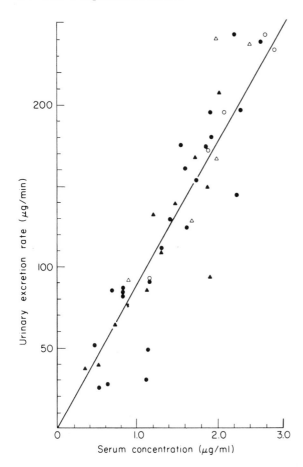

Fig. 1.6 Relationship between urinary excretion rates of tetracycline and serum concentrations of the drug determined at the midpoints of each urine collection interval after oral administration of a 250 mg dose to five healthy adults. Two different oral preparations (●, ▲) were given to each subject. The open symbols (O, Δ) denote the maximum excretion rate for each preparation. The data are described by Eq. (1.26); the slope of the line is equal to the average renal clearance of tetracycline in the group. (Data from Ref. 6.)

The term $\int_0^\infty C\, dt$ or AUC represents the total area under the drug concentration in plasma versus time curve plotted on rectilinear graph paper (see Fig. 1.7). This method has been used to estimate renal clearance (see Fig. 1.8) but is not ideal because it is difficult to collect urine for long periods to get an accurate estimate of X_u^∞, particularly for drugs with long half-lives.

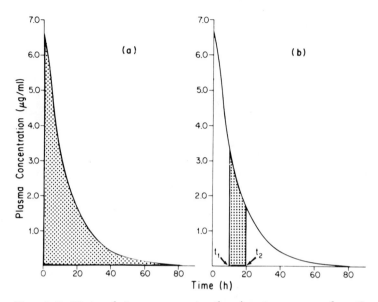

Fig. 1.7 Plots of drug concentration in plasma as a function of time after intravenous administration illustrating, by the shaded region, (a) $\int_0^\infty C\,dt$, the total area under the curve, AUC, and (b) $\int_{t_1}^{t_2} C\,dt$, the partial area under the curve from t_1 to t_2.

Use of Eqs. (1.27) and (1.28) for calculating renal clearance requires the measurement of areas under the drug concentration in plasma versus time curves. Several methods are available for determining the area under a curve. For each of these methods it is essential to obtain a sufficient number of blood samples to characterize adequately the curve or a portion thereof. A planimeter, which is an instrument for mechanically measuring the area of plane figures, is often used to measure the area under the curve (drawn on rectilinear graph paper). Another procedure, known as the cut and weigh method, is to cut out the area under the entire curve on rectilinear graph paper and to weigh it on an analytical balance. The weight thus obtained is converted to the proper units by dividing it by the weight of a unit area of the same paper. A third method to determine the area under the curve is to estimate it by means of the trapezoidal rule (see Appendix D). Other methods are described by Yeh and Kwan [7].

An exact mathematical method for determining the total area under the plasma concentration-time curve is to convert Eq. (1.10) to its exponential form and integrate over the time interval zero to infinity. Equation (1.10) expressed as natural logarithms is

$$\ln C = \ln C_0 - Kt \qquad\qquad (1.29)$$

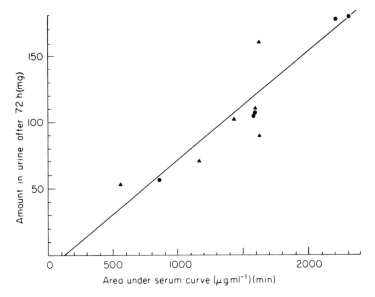

Fig. 1.8 Relationship between cumulative amount of tetracycline excreted after 72 h and the total area under the tetracycline concentration
in serum versus time curve after oral administration of a 250 mg dose to
five healthy adults. Two different oral preparations (●,▲) were given
to each subject. The data are described by Eq. (1.28); the slope of
the line is equal to the average renal clearance of tetracycline in the
group. (Data from Ref. 6.)

Therefore,

$$C = C_0 e^{-Kt} \qquad (1.30)$$

Integration from time zero to time infinity yields

$$AUC = -\left.\frac{C_0}{K} e^{-Kt}\right|_0^\infty = \frac{C_0}{K} \qquad (1.31)$$

Therefore, the total area under the plasma drug concentration-time
curve is the plasma concentration at time zero, obtained by extrapolation, divided by the apparent first-order elimination rate constant of
the drug. Since most drugs do not distribute instantaneously between
plasma and tissues, Eq. (1.31) will usually underestimate the total
area under the drug concentration in plasma versus time plot after
intravenous administration. This error may be negligible or substantial, depending on the distribution and elimination characteristics
of the drug.

Systemic Clearance

It has been shown that the product of the urinary excretion rate constant k_e and V is equal to renal clearance [Eq. (1.25)]. The product of the elimination rate constant K and V also yields a clearance term, which has alternatively been called plasma clearance, total body clearance, or systemic clearance. We will use the last-mentioned term and the designation Cl_s. It can be shown that the systemic clearance is given by the ratio of the intravenous dose to the total area under the drug concentration versus time curve. Since $Cl_r = k_e V$ [according to Eq. (1.25)], we can transform Eq. (1.28) to the expression

$$V = \frac{X_u^\infty}{k_e \cdot AUC} \tag{1.32}$$

Since we can show by rearranging Eq. (1.20) that

$$\frac{X_u^\infty}{k_e} = \frac{X_0}{K} \tag{1.33}$$

it follows that

$$Cl_s = VK = \frac{X_0}{AUC} \tag{1.34}$$

where X_0 is the intravenous dose.

Systemic clearance represents the sum of the clearances of all individual processes involved in the elimination of drug from the body. It is particularly useful for comparing data obtained using different compartmental models and for relating pharmacokinetic and physiologic processes. A comprehensive discussion of clearance is presented in Chap. 8.

Another particularly useful relationship, from which the apparent volume of distribution can be estimated, is obtained by rearranging Eq. (1.34):

$$V = \frac{X_0}{K \cdot AUC} \tag{1.35}$$

This relationship is used very widely for calculating the apparent volume of distribution. The validity of Eq. (1.35) is not dependent on instantaneous distribution of drug between plasma and tissues, as is the case for Eq. (1.11). Accordingly, Eq. (1.35) can be applied in principle to many compartmental models. When applied to one-compartmental models, it is often called the area method for estimating apparent volume of distribution and V is sometimes written as V_{area}.

Metabolite Concentrations in the Plasma

Scheme 2 illustrates parallel routes of drug elimination; one is urinary, the kinetics of which have been discussed, and the other is metabolism.

Scheme 2

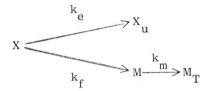

In this scheme X, X_u, and k_e are as defined previously, M is the amount of metabolite in the body, and M_T is the total amount of metabo- lite eliminated by renal and/or biliary pathways as well as by metabo- lism (i.e., where the primary metabolite M is further biotransformed). The constants k_f and k_m are the respective apparent first-order rate constants for metabolite formation and elimination. The time course of metabolite levels in the body is a function of the rates of formation and elimination of the metabolite:

$$\frac{dM}{dt} = k_f X - k_m M \tag{1.36}$$

The Laplace transform of this equation (see Appendix A) is

$$s\overline{M} = k_f \overline{X} - k_m \overline{M} \tag{1.37}$$

Solving for $\overline{M}$ and substituting for $\overline{X}$ from Eq. (1.4) yields

$$\overline{M} = \frac{k_f X_0}{(s + k_m)(s + K)} \tag{1.38}$$

which when solved for M, employing a table of Laplace transforms, gives

$$M = \frac{k_f X_0}{K - k_m}(e^{-k_m t} - e^{-Kt}) \tag{1.39}$$

This equation permits calculation of the amount of metabolite in the body at any time after intravenous injection of a dose X_0 of a drug. Dividing both sides of this equation by the apparent volume of distribu- tion of the metabolite V_m yields

$$C_m = \frac{k_f X_0}{V_m(K - k_m)}(e^{-k_m t} - e^{-Kt}) \tag{1.40}$$

which describes the plasma concentration of metabolite C_m versus time curve following the intravenous administration of parent drug.

It is informative to consider two different cases, one in which k_m is greater than K and the other where K is greater than k_m. At one time the general assumption was that k_m was always greater than K since metabolites were considered to be more polar and hence more readily eliminated from the body than the parent drug. This assumption may be true when polar conjugates such as glucuronides and glycine conjugates are the major metabolites of a drug. However, the assumption is often not true when biotransformation results in acetylation or oxidation. If k_m is larger than K, then at some time after drug administration $e^{-k_m t}$ will approach zero, whereas e^{-Kt} still has a finite value resulting in Eq. (1.40) reducing to

$$C_m \simeq \frac{k_f X_0}{V_m (k_m - K)} e^{-Kt}$$
(1.41)

which when written in logarithmic form becomes

$$\log C_m \simeq \log \frac{k_f X_0}{V_m (k_m - K)} - \frac{Kt}{2.303}$$
(1.42)

Therefore, a plot of log plasma concentration of metabolite versus time will eventually become linear and parallel to the curve of log plasma concentration of unchanged drug versus time (i.e., both will have a slope of $-K/2.303$), as illustrated by Fig. 1.9. From a practical point of view, this will be obvious only when k_m is several times larger than K.

Conversely, if K is larger than k_m, metabolite concentration in the plasma will decline more slowly than the concentration of unchanged drug. In this instance the equation analogous to (1.42) is

$$\log C_m \simeq \log \frac{k_f X_0}{V_m (K - k_m)} - \frac{k_m t}{2.303}$$
(1.43)

The terminal slope of a plot of the logarithm of metabolite concentration versus time is $-k_m/2.303$ (Fig. 1.10). Again the linear segment will be obvious only when K is several times larger than k_m. In either instance (i.e., when $k_m > K$ or when $K > k_m$), the closer K and k_m are, the more difficult it is to delineate a linear segment of the curve. It is important to point out that by simply following metabolite concentration in the plasma as a function of time and obtaining a linear portion of a curve, one does not know whether the slope yields k_m or K. To resolve this dilemma, either the apparent first-order elimination rate constant of the drug, K, must be known, or in some limited circumstances the metabolite can be administered as such and its elimination

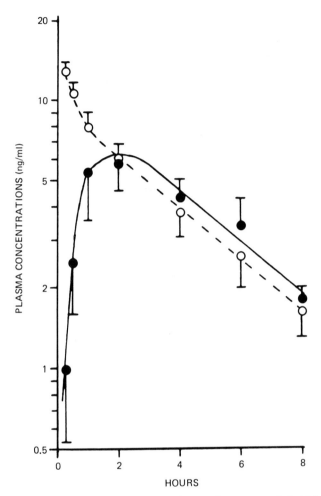

Fig. 1.9 Plasma concentrations of propranolol (O) and propranolol glucuronide (●) after a 0.05 mg/kg intravenous dose of propranolol to five normal volunteers. After about 4 h the concentrations of parent drug and metabolite decline in parallel since the metabolite has a shorter half-life than propranolol. (From Ref. 8.)

rate constant determined. Regardless of which rate constant (K or k_m) is determined from the terminal linear segment of the curve, the other rate constant can be estimated by the method of residuals (see Appendix C for a discussion of this method).

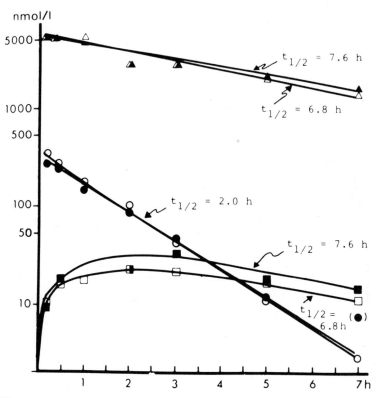

Fig. 1.10 Individual plasma concentrations of metoprolol (●,○), α-hydroxymetoprolol, a metabolite, formed after administration of metoprolol (■,□), and α-hydroxymetoprolol after administration of the metabolite per se (▲,△) in two dogs. The half-life of the metabolite is considerably longer than the half-life of the parent drug. (From Ref. 9. © 1979 Plenum Publishing Corp.)

Metabolite Excretion in the Urine

Urinary excretion data for a metabolite may be employed to determine the elimination kinetics of the parent drug and of the metabolite. According to Scheme 3

Scheme 3

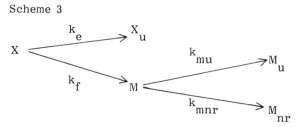

the differential equation describing the appearance of metabolite in
the urine is given by

$$\frac{dM_u}{dt} = k_{mu}M \qquad (1.44)$$

where M_u is the amount of metabolite in the urine. M_{nr} is the
amount of metabolite eliminated by all processes other than renal
elimination. The constant k_{mu} is the apparent first-order rate constant for the excretion of metabolite in the urine, and k_{mnr} is the
sum of all apparent first-order rate constants for the elimination of
metabolite other than by renal excretion. The elimination rate constant
of the metabolite k_m is the sum of these two rate constants (i.e.,
$k_m = k_{mu} + k_{mnr}$).

The Laplace transform of (1.44) is

$$s\overline{M}_u = k_{mu}\overline{M} \qquad (1.45)$$

Substitution for $\overline{M}$ from (1.38) and solving for $\overline{M}_u$ yields

$$\overline{M}_u = \frac{k_{mu}k_f X_0}{s(s + k_m)(s + K)} \qquad (1.46)$$

Solving for M_u employing a table of Laplace transforms results in the
following relationship between metabolite levels in the urine and time:

$$M_u = k_{mu}k_f X_0 \left[\frac{1}{k_m K} + \frac{e^{-k_m t}}{k_m(k_m - K)} - \frac{e^{-Kt}}{K(k_m - K)} \right] \qquad (1.47)$$

Rearrangement of (1.47) yields

$$M_u = \frac{k_{mu}k_f X_0}{k_m K} \left[1 + \frac{1}{k_m - K}(Ke^{-k_m t} - k_m e^{-Kt}) \right] \qquad (1.48)$$

At time $t = \infty$, M_u equals M_u^∞, the amount of metabolite in the urine
at infinity, which is given by

$$M_u^\infty = \frac{k_{mu}k_f X_0}{k_m K} \qquad (1.49)$$

Substituting M_u^∞ for the term $k_{mu}k_f X_0/k_m K$ in (1.48) and rearranging
yields

$$M_u^\infty - M_u = \frac{M_u^\infty}{k_m - K}(k_m e^{-Kt} - Ke^{-k_m t}) \qquad (1.50)$$

A second biexponential relationship may be obtained by substituting in (1.44) the value of M from (1.39). This gives the rate expression

$$\frac{dM_u}{dt} = \frac{k_{mu}k_f X_0}{k_m - K}(e^{-Kt} - e^{-k_m t}) \qquad (1.51)$$

Assuming that k_m is greater than K, a plot of either log $(M_u^\infty - M_u)$ versus time or log (dM_u/dt) versus time will result in a biexponential curve (Fig. 1.11). The apparent first-order elimination rate constant K of the parent drug can be estimated from the slope of the terminal linear portion of each curve, which equals $-K/2.303$. Figure 1.12 shows the correlation between the half-life of antipyrine determined by following the decline of drug concentrations in plasma and that determined from a semilogarithmic plot of the urinary excretion rate

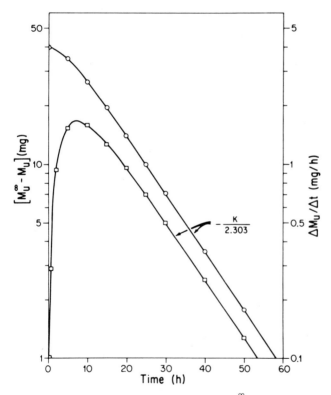

Fig. 1.11 Semilogarithmic plots of $[M_u^\infty - M_u]$ (O) and $\Delta M_u/\Delta t$ (□) versus time after intravenous administration of a drug. The data are described by Eqs. (1.50) and (1.51), respectively, for a situation where k_m is greater than K.

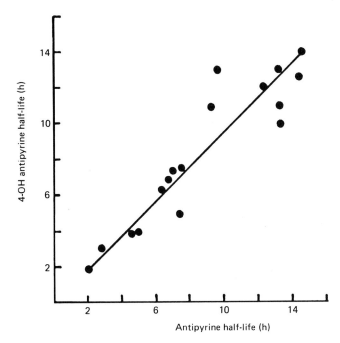

Fig. 1.12 Correlation between the half-life of antipyrine determined by following the decline of drug concentrations in plasma and that determined from a semilogarithmic plot of the urinary excretion rate of an antipyrine metabolite, 4-hydroxyantipyrine, versus time in individual patients. It is evident that the elimination rate constant of the metabolite, k_m, is significantly larger than the elimination rate constant of antipyrine, K. n = 17, r = 0.89, P < 0.001. (From Ref. 10.)

of an antipyrine metabolite, 4-hydroxyantipyrine, versus time in individual patients. Application of the method of residuals (see Appendix C) in both instances will enable estimation of k_m, the apparent first-order elimination rate constant of the metabolite. If, however, K is larger than k_m, k_m can be determined from the slopes of the terminal linear phases of these plots and K can be determined from the slopes of the residual lines. Without prior knowledge of either K or k_m, one cannot tell whether the slope of the terminal linear segment of the urinary excretion-time plots yields K or k_m.

   With regard to the use of (1.50) and (1.51) for evaluating the elimination kinetics of a drug and its metabolite, the same factors must be considered as discussed for the analogous equations (1.15) and (1.21) for urinary excretion of parent drug. As with (1.15), experimentally determined urinary excretion rates of metabolite in (1.51) are not instantaneous rates but average rates over a finite period of time (see Appendix F). With respect to (1.50), the determination of M_u^∞ requires urine collection to be carried out until no further metabolite can be detected in the urine. This may present difficulties if the parent drug or metabolite has a long half-life.

Determination of Metabolite–Associated Rate Constants

Scheme 3 suggests that three rate constants are of interest in characterizing the time course of metabolite in the body: the formation rate constant k_f, the overall rate constant for elimination of metabolite k_m (i.e., the sum of k_{mu} and k_{mnr}), and the rate constant for renal excretion of metabolite k_{mu}. The formation rate constant is usually estimated by determining the total amount of metabolite ultimately excreted in the urine. Equation (1.49) can be rearranged to give

$$k_f = \frac{k_m KM_u^\infty}{k_{mu} X_0} \qquad (1.52)$$

If the metabolite is eliminated solely by renal excretion (i.e., $k_m = k_{mu}$), then

$$k_f = \frac{KM_u^\infty}{X_0} \qquad (1.53)$$

Hence the ratio of total amount of metabolite ultimately excreted in the urine to the intravenous dose, times the rate constant for elimination of parent drug, is equal to the formation rate constant if the metabolite is subject to neither further metabolism nor nonrenal elimination in the body.

Kaplan et al. [11] have proposed a more general method for estimating k_f. This method is often limited to animal studies, for it requires the administration of the metabolite. To determine k_f in Scheme 3, one must give the parent drug intravenously and determine its elimination rate constant K, as well as the area under the metabolite concentration in plasma versus time curve resulting from this administration. Then one must administer intravenously a dose of metabolite that is equimolar to the dose of drug and again determine the area under the metabolite concentration versus time curve. The estimate of k_f is given by the relationship

$$k_f = \frac{K[\int_0^\infty C_m \, dt]_X}{\int_0^\infty C_m \, dt} \qquad (1.54)$$

where $[\int_0^\infty C_m \, dt]_X$ and $\int_0^\infty C_m \, dt$ represent the total areas under the metabolite concentration-time curves after administration of the drug and metabolite, respectively.

Several relationships have been described for the determination of the rate constant for overall elimination of metabolite from the body, k_m [see Eqs. (1.40), (1.50), and (1.51)]. The rate constant may be estimated from either the slopes of the linear portions of the appropriate semilogarithmic plots or the residual curves derived from such plots (see Appendix C). Other methods have been proposed for estimating k_m [12] but seem to offer no particular advantage.

No general method appears to be available for estimating the rate constant for renal excretion of metabolite, k_{mu}, other than to administer the metabolite intravenously and carry out the appropriate measurements. This is usually not possible in humans. On the other hand, the renal clearance of the metabolite Cl_{rm} is relatively easily determined after administering the parent drug by determining metabolite concentrations in plasma and urine and applying equations analogous to Eqs. (1.23), (1.27), or (1.28); for example,

$$Cl_{rm} = \frac{dM_u/dt}{C_m} \tag{1.55}$$

or

$$Cl_{rm} = \frac{M_u^\infty}{[\int_0^\infty C_m \, dt]_X} \tag{1.56}$$

Interpretation of Total Radioactivity Data

Many studies in laboratory animals and some studies in humans involve the administration of radiolabeled drug. Often, the results of such studies are expressed in terms of total radioactivity in plasma. Sometimes, drug studies are initiated before a specific assay is available and the results are reported in terms of the concentration of apparent drug in plasma. In either case, great care must be exercised in attempting to carry out a pharmacokinetic analysis of such data. The concentration of total radioactivity or apparent drug in plasma, C_T, must be viewed as the sum of the concentrations of parent drug, C, and all metabolites that are detected by the assay method, C_{MT}. The time course of unmetabolized drug after intravenous administration is given by

$$C = \frac{X_0}{V} e^{-Kt} \tag{1.57}$$

Equation (1.40) describes the time course of a single metabolite in the plasma after intravenous administration of parent drug. This equation applies to each primary metabolite arising from the administered drug. Consequently, the plasma concentrations of all primary metabolites can be expressed by

$$C_{MT} = \sum_{i=1}^{n} \frac{(k_f)_i X_0}{(V_m)_i [K - (k_m)_i]} (e^{-(k_m)_i t} - e^{-Kt}) \qquad (1.58)$$

Combining Eqs. (1.57) and (1.58) and rearranging terms, we can show that

$$C_T = X_0 \left\{ \sum_{i=1}^{n} \frac{(k_f)_i e^{-(k_m)_i t}}{(V_m)_i [K - (k_m)_i]} \right.$$

$$\left. + \left[\frac{1}{V} - \sum_{i=1}^{n} \frac{(k_f)_i}{(V_m)_i [K - (k_m)_i]} \right] e^{-Kt} \right\} \qquad (1.59)$$

where $(k_f)_i$, $(V_m)_i$, and $(k_m)_i$ are the apparent first-order formation rate constant, the apparent volume of distribution, and the apparent first-order elimination rate constant, respectively, for each of the n primary metabolites, V is the apparent volume of parent drug, K is the apparent first-order rate constant for drug elimination, and X_0 is the intravenous dose of drug.

If the individual rate constant for elimination of every primary metabolite is greater than the elimination rate constant of administered drug [i.e., $(k_m)_i > K$], a semilogarithmic plot of total radioactivity or apparent drug concentration in plasma versus time will yield a biexponential curve and the slope of the terminal segment is equal to $-K/2.303$. The same applies to plots of urinary excretion rates of total radioactivity versus time [i.e., log $d(X_T)_u/dt$ versus t] and to sigma-minus plots for total radioactivity (i.e., log $[(X_T)_u^{\infty} - (X_T)_u]$ versus t.

Hence under special circumstances which can be neither predicted nor assumed, one may find that the half-life of elimination of total radioactivity is equal to the elimination half-life of parent drug. Since one is not certain of the chemical species being measured by counting total radioactivity, no other pharmacokinetic parameter, including apparent volume of distribution, can be calculated. Perhaps the most useful pharmacokinetic information that may be derived unambiguously from studies based on total radioactivity is that the drug administered must have a biologic half-life equal to or less than the apparent half-life of elimination of total radioactivity.

INTRAVENOUS INFUSION

Drug Concentration in the Plasma

If a drug is administered intravenously at a constant rate, the following differential equation may be written for the change in amount of drug in the body with time:

$$\frac{dX}{dt} = k_0 - KX \tag{1.60}$$

where k_0 is the rate of drug infusion, expressed in amount per unit time. The Laplace transform of (1.60) is

$$s\overline{X} = \frac{k_0}{s} - K\overline{X} \tag{1.61}$$

Rearrangement yields

$$\overline{X} = \frac{k_0}{s(s + K)} \tag{1.62}$$

Solving (1.62), employing a table of Laplace transforms, gives the following relationship between the amount of drug in the body and time:

$$X = \frac{k_0}{K}(1 - e^{-Kt}) \tag{1.63}$$

which can be written in concentration terms:

$$C = \frac{k_0}{VK}(1 - e^{-Kt}) \tag{1.64}$$

During continuous constant rate intravenous infusion drug concentrations in plasma increase according to Eq. (1.64) but eventually approach a constant value (i.e., as $t \to \infty$, $e^{-Kt} \to 0$ and $C \to k_0/VK$). This constant drug concentration or plateau is sometimes called infusion equilibrium but is actually a steady-state situation since at this concentration the elimination rate equals the infusion rate and $dC/dt = 0$. The steady-state concentration in plasma C_{ss} is given by

$$C_{ss} = \frac{k_0}{VK} \tag{1.65}$$

After infusing a drug for a period of time equal to four biologic half-lives, drug concentrations in plasma are within 10% of steady state. Infusion for a period of time equal to seven half-lives results in concentrations within 1% of steady state. Drug concentration in plasma at steady state is directly proportional to the infusion rate and inversely proportional to the systemic clearance (i.e., the product of

V and K) of the drug. The systemic clearance of a drug is readily calculated from the ratio of infusion rate to steady-state drug concentration in plasma:

$$Cl_s = VK = \frac{k_0}{C_{ss}} \tag{1.66}$$

The elimination rate constant and half-life of a drug may also be calculated from data collected during infusion to steady state. Substitution for k_0/VK in Eq. (1.64) according to Eq. (1.65) yields

$$C = C_{ss}(1 - e^{-Kt}) \tag{1.67}$$

Upon rearrangement it can be shown that

$$\frac{C_{ss} - C}{C_{ss}} = e^{-Kt} \tag{1.68}$$

Therefore,

$$\log \frac{C_{ss} - C}{C_{ss}} = -\frac{Kt}{2.303} \tag{1.69}$$

A semilogarithmic plot of $(C_{ss} - C)/C_{ss}$ versus time yields a straight line with a slope of $-K/2.303$. The elimination rate constant may be estimated directly from the slope. The half-life may be estimated either directly from the semilogarithmic plot or from K by rearranging Eq. (1.12),

$$t_{1/2} = \frac{0.693}{K} \tag{1.70}$$

The elimination rate constant may also be determined using the declining drug concentration in plasma versus time data collected after stopping the infusion. The differential equation describing these data is simply

$$\frac{dC}{dt} = -KC \tag{1.71}$$

The Laplace transform of Eq. (1.71) is given by

$$s\overline{C} - C_{max} = -K\overline{C} \tag{1.72}$$

where C_{max} is the drug concentration in plasma when the infusion was terminated, (i.e., the initial condition for the postinfusion period).
On rearranging Eq. (1.72), we obtain

$$\overline{C} = \frac{C_{max}}{s + K} \tag{1.73}$$

Solving Eq. (1.73) for C using a table of Laplace transforms gives

$$C = C_{max} e^{-Kt'} \tag{1.74}$$

or, in logarithmic form,

$$\log C = \log C_{max} - \frac{Kt'}{2.303} \tag{1.75}$$

where t' is the time after stopping the infusion. The time during which infusion took place is generally designated as T. If the infusion has been carried out for a sufficiently long period such that T > seven biologic half-lives, $C_{max} = C_{ss} = k_0/VK$. If the infusion were terminated before reaching steady state, $C_{max} = k_0(1 - e^{-KT})/VK$. Depending on the infusion time, Eq. (1.75) may be transformed to either

$$\log C = \log \frac{k_0}{VK} - \frac{Kt'}{2.303} \tag{1.76}$$

or

$$\log C = \log \frac{k_0}{VK}(1 - e^{-KT}) - \frac{Kt'}{2.303} \tag{1.77}$$

In either case a semilogarithmic plot of postinfusion drug concentration in plasma versus time t' will yield a straight line with a slope equal to $-K/2.303$. The time course of drug concentrations in plasma during and after constant rate intravenous infusions is shown in Fig. 1.13.

Data obtained from infusion studies are also useful for estimating the apparent volume of distribution of a drug. For example, we can show on rearranging Eq. (1.65) that

$$V = \frac{k_0}{C_{ss}K} \tag{1.78}$$

Alternatively, if the infusion is terminated before attaining steady state, then

$$V = \frac{k_0(1 - e^{-KT})}{C_{max}K} \tag{1.79}$$

where C_{max} is the drug concentration in plasma when the infusion was stopped and T is the infusion time. The validity of Eq. (1.79) requires the assumption of a one-compartment model, but Eq. (1.78) is a general relationship that applies to many situations.

If drug concentration versus time data are obtained during as well as after constant rate intravenous infusion, one can calculate systemic clearance Cl_s and apparent volume of distribution V from the

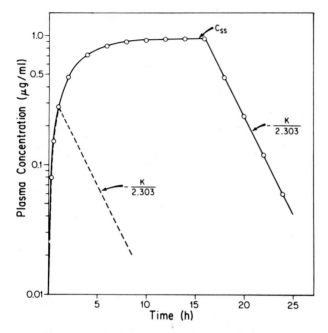

Fig. 1.13 Drug concentrations (log scale) in plasma during and after constant rate intravenous infusion to steady state. The dashed line denotes the decline of drug concentration in plasma after an infusion period shorter than the time required to reach steady state.

total area under the concentration versus time curve. The area under the up-curve is obtained by integrating Eq. (1.64) from $t = 0$ to $t = T$. The area under the down-curve is obtained by integrating Eq. (1.74) from $t' = 0$ to $t' = \infty$. Combining these areas and simplifying terms yields

$$AUC = \frac{k_0 T}{VK} \qquad (1.80)$$

Therefore,

$$Cl_s = VK = \frac{k_0 T}{AUC} \qquad (1.81)$$

and

$$V = \frac{k_0 T}{K \cdot AUC} \qquad (1.82)$$

where T is the infusion time. Equations (1.81) and (1.82) apply irrespective of infusion time and do not require attainment of steady state. Both are general expressions that may be used for many pharmacokinetic models.

Simultaneous Rapid Intravenous Injection and Intravenous Infusion

Since the time required to reach steady state will be very long for a drug with a long half-life, it is often desirable in such cases to administer an intravenous loading dose just before starting the intravenous infusion. The loading dose should be large enough to yield the desired steady-state drug concentration in plasma, C_{ss}, immediately upon injection. The infusion rate should be fast enough to maintain this concentration. If we know the drug concentration we wish to maintain, the appropriate infusion rate is given by rearrangement of Eq. (1.65) (i.e., $k_0 = C_{ss}VK$). Recalling that V is the proportionality constant relating drug concentration in plasma to total amount of drug in the body, one concludes for a one-compartment model that the loading dose X_0 equals $C_{ss}V$. Using this dosage regimen, we can show that the amount of drug in the body is constant until the infusion is stopped.

The equation describing the time course of the amount of drug in the body following simultaneous intravenous injection of a loading dose and initiation of a constant rate intravenous infusion is the sum of the two equations describing each process [i.e., Eqs. (1.5) and (1.63)]. Therefore,

$$X = X_0 e^{-Kt} + \frac{k_0}{K}(1 - e^{-Kt}) \tag{1.83}$$

Substituting $C_{ss}V$ for X_0 and $C_{ss}VK$ for k_0 and rearranging terms yields

$$X = C_{ss}V \tag{1.84}$$

Hence the amount of drug in the body is constant throughout the time course of drug administration.

Urinary Excretion Data

Drug elimination kinetics may also be evaluated from urinary excretion data obtained during constant rate intravenous infusion. The differential equation for the rate of appearance of unmetabolized drug in the urine during infusion is the same as that describing urinary excretion of drug following an intravenous bolus injection [i.e., $dX_u/dt = k_e X$; Eq. (1.14)]. The Laplace transform of this expression is $s\bar{X}_u = k_e\bar{X}$ [Eq. (1.17)]. Substituting for $\bar{X}$ according to Eq. (1.62) and rearranging terms yields

$$\overline{X}_u = \frac{k_e k_0}{s^2 (s + K)} \tag{1.85}$$

Solving for X_u (see Appendix A) gives the following relationship between the cumulative amount of drug in the urine and time:

$$X_u = \frac{k_e k_0}{K} t - \frac{k_e k_0}{K^2} (1 - e^{-Kt}) \tag{1.86}$$

When the drug has been infused for a sufficient period so as to approach steady state in the plasma, the term e^{-Kt} approaches zero and Eq. (1.86) reduces to

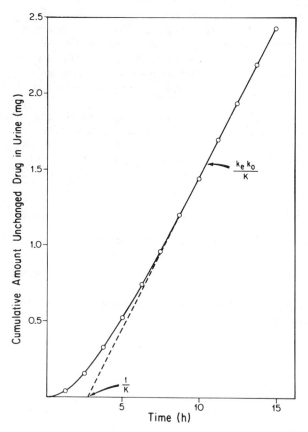

Fig. 1.14 Cumulative amount of unmetabolized drug excreted in the urine as a function of time during constant rate intravenous infusion. The data are described by Eq. (1.86).

$$X_u = \frac{k_e k_0}{K} t - \frac{k_e k_0}{K^2} \quad (1.87)$$

Accordingly, a plot of the cumulative amount of excreted drug versus time is curvilinear initially but eventually becomes linear (see Fig. 1.14). The slope of the linear region is $k_e k_0/K$. Extrapolation of the linear segment of the curve to the time axis yields an intercept equal to $1/K$, since according to Eq. (1.87), $t = 1/K$ when $X_u = 0$. In principle, a plot of cumulative amount of drug excreted during infusion to steady state versus time permits us to estimate both the overall elimination rate constant and the excretion rate constant of a drug.

FIRST-ORDER ABSORPTION

Drug Concentrations in the Plasma

A very large number of plasma concentration-time curves obtained after extravascular (e.g., oral, intramuscular, rectal, etc.) administration of drugs can be described by a one-compartment model with first-order absorption and elimination, despite the fact that first-order absorption is often difficult to rationalize rigorously based on theoretical principles. The equations describing this type of model are analogous to those developed for metabolite concentrations in the plasma and urine. For a drug that enters the body by an apparent first-order absorption process, is eliminated by a first-order process, and distributes in the body according to a one-compartment model, the following differential equation applies:

$$\frac{dX}{dt} = k_a X_a - KX \quad (1.88)$$

where X and K are as defined previously, k_a is the apparent first-order absorption rate constant, and X_a is the amount of drug at the absorption site. The Laplace transform of (1.88) is

$$s\overline{X} = k_a \overline{X}_a - K\overline{X} \quad (1.89)$$

The rate of loss of drug from the absorption site is

$$\frac{dX_a}{dt} = -k_a X_a \quad (1.90)$$

The Laplace transform of which is

$$s\overline{X}_a - FX_0 = -k_a \overline{X}_a \quad (1.91)$$

where F is the fraction of the administered dose X_0 that is absorbed following extravascular administration. Solving (1.91) for $\overline{X}_a$, substituting this value for $\overline{X}_a$ in (1.89), and solving for $\overline{X}$ yields

$$\overline{X} = \frac{k_a FX_0}{(s + K)(s + k_a)} \tag{1.92}$$

By employing a table of Laplace transforms, the following biexponential relationship between the amount of drug in the body and time results:

$$X = \frac{k_a FX_0}{k_a - K} (e^{-Kt} - e^{-k_a t}) \tag{1.93}$$

which in concentration terms is

$$C = \frac{k_a FX_0}{V(k_a - K)} (e^{-Kt} - e^{-k_a t}) \tag{1.94}$$

A survey of the literature indicates that for most drugs administered extravascularly in conventional dosage forms, the absorption rate constant is significantly larger than the elimination rate constant. As a result, at some time after administration the term $e^{-k_a t}$ approaches zero, whereas the term e^{-Kt} is finite, and (1.94) reduces to

$$C = \frac{k_a FX_0}{V(k_a - K)} e^{-Kt} \tag{1.95}$$

This equation describes the postabsorptive phase (i.e., the time when absorption no longer occurs) of a plasma concentration-time curve. Equation (1.95) written in common logarithms is

$$\log C = \log \frac{k_a FX_0}{V(k_a - K)} - \frac{Kt}{2.303} \tag{1.96}$$

A plot of the logarithm of drug concentration in plasma versus time yields a biexponential curve, the terminal portion of which is linear and described by (1.96) (Fig. 1.15). Therefore, an estimate of the elimination rate constant can be obtained from the slope of this terminal linear segment, which is equal to $-K/2.303$. The absorption rate constant may be calculated by the method of residuals (see Appendix C). This graphical approach for estimating k_a and K is useful only if the two rate constants are substantially different. In our experience the method works best if $k_a/K \geq 3$. If this is not the case, the rate constants are best estimated by fitting the concentration-time data to Eq. (1.94) with the aid of a nonlinear least-squares regression program and a digital computer (see Appendix H).

Some drugs are absorbed very slowly, usually because of limited solubility in the fluids at the site of administration—or by design. Other drugs are eliminated from the body very rapidly. In either case absorption may be relatively slow compared to elimination and the ab-

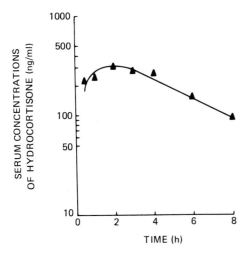

Fig. 1.15 Hydrocortisone concentrations in serum after rectal administration of a retention enema to a healthy subject. The data are described by Eq. (1.94) for the situation where k_a is greater than K.
(From Ref. 13, subject 6.)

sorption rate constant may be smaller than the elimination rate constant.
This situation is observed often after the administration of drugs in
sustained-release dosage forms. In such cases the time course of drug
concentration in plasma is described by Eq. (1.94), but the slope of
the linear segment of the semilogarithmic plot of concentration versus
time is equal to $-k_a/2.303$ rather than $-K/2.303$ and the elimination
rate constant must be determined by the method of residuals (see Appendix C). This circumstance is frequently called the flip-flop phenomenon. The determination of whether the linear segment of a semilogarithmic plot of drug concentration in plasma versus time after extravascular administration is related to the elimination rate constant or
to the absorption rate constant must be based on an independent estimation of the elimination rate constant either after intravenous administration of the drug or, in some circumstances, after administration of
a dosage form from which the drug is more rapidly absorbed (e.g.,
a solution).

The time course of concentration in plasma of certain drugs suggests a time lag between oral administration and the apparent onset of
absorption. This lag may be the result of delayed release of drugs
from the dosage form or of a combination of negligible absorption from
the stomach and slow gastric emptying. One usually concludes the ex-
istence of a time lag if the intersection of the extrapolations of the
terminal exponential phase and residual line occurs at a time greater

than zero. If there is no lag time, both extrapolations intersect the log concentration axis at the same point. When a lag is evident, the appropriate equation to describe the time course of drug concentrations in plasma is

$$C = \frac{k_a FX_0}{V(k_a - K)} [e^{-K(t-t_0)} - e^{-k_a(t-t_0)}]$$
(1.97)

where t_0 is the lag time.

Drug concentration in plasma versus time data after oral administration can provide estimates of the apparent absorption and elimination rate constants of a drug but usually cannot provide unambiguous estimates of systemic clearance or apparent volume or distribution. Integration of Eq. (1.94) from time zero to time infinity yields

$$AUC = \frac{k_a FX_0}{V(k_a - K)} \left(\frac{1}{K} - \frac{1}{k_a} \right)$$
(1.98)

where $k_a FX_0 / V(k_a - K)$ is the intersection of the extrapolation of the terminal exponential phase on the log concentration axis (assuming no lag time). Rearrangement of Eq. (1.98) yields

$$AUC = \frac{FX_0}{VK}$$
(1.99)

It follows that the systemic clearance is given by

$$Cl_s = VK = \frac{FX_0}{AUC}$$
(1.100)

and the apparent volume of distribution by

$$V = \frac{FX_0}{K \cdot AUC}$$
(1.101)

where FX_0 is the amount of drug absorbed or more precisely the amount of drug reaching the systemic circulation. Cl_s and V can be estimated only by assuming absorption to be complete (i.e., by assuming that F = 1). If this is not the case, the ratio of administered dose to AUC is not Cl_s but Cl_s/F and the ratio of administered dose to the product of K and AUC is not V but V/F.

Some literature reports have incorrectly estimated V after oral administration by extrapolating the terminal linear phase of the log concentration versus time plot to the log concentration axis and by assuming that the intercept is equal to the administered dose divided by the apparent volume of distribution. As cited above, this intercept is equal to $k_a FX_0 / V(k_a - K)$ rather than to X_0/V.

Determination of C_{max} and t_{max}

Mathematical relationships can be developed to estimate the time at which a peak plasma concentration of drug should be observed and the maximum plasma concentration at this time following first-order input into the body. Expanding Eq. (1.94) yields

$$C = \frac{k_a FX_0}{V(k_a - K)} e^{-Kt} - \frac{k_a FX_0}{V(k_a - K)} e^{-k_a t} \qquad (1.102)$$

which when differentiated with respect to time gives

$$\frac{dC}{dt} = \frac{k_a^2 FX_0}{V(k_a - K)} e^{-k_a t} - \frac{k_a KFX_0}{V(k_a - K)} e^{-Kt} \qquad (1.103)$$

When the plasma concentration reaches a maximum (C_{max}) at time t_{max}, $dC/dt = 0$. Therefore,

$$\frac{k_a^2 FX_0}{V(k_a - K)} e^{-k_a t_{max}} = \frac{k_a KFX_0}{V(k_a - K)} e^{-Kt_{max}} \qquad (1.104)$$

which reduces to

$$\frac{k_a}{K} = \frac{e^{-Kt_{max}}}{e^{-k_a t_{max}}} \qquad (1.105)$$

Taking the logarithm of both sides of Eq. (1.105) and solving for t_{max} yields

$$t_{max} = \frac{2.303}{k_a - K} \log \frac{k_a}{K} \qquad (1.106)$$

For a given drug, as the absorption rate constant increases, the time required for the maximum plasma concentration to be reached decreases.

The maximum plasma concentration is described by substituting t_{max} for t in Eq. (1.94):

$$C_{max} = \frac{k_a FX_0}{V(k_a - K)} (e^{-Kt_{max}} - e^{-k_a t_{max}}) \qquad (1.107)$$

However, a simpler expression can be obtained. From (1.105) it can be shown that

$$e^{-k_a t_{max}} = \frac{K}{k_a} e^{-K t_{max}} \tag{1.108}$$

Substituting for $e^{-k_a t_{max}}$, according to (1.108), in (1.107) yields

$$C_{max} = \frac{k_a F X_0}{V(k_a - K)} \frac{k_a - K}{k_a} e^{-K t_{max}} \tag{1.109}$$

which is readily simplified to

$$C_{max} = \frac{F X_0}{V} e^{-K t_{max}} \tag{1.110}$$

The values of C_{max} and t_{max} under the special circumstance when $k_a = K$ is of mathematical interest and will be considered briefly. Under these conditions, Eq. (1.92) can be written as

$$\bar{X} = \frac{K F X_0}{(s + K)^2} \tag{1.111}$$

Hence

$$X = K F X_0 t e^{-Kt} \tag{1.112}$$

$$C = \frac{K F X_0 t e^{-Kt}}{V} \tag{1.113}$$

and

$$\log C = \log \frac{K F X_0 t}{V} - \frac{Kt}{2.303} \tag{1.114}$$

Equation (1.114) indicates that when $k_a = K$, a semilogarithmic plot of C versus t will contain no linear segments.

Differentiating Eq. (1.113) with respect to time yields

$$\frac{dC}{dt} = \frac{K F X_0}{V} e^{-Kt} - \frac{K^2 F X_0}{V} t e^{-Kt} \tag{1.115}$$

At t_{max}, $C = C_{max}$ and $dC/dt = 0$. Therefore,

$$\frac{K F X_0}{V} e^{-K t_{max}} = \frac{K^2 F X_0}{V} t_{max} e^{-K t_{max}} \tag{1.116}$$

which simplifies to

$$t_{max} = \frac{1}{K} \tag{1.117}$$

Substituting t_{max} for t in Eq. (1.113) according to (1.117) gives

$$C_{max} = \frac{KFX_0}{V} \frac{1}{K} e^{-K(1/K)} \tag{1.118}$$

which simplifies to

$$C_{max} = \frac{FX_0}{V} e^{-1} = \frac{0.37FX_0}{V} \tag{1.119}$$

Urinary Excretion Data

Pharmacokinetic evaluation of urinary excretion data obtained after extravascular administration involves relationships similar to those described for evaluating such data after intravenous bolus injection. Substituting for X in Eq. (1.14) according to (1.93) yields

$$\frac{dX_u}{dt} = \frac{k_e k_a FX_0}{k_a - K} (e^{-Kt} - e^{-k_a t}) \tag{1.120}$$

The Laplace transform of Eq. (1.14) is $s\overline{X}_u = k_e\overline{X}$ [Eq. (1.17)]. Substituting for $\overline{X}$ according to Eq. (1.92) gives

$$\overline{X}_u = \frac{k_e k_a FX_0}{s(s + K)(s + k_a)} \tag{1.121}$$

which, when solved for X_u, yields

$$X_u = \frac{k_e k_a FX_0}{K} \left[\frac{1}{k_a} + \frac{e^{-Kt}}{K - k_a} - \frac{Ke^{-k_a t}}{k_a(K - k_a)} \right] \tag{1.122}$$

Equation (1.122) describes the time course of the cumulative amount of intact drug in the urine. At time infinity, (1.122) reduces to

$$X_u^{\infty} = \frac{k_e FX_0}{K} \tag{1.123}$$

Substitution of X_u^{∞} for $k_e FX_0/K$ in (1.122) and rearrangement yields

$$X_u^{\infty} - X_u = \frac{X_u^{\infty}}{k_a - K} (k_a e^{-Kt} - Ke^{-k_a t}) \tag{1.124}$$

Therefore, a plot of log (dX_u/dt) versus time or log $(X_u^\infty - X_u)$ versus time, according to Eq. (1.120) or (1.124), respectively, will result in a biexponential curve. If k_a is larger than K, the slope of the terminal linear segment of the curve will yield an estimate of the first-order elimination rate constant of parent drug. However, if the opposite is true (i.e., $K > k_a$), the constant obtained from the slope will be the absorption rate constant. If urine samples are obtained soon enough following drug administration, an estimate of k_a (when $k_a > K$) or K (when $K > k_a$) may be obtained by the method of residuals (see Appendix C). However, collection of a sufficient number of urine samples during the absorption phase to enable a pharmacokinetic analysis of this phase is often difficult unless the drug is absorbed slowly.

Metabolite Concentrations in Plasma and Urine

Metabolite concentrations in plasma and urine following oral or intramuscular drug administration may be used under certain conditions to obtain an estimate of the apparent first-order elimination rate constant of a drug. As illustrated in Scheme 4,

Scheme 4

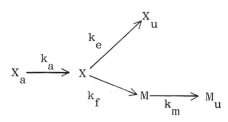

three steps are involved in the appearance of the metabolite in the urine: absorption of the drug, conversion of the drug to a metabolite, and elimination of the metabolite. Considering the principles developed in analyzing metabolite concentrations in the plasma and urine following intravenous injection, it is apparent that the time course of metabolite in the plasma or urine following first-order absorption would be described by a triexponential equation (i.e., a third exponential term is required for the absorption step). Assuming that both k_a and k_m are significantly larger than K, a plot of log C_m, log (dM_u/dt), or log $(M_u^\infty - M_u)$ versus time yields a triexponential curve which at some time becomes linear. An estimate of K may be made from the slope of this terminal linear segment, which is equal to $-K/2.303$.

APPARENT ZERO-ORDER ABSORPTION

The gastrointestinal absorption of drugs is complex and involves several rate processes, including dissolution, absorption from different sites, and gastric emptying, that occur both simultaneously and sequentially. Despite this complexity the rate of appearance of drug in the systemic circulation after oral administration can usually be described by simple first-order kinetics.

Although the assumption of first-order absorption in pharmacokinetics is almost axiomatic, there are several exceptions. Under certain conditions, it has been found that the absorption of certain drugs may be better described by assuming zero-order (constant rate) rather than first-order kinetics (see Fig. 1.16).

The equation describing drug concentration in plasma under these conditions is derived in Appendix B and is given by

$$C = \frac{k_0(e^{KT} - 1)e^{-Kt}}{VK} \qquad (1.125)$$

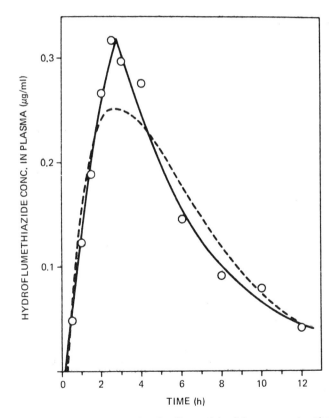

Fig. 1.16 Average hydroflumethiazide concentrations in plasma after a single 100 mg oral dose to 12 healthy subjects. The solid line represents the best fit of the data assuming zero-order abosrption [Eq. (1.125)], and the dashed line represents the best fit assuming first-order absorption [Eq. (1.94)]. (From Ref. 16).

where k_0 is the apparent zero-order absorption rate constant and t is time after drug administration. During absorption, T = t. After absorption apparently ceases, T is a constant corresponding to the absorption time. In the postabsorption phase t = T + t', where t' is the time from the start of the postabsorption phase. Equation (1.125) describes the entire time course of drug concentration in plasma and applies equally to drug concentrations in plasma during and after constant rate intravenous infusion. During the absorption phase $C = k_0(1 - e^{-Kt})/VK$, which is the same as Eq. (1.64) since T = t. The maximum drug concentration in plasma occurs at the end of the absorption phase when t = T. Thus $C_{max} = k_0(1 - e^{-KT})/VK$. During the postabsorption period drug concentrations decline according to Eq. (1.74) since $(e^{KT} - 1)e^{-K(T+t')} = (1 - e^{-KT})e^{-Kt'}$.

The pharmacokinetic parameters required to describe the time course of drug concentrations in plasma (i.e., k_0/V, K, and T) are best estimated by fitting the concentration-time data to Eq. (1.125) with the aid of a nonlinear least-squares regression program and a digital computer (see Appendix H).

REFERENCES

1. J. G. Gambertoglio, W. J. C. Amend, Jr., and L. Z. Benet. Pharmacokinetics and bioavailability of prednisone and prednisolone in healthy volunteers: A review. *J. Pharmacokinet. Biopharm.* *8*:1 (1980).

2. T. J. Mellinger and J. G. Bohorfousch. Pathways and tissue distribution of dipyridamole. *Arch. Int. Pharmacodyn.* *156*:380 (1965).

3. A. Goldstein. *Biostatistics—An Introductory Text.* Macmillan, New York, 1964.

4. G. R. Wilkinson and A. H. Beckett. Absorption, metabolism and excretion of the ephedrines in man: I. The influence of urinary pH and urine volume output. *J. Pharmacol. Exp. Ther.* *162*:139 (1968).

5. J. A. Taylor. Pharmacokinetics and biotransformation of chlorpropamide in man. *Clin. Pharmacol. Ther.* *13*:710 (1972).

6. W. H. Barr, L. M. Gerbracht, K. Letcher, M. Plaut, and N. Strahl. Assessment of the biologic availability of tetracycline products in man. *Clin. Pharmacol. Ther.* *13*:97 (1972).

7. K. C. Yeh and K. C. Kwan. A comparison of numerical integrating algorithms by trapezoid, Lagrange, and spline approximation. *J. Pharmacokinet. Biopharm.* *6*:79 (1978).

8. T. Walle, T. C. Fagan, E. C. Conradi, U. K. Walle, and T. E. Gaffney. Presystemic and systemic glucuronidation of propranolol. *Clin. Pharmacol. Ther.* *26*:167 (1979).

9. C. G. Regardh, L. Elk, and K. J. Hoffmann. Plasma levels and β-blocking effect of α-hydroxymetoprolol—metabolite of metoprolol—in the dog. *J. Pharmacokinet. Biopharm.* 7:471 (1979).

10. D. H. Huffman, D. W. Shoeman, and D. L. Azarnoff. Correlation of the plasma elimination of antipyrine and the appearance of 4-hydroxyantipyrine in the urine of man. *Biochem. Pharmacol.* 23:197 (1974).

11. S. A. Kaplan, M. L. Jack, S. Cotler, and K. Alexander. Utilization of area under the curve to elucidate the disposition of an extensively biotransformed drug. *J. Pharmacokinet. Biopharm.* 1:201 (1973).

12. A. J. Cummings, B. K. Martin, and G. S. Park. Kinetic considerations relating to the accrual and elimination of drug metabolites. *Br. J. Pharmacol. Chemother.* 29:136 (1967).

13. J. J. Lima and W. J. Jusko. Bioavailability of hydrocortisone retention enemas in relation to absorption kinetics. *Clin. Pharmacol. Ther.* 28:262 (1980).

14. P. J. McNamara, W. A. Colburn, and M. Gibaldi. Absorption kinetics of hydroflumethiazide. *J. Clin. Pharmacol.* 18:190 (1978).

2
Multicompartment Models

Most drugs entering the systemic circulation require a finite time to distribute fully throughout the available body space. This fact is particularly obvious upon rapid intravenous injection. During this distributive phase, drug concentration in the plasma will decrease more rapidly than in the postdistributive phase. Whether or not such a distributive phase is apparent depends on the frequency with which blood samples are taken. A distributive phase may last for only a few minutes, for hours, or even for days.

If drug distribution is related to blood flow, highly perfused organs and tissues such as the liver and kidney should be in rapid distribution equilibrium with the blood. The blood and all readily accessible fluids and tissues may often be treated kinetically as a common homogeneous unit generally referred to as the central compartment. As discussed in Chap. 1 with respect to the one-compartment model, kinetic homogeneity does not necessarily mean that the drug concentrations in all tissues of the central compartment at any given time are the same. However, it does assume that any change that occurs in the plasma level of a drug quantitatively reflects a change that occurs in central compartment tissue levels.

Following the intravenous injection of a drug that exhibits multicompartment pharmacokinetics, the levels of drug in all tissues and fluids associated with the central compartment should decline more rapidly during the distributive phase than during the postdistributive phase (Fig. 2.1). In contrast, drug levels in poorly perfused tissues (e.g., muscle, lean tissue, and fat) first increase, reach a maximum, and then begin to decline during the distributive phase (Fig. 2.2). After some time, a pseudodistribution equilibrium is attained between the tissues and fluids of the central compartment and the poorly perfused or less readily accessible tissues. Once pseudodistribution equilibrium has been established, loss of drug from the plasma is described by a monoexponential process indicating kinetic homogeneity with respect to drug levels in all fluids and tissues of the body. The

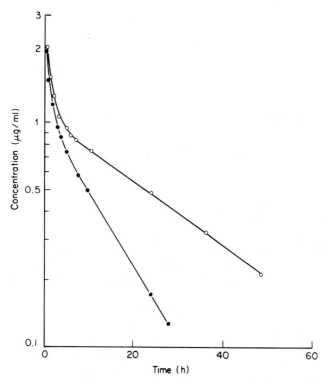

Fig. 2.1 Multiexponential decline of griseofulvin concentration in plas-ma following intravenous administration of the drug to two healthy volunteers. (Data from Ref. 1.)

access of drug to the various poorly perfused tissues may occur at different rates. Frequently, however, for a given drug these rates would appear to be very similar and, therefore, cannot be differen-tiated based solely on plasma concentration-time data. Consequently, all poorly perfused tissues are often "lumped" into a single peripheral compartment. It must be realized however, that the time course of drug levels in a hypothetical peripheral compartment, as inferred from the mathematical analysis of plasma concentration data, may not ex-actly correspond to the actual time course of drug levels in any real tissue. The peripheral compartments of pharmacokinetic models are, at best, hybrids of several functional physiologic units.

The particular compartment (i.e., central or peripheral) with which some tissue or part of a tissue may be associated often depends on the properties of the particular drug being studied. For example, the brain is a highly perfused organ. However, it is clearly separated from the blood by an apparent barrier with lipid characteristics. Therefore, for lipid-soluble drugs the brain would probably be in the central compartment, whereas for more polar drugs the brain would probably be considered as part of a peripheral compartment. Hence, depending on the drug, the brain may be in the peripheral or in the central compartment.

As with the one-compartment model, drug elimination in multicompartment systems is assumed to occur in a first-order fashion. Transfer of drug between body compartments is also assumed to occur by first-order processes.

Following intravenous injection many drugs require more than one exponential term to characterize the resulting decline in plasma concentrations as a function of time. The number of exponentials needed to

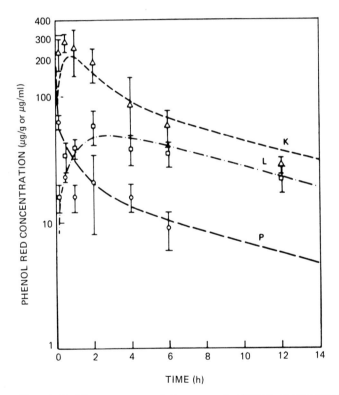

Fig. 2.2 Time course of tissue and plasma concentrations of phenol red in the dogfish shark after intravenous injection of the compound. Phenol red is so polar that even highly perfused organs such as the kidney and liver take on the characteristics of a peripheral compartment. △ kidney, □ liver, ○ plasma. (From Ref. 2 © 1976 Plenum Publishing Corp.)

describe adequately such a plasma concentration versus time curve determines the number of kinetically "homogeneous" compartments that a drug confers on the body. There are several types of n-compartment systems for any n-exponential curve. They differ in that elimination may be assumed to occur either from the central compartment, from one of the peripheral compartments, or from any combination of the central or peripheral compartments. Therefore, there are three types of two-compartment models and seven types of three-compartment models which are mathematically indistinguishable on the basis of the usually available experimental data (drug concentrations in the plasma and/or urinary excretion data). In the absence of information to the contrary, it is usually assumed that drug elimination takes place exclusively from the central compartment. All subsequent equations are based on this assumption unless otherwise stated. The basis of this assumption is that the major sites of biotransformation and excretion (i.e., the liver and kidneys) are well perfused with blood and are therefore presumed to be rapidly accessible to drug in the systemic circulation.

INTRAVENOUS INJECTION

Drug Concentrations in the Plasma

Following the rapid intravenous injection of a drug that distributes in the body according to an n-compartment system with elimination occurring from the central compartment, the disposition function for the central compartment $d_{s,c}$ is given by (see Appendix B)

$$d_{s,c} = \frac{\prod\limits_{i=2}^{n} (s + E_i)}{\prod\limits_{i=1}^{n} (s + \lambda_i)} \tag{2.1}$$

where n is the number of driving force compartments (i.e., compartments having exit rate constants), s is the Laplace operator, E_i is the sum of the exit rate constants from the ith compartment (e.g., $E_1 = k_{10} + k_{12}$ and $E_2 = k_{21}$ in Fig. 2.3), and λ_i is a disposition rate constant which may be expressed in terms of the individual intercompartmental transfer rate constants and elimination rate constants. When a drug is administered as an intravenous bolus, the input function in_s is

$$in_s = X_0 \tag{2.2}$$

where X_0 is the intravenous dose. The Laplace transform for the amount of drug in the central compartment $a_{s,c}$ is given by the product

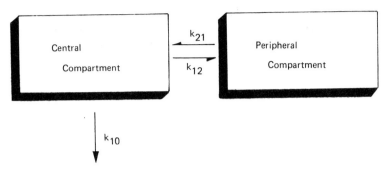

Fig. 2.3 Schematic representation of the body as a two-compartment open model. Drug elimination is restricted to the central compartment.

of the input and disposition functions (2.1) and (2.2), respectively. Therefore,

$$a_{s,c} = X_0 \frac{\prod\limits_{i=2}^{n} (s + E_i)}{\prod\limits_{i=1}^{n} (s + \lambda_i)} \tag{2.3}$$

Equation (2.3) may be solved for X_c, the amount of drug in the central compartment, by taking the anti-Laplace of this equation employing the general method of partial fractions (see Appendix B).

$$X_c = X_0 \sum_{\ell=1}^{n} \frac{\prod\limits_{i=2}^{n} (E_i - \lambda_\ell)}{\prod\limits_{\substack{i=1 \\ i \neq \ell}}^{n} (\lambda_i - \lambda_\ell)} e^{-\lambda_\ell t} \tag{2.4}$$

Although the central compartment is obviously not homogeneous, by assuming that the ratio of drug concentrations in the various tissues and fluids of the central compartment is constant (i.e., there is very rapid distribution between the plasma and the fluids and tissues of the central compartment), a linear relationship exists between the drug concentration in the plasma C and the amount of drug in the central compartment. That is,

$$X_c = V_c C \tag{2.5}$$

where V_c is the apparent volume of the central compartment. This relationship enables the conversion of (2.4) from an amount-time to a concentration-time equation which can be expressed as

$$C = \frac{X_0}{V_c} \sum_{\ell=1}^{n} \frac{\prod\limits_{i=2}^{n} (E_i - \lambda_\ell)}{\prod\limits_{\substack{i=1 \\ i \neq \ell}}^{n} (\lambda_i - \lambda_\ell)} e^{-\lambda_\ell t} \qquad (2.6)$$

or

$$C = \sum_{\ell=1}^{n} A_\ell e^{-\lambda_\ell t} \qquad (2.7)$$

where

$$A_\ell = \frac{X_0}{V_c} \frac{\prod\limits_{i=2}^{n} (E_i - \lambda_\ell)}{\prod\limits_{\substack{i=1 \\ i \neq \ell}}^{n} (\lambda_i - \lambda_\ell)} \qquad (2.8)$$

A plot of the logarithm of drug plasma concentration versus time according to (2.7) will yield a multiexponential curve (Fig. 2.4). The disposition constants λ_1 to λ_{n-1} are by definition larger than λ_n; therefore, at some time the terms $A_1 e^{-\lambda_1 t}$ to $A_{n-1} e^{-\lambda_{n-1} t}$ will approach zero, whereas $A_n e^{-\lambda_n t}$ will still have a finite value. Equation (2.7) will then reduce to

$$C = A_n e^{-\lambda_n t} \qquad (2.9)$$

which in common logarithms is

$$\log C = \log A_n - \frac{\lambda_n t}{2.303} \qquad (2.10)$$

Hence an estimate of λ_n can be obtained from the slope, $-\lambda_n/2.303$, of the terminal exponential phase, and the biologic half life $t_{1/2}$ can be determined either directly from the terminal phase or by employing the following relationship:

$$t_{1/2} = \frac{0.693}{\lambda_n} \qquad (2.11)$$

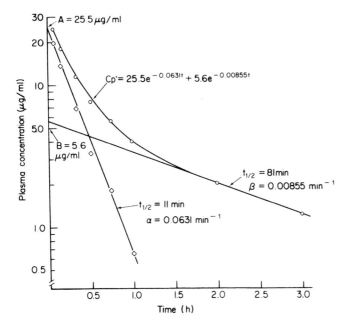

Fig. 2.4 Plasma levels of pralidoxime after intravenous administration of the iodine salt to a healthy volunteer. The data (O) are described by a biexponential equation; the method of residuals has been applied. In the notation of the text, A, B, α, β, and C_p correspond to A_1, A_2, λ_1, λ_2, and C, respectively. O Experimental values, $\Diamond$ residuals. (Data from Ref. 3, subject 2663, dose = 10 mg/kg.)

The zero-time intercept obtained by extrapolation of the terminal linear phase to t = 0 is A_n. Successive application of the method of residuals (Appendix C) will yield linear segment(s) with slope(s) and intercept(s) from which the remaining value(s) of λ and A can be determined.

The constants A_ℓ and λ_ℓ may be obtained graphically as shown in Fig. 2.4 or with the aid of a digital computer. The best approach is to fit the entire plasma concentration-time curve by means of a digital computer program which provides a nonlinear regression analysis of the curve (Appendix H). Once these experimental constants are obtained, other pharmacokinetic parameters can be readily generated.

At time t = 0, (2.7) becomes

$$C_0 = \sum_{\ell=1}^{n} A_\ell \tag{2.12}$$

where C_0 is the zero-time plasma concentration. Substituting the value of A_ℓ from (2.8) into (2.12) yields

$$C_o = \frac{X_0}{V_c} \sum_{\ell=1}^{n} \frac{\prod\limits_{i=2}^{n} (E_i - \lambda_\ell)}{\prod\limits_{\substack{i=1 \\ i \neq \ell}}^{n} (\lambda_i - \lambda_\ell)} \tag{2.13}$$

which simplifies to

$$C_0 = \frac{X_0}{V_c} \tag{2.14}$$

for any multicompartment model. Substitution of $\sum_{\ell=1}^{n} A_\ell$ for C_0, according to (2.12), into (2.14), and rearrangement yields the following expression, from which the apparent volume of the central compartment can be estimated:

$$V_c = \frac{X_0}{\sum\limits_{\ell=1}^{n} A_\ell} \tag{2.15}$$

where X_0 is the intravenous dose.

Drug Levels in a Peripheral or "Tissue" Compartment

The differential equation describing the rate of change in the amount of drug in a peripheral compartment X_{pj} is

$$\frac{dX_{pj}}{dt} = k_{1j} X_c - E_j X_{pj} \tag{2.16}$$

where k_{1j} is the first-order intercompartmental transfer rate constant from the central to the peripheral compartment. The value of j varies from 2 to n. The Laplace transform of (2.16) (see Appendix B) is given by

$$s(a_{s,p}) = k_{1j}(a_{s,c}) - E_j(a_{s,p}) \tag{2.17}$$

Solving for $a_{s,p}$ and substituting the value of $a_{s,c}$ as given in (2.3) yields

$$a_{s,p} = X_0 \frac{k_{1j}}{s + E_j} \frac{\prod\limits_{i=2}^{n} (s + E_i)}{\prod\limits_{i=1}^{n} (s + \lambda_i)} \tag{2.18}$$

the anti-Laplace of which is (see Appendix B)

$$X_{pj} = X_0 \sum_{\ell=1}^{n} \frac{k_{1j}}{E_j - \lambda_\ell} \frac{\displaystyle\prod_{i=2}^{n} (E_i - \lambda_\ell)}{\displaystyle\prod_{\substack{i=1 \\ i \neq \ell}}^{n} (\lambda_i - \lambda_\ell)} e^{-\lambda_\ell t} \qquad (2.19)$$

This equation describes the time course of the amount of drug in the peripheral compartment following intravenous administration. It is obvious from (2.19) that after a sufficiently long period of time the exponential terms $e^{-\lambda_1 t}$ to $e^{-\lambda_{n-1} t}$ will approach zero and (2.19) reduces to

$$X_{pj} = X_0 \frac{k_{1j}}{E_j - \lambda_n} \frac{\displaystyle\prod_{i=2}^{n} (E_i - \lambda_n)}{\displaystyle\prod_{\substack{i=1 \\ i \neq \ell}}^{n} (\lambda_i - \lambda_n)} e^{-\lambda_n t} \qquad (2.20)$$

Hence the slope of the terminal exponential phase of a semilogarithmic plot of tissue level versus time equals $-\lambda_n/2.303$. Therefore, in the postdistributive phase, plasma and peripheral compartment levels decline in parallel. This is illustrated in Fig. 2.5.

Urinary Excretion Data

It may be possible to obtain from urinary excretion data the pharmacokinetic parameters of a drug that confers on the body the pharmacokinetic characteristics of a multicompartment model. For a drug eliminated from the body partly by nonrenal processes a scheme analogous to Scheme 1 of Chap. 1 can be drawn:

Scheme 1

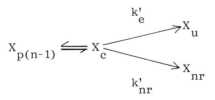

where X_u and X_{nr} are the respective cumulative amounts of unchanged drug eliminated in the urine and drug eliminated by all nonrenal path-

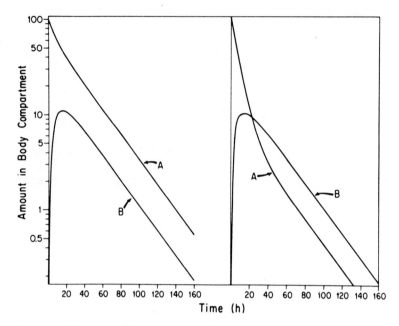

Fig. 2.5 Semilogarithmic plots of the amounts of drug in the central (A) and peripheral (B) compartments following intravenous adminis- tration of two drugs, each of which confer the pharmacokinetic charac- teristics of a two-compartment open model on the body, but which have different distribution characteristics.

ways to time t. The elimination rate constant from the central compart- ment, k_{10}, is the sum of the individual rate constants that character- ize the parallel elimination processes. Therefore, $k_{10} = k_e' + k_{nr}'$, where k_e' is the apparent first-order rate constant for renal excretion and k_{nr}' is the sum of all other apparent first-order elimination rate constants for drug elimination by nonrenal pathways.

The excretion rate of intact drug, dX_u/dt, can be defined as

$$\frac{dX_u}{dt} = k_e' X_c \qquad (2.21)$$

where X_c is as defined previously. Substitution for X_c, according to (2.4), into (2.21) yields

$$\frac{dX_u}{dt} = k_e' X_0 \sum_{\ell=1}^{n} \frac{\prod\limits_{i=2}^{n} (E_i - \lambda_\ell)}{\prod\limits_{\substack{i=1 \\ i \neq \ell}}^{n} (\lambda_i - \lambda_\ell)} e^{-\lambda_\ell t} \qquad (2.22)$$

or

$$\frac{dX_u}{dt} = \sum_{\ell=1}^{n} A'_{\ell} e^{-\lambda_{\ell} t} \tag{2.23}$$

where

$$A'_{\ell} = k'_e X_0 \frac{\displaystyle\prod_{i=2}^{n} (E_i - \lambda_{\ell})}{\displaystyle\prod_{\substack{i=1 \\ i \neq \ell}}^{n} (\lambda_i - \lambda_{\ell})} \tag{2.24}$$

A semilogarithmic plot of excretion rate of unmetabolized drug versus time according to (2.23) will yield a multiexponential curve (Fig. 2.6). As with the semilogarithmic plasma concentration-time plot, λ_n can be obtained from the slope, $-\lambda_n/2.303$, of the terminal exponential phase, and the biologic half-life $t_{1/2}$ can be determined either directly from the terminal phase or from λ_n by (2.11). A'_n can be obtained by extrapolation of the terminal linear phase to time zero. Application of the method of residuals (Appendix C) permits estimates of the remaining value(s) of λ and A'. As with plasma concentration-time data, the constants λ_ℓ and A'_ℓ can be better obtained with the aid of a digital computer (Appendix H). It must be emphasized that the terminal slope of the log excretion rate versus time curve is a function of the overall elimination rate constant λ_n and not of the urinary excretion rate constant k'_e. However, k'_e can be calculated once the experimental constants λ_ℓ and A'_ℓ are obtained. The sum of the zero-time intercepts is given by

$$\sum_{\ell=1}^{n} A'_{\ell} = k'_e X_0 \sum_{\ell=1}^{n} \frac{\displaystyle\prod_{i=2}^{n} (E_i - \lambda_{\ell})}{\displaystyle\prod_{\substack{i=1 \\ i \neq \ell}}^{n} (\lambda_i - \lambda_{\ell})} \tag{2.25}$$

This equation can be simplified to

$$\sum_{\ell=1}^{n} A'_{\ell} = k'_e X_0 \tag{2.26}$$

which when rearranged yields the following expression for k'_e:

$$k'_e = \frac{\displaystyle\sum_{\ell=1}^{n} A'_{\ell}}{X_0} \tag{2.27}$$

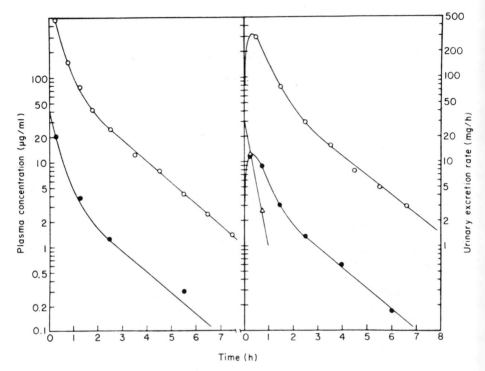

Fig. 2.6 Plasma concentrations (○) and urinary excretion rates (●) of ampicillin (left) after intravenous injection of ampicillin itself or of its prodrug, hetacillin (right). The triangles (right) indicate hetacillin concentrations in plasma. (Data from Ref. 4.)

Therefore, by knowing the intravenous dose and the values of A'_ℓ, the urinary excretion rate constant of intact drug can be determined.

An alternative approach, the sigma-minus method, is also available, from which the parameters of a multicompartment model can be evaluated based on urinary excretion data. The Laplace transform of (2.21) for the amount of drug in the urine $a_{s,u}$ is

$$s(a_{s,u}) = k'_e(a_{s,c}) \qquad (2.28)$$

Substitution for $a_{s,c}$ from (2.3) and rearrangement yields

$$a_{s,u} = k'_e X_0 \frac{\prod\limits_{i=2}^{n} (s + E_i)}{\prod\limits_{i=1}^{n} s(s + \lambda_i)} \qquad (2.29)$$

Solving (2.29) (see Appendix B) produces the following relation-ship between the amount of drug in the urine and time:

$$X_u = k_e' X_0 \frac{\prod\limits_{i=2}^{n} E_i}{\prod\limits_{i=1}^{n} \lambda_i} + k_e' X_0 \sum_{\ell=1}^{n} \frac{\prod\limits_{i=2}^{n} (E_i - \lambda_\ell)}{\prod\limits_{\substack{i=1 \\ i \neq \ell}}^{n} -\lambda_\ell (\lambda_i - \lambda_\ell)} e^{-\lambda_\ell t} \qquad (2.30)$$

where X_u is the cumulative amount of unchanged drug excreted in the urine to time t. The amount of unmetabolized drug ultimately elim-inated in the urine, X_u^∞, can be determined by setting time in (2.30) equal to infinity:

$$X_u^\infty = k_e' X_0 \frac{\prod\limits_{i=2}^{n} E_i}{\prod\limits_{i=1}^{n} \lambda_i} \qquad (2.31)$$

Substitution of X_u^∞ for $k_e' X_0 \prod_{i=2}^{n} E_i / \prod_{i=1}^{n} \lambda_i$ in (2.30) and rearrangement yields

$$X_u^\infty - X_u = k_e' X_0 \sum_{\ell=1}^{n} \frac{\prod\limits_{i=2}^{n} (E_i - \lambda_\ell)}{\prod\limits_{\substack{i=1 \\ i \neq \ell}}^{n} \lambda_\ell (\lambda_i - \lambda_\ell)} e^{-\lambda_\ell t} \qquad (2.32)$$

or

$$X_u^\infty - X_u = \sum_{i=\ell}^{n} A_\ell'' e^{-\lambda_\ell t} \qquad (2.33)$$

where

$$A_\ell'' = k_e' X_0 \frac{\prod\limits_{i=2}^{n} (E_i - \lambda_\ell)}{\prod\limits_{\substack{i=1 \\ i \neq \ell}}^{n} \lambda_\ell (\lambda_i - \lambda_\ell)} \qquad (2.34)$$

A plot of the logarithm of the amount of unchanged drug remaining to be excreted versus time is multiexponential (Fig. 2.7), and the slope

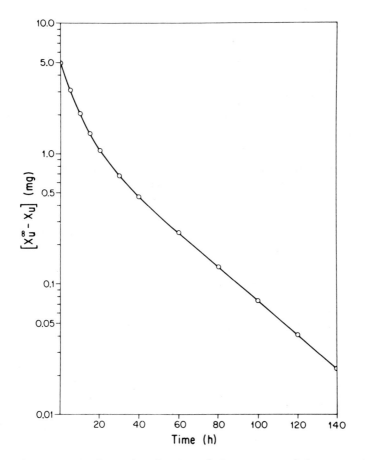

Fig. 2.7 Semilogarithmic plot of the amount of drug remaining to be excreted following intravenous administration of a drug. The data are described by Eq. (2.33), where n = 2.

of the terminal exponential phase is $-\lambda_n/2.303$, the same slope as a plot of log C versus t or a plot of log (dX_u/dt) versus t. The zero-time intercept of the extrapolated terminal linear phase yields A_n''. The other values of λ_ℓ and A_ℓ'' can be obtained from the slope(s) and intercept(s), respectively, of the residual line(s).

The general merits of these two urinary excretion methods, the excretion rate method and sigma-minus method, have been discussed in Chap. 1. It is important to emphasize that the value of urinary excretion data to obtain the pharmacokinetic parameters of a multicompartment model may be limited. In order to perform a multicompartment analysis of urinary excretion data, urine must be collected

with sufficient frequency to enable the characterization of the distributive phase. Since it is difficult to collect urine samples at a frequency
of greater than every half-hour, the drug being examined must have
a significant distributive phase. This problem is usually not encountered with plasma-level data because plasma samples can generally
be collected with almost any desired frequency.

Renal Clearance

One can characterize the kinetics of renal excretion of a drug by a
clearance value as well as by an excretion rate constant. The concept
of clearance is discussed in Chap. 8. Renal clearance, as defined in
Chap. 1, is the volume of blood flowing through the kidney per unit
time from which all drug is extracted and excreted. In pharmacokinetic terms, renal clearance Cl_r is the urinary excretion rate divided
by the blood or plasma concentration of drug at the midpoint of the
urine collection period:

$$Cl_r = \frac{dX_u/dt}{C} \tag{2.35}$$

Replacement of dX_u/dt by $k_e'X_c$, according to (2.21), yields

$$Cl_r = \frac{k_e'X_c}{C} \tag{2.36}$$

Recognizing that X_c/C equals V_c [Eq. (2.5)], the following expression
for renal clearance can be obtained:

$$Cl_r = k_e'V_c \tag{2.37}$$

Therefore, renal clearance equals the product of the renal excretion
rate constant k_e' and the apparent volume of the central compartment
V_c. If renal clearance is determined independently by (2.35) and if
an estimate of V_c is available, (2.37) may be employed to calculate k_e'.
This method for determining k_e' has an advantage over the method
which employs (2.27) in that estimates of the zero-time intercepts of
an excretion rate plot, A_λ', may be difficult to obtain.

Probably a more satisfactory method for determining clearance than
the one-point determination obtained by employing (2.35) would be to
rearrange Eq. (2.35) (i.e., $dX_u/dt = Cl_rC$) and to plot excretion rate
versus the plasma concentration at the midpoint of each urine collection
period. The slope of such a plot equals renal clearance. The utilization of rate plots is discussed in Appendix F.

Recognizing that renal clearance as defined by (2.35) equals k_eV
for a one-compartment model [Eq. (1.25)] and $k_e'V_c$ for a multicompartment model, it can be readily shown that (1.27) and (1.28) also apply
to multicompartment models:

$$(X_u)_{t_1}^{t_2} = Cl_r \int_{t_1}^{t_2} C \, dt \tag{2.38}$$

and

$$Cl_r = \frac{X_u^\infty}{\int_0^\infty C \, dt} = \frac{X_u^\infty}{AUC} \tag{2.39}$$

respectively. The term $(X_u)_{t_1}^{t_2}$ is the amount of unmetabolized drug eliminated in the urine during the time interval t_1 to t_2, and $\int_{t_1}^{t_2} C \, dt$ is the area under the blood or plasma concentration versus time curve during the same time interval t_1 to t_2. $\int_0^\infty C \, dt$ or AUC represents the total area under the drug concentration in the blood or plasma-time curve. Therefore, by employing (2.38), an estimate of the renal clearance of a drug, which distributes in the body according to a multicompartment model, may be obtained from the slope of a plot of the amounts of unmetabolized drug eliminated in the urine during time intervals t_1 to t_2 $[(X_u)_{t_1}^{t_2}]$ versus the areas under the plasma concentration-time curve (plotted on rectilinear graph paper) during the same time intervals ($\int_{t_1}^{t_2} C \, dt$). The average renal clearance of a drug can be determined using (2.39) if the total amount of unmetabolized drug eliminated in the urine and the area under the plasma concentration-time curve from time zero to infinity are known.

The total area under the curve as required by (2.39) for the calculation of renal clearance can be readily determined employing the relationship

$$AUC = \sum_{\ell=1}^{n} \frac{A_\ell}{\lambda_\ell} \tag{2.40}$$

which results from the integration of (2.7) from time zero to infinity.

Systemic Clearance

Systemic clearance Cl_s or total body clearance is the sum of clearances for all processes involved in the elimination of a drug from the body and can be given by an expression analogous to (2.35), the equation for renal clearance:

$$Cl_s = \frac{dX_E/dt}{C} \tag{2.41}$$

where dX_E/dt is the rate of drug elimination by all routes of elimination. Solving (2.41) for dX_E/dt and integrating the resulting expression from time zero to infinity yields

$$(X_E)_0^\infty = Cl_s \int_0^\infty C\ dt = Cl_s \cdot AUC \tag{2.42}$$

where $(X_E)_0^\infty$ is the total amount of drug eliminated, which must be equal to the dose X_0 of drug administered when the drug is given intravenously. Therefore, substitution of X_0 for $(X_E)_0^\infty$ in (2.42) and rearrangement provides the following expression for clearance:

$$Cl_s = \frac{X_0}{AUC} \tag{2.43}$$

Clearance is extensively discussed in Chap. 8.

Metabolite Levels in the Plasma

The formation of a metabolite that distributes in the body according to a multicompartment model following the intravenous administration of a drug which also distributes according to a multicompartment model is illustrated in Scheme 2:

Scheme 2

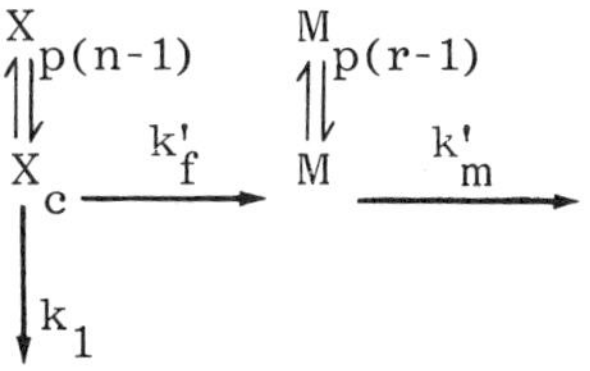

X_p and X_c are as defined previously; M and M_p are the amounts of metabolite in the central and peripheral body compartments, respectively; the constants k_f' and k_m' are the apparent first-order formation and elimination rate constants, respectively, of the metabolite; and k_1 is the sum of all apparent first-order elimination rate constants for all processes other than metabolism. In this scheme $k_{10} = k_1 + k_f'$, where k_{10} is the elimination rate constant from the central compartment for parent drug.

The disposition functions for the drug, $d_{s,c}$, and metabolite, $d_{s,m}$, in their respective central compartments (see Appendix B) are

$$d_{s,c} = \frac{\displaystyle\prod_{i=2}^{n} (s + E_i)}{\displaystyle\prod_{i=1}^{n} (s + \lambda_i)}$$

[Eq. (2.1)] and

$$d_{s,m} = \frac{\prod\limits_{j=2}^{r} (s + E_j)}{\prod\limits_{j=1}^{r} (s + \gamma_j)} \tag{2.44}$$

respectively, where E_i and λ_i are as defined previously, E_j is the sum of the exit rate constants from the jth compartment for the metabolite, and γ_j is a disposition rate constant associated with the blood or plasma concentration-time curve following an intravenous bolus injection of metabolite and is analogous to λ_i. The Laplace transform for the amount of drug in the central compartment, $a_{s,c}$, following intravenous injection is given by

$$a_{s,c} = X_0 \frac{\prod\limits_{i=2}^{n} (s + E_i)}{\prod\limits_{i=1}^{n} (s + \lambda_i)}$$

[Eq. (2.3)]. The input function into the central compartment for the metabolite, $in_{s,m}$, is given by

$$in_{s,m} = k_f'(a_{s,c}) \tag{2.45}$$

Therefore, the Laplace transform for the amount of metabolite in the central compartment, $a_{s,m}$, following the intravenous injection of a drug is given by the product of (2.44) and (2.45):

$$a_{s,m} = k_f'(a_{s,c}) \frac{\prod\limits_{j=2}^{r} (s + E_j)}{\prod\limits_{j=1}^{r} (s + \gamma_j)} \tag{2.46}$$

Substitution for $a_{s,c}$, according to (2.3), in (2.46) yields

$$a_{s,m} = k_f' X_0 \frac{\prod\limits_{i=2}^{n} (s + E_i) \prod\limits_{j=2}^{r} (s + E_j)}{\prod\limits_{i=1}^{n} (s + \lambda_i) \prod\limits_{j=1}^{r} (s + \gamma_j)} \tag{2.47}$$

Taking the anti-Laplace of (2.47) and writing a general equation for the concentration of metabolite in the plasma, C_m, gives

$$C_m = \sum_{\ell=1}^{n} A_\ell e^{-\lambda_\ell t} + \sum_{u=1}^{r} B_u e^{-\gamma_u t} \qquad (2.48)$$

Equation (2.48) indicates that a minimum of five exponential terms are required to describe the time course of a relatively slowly distributing metabolite which is formed after intravenous administration of a drug with multicompartment characteristics. In fact, metabolite concentration-time curves rarely require more than two or three exponential terms to describe them, reflecting a lack of discrimination of individual rate processes. A rigorous analysis of metabolite concentration-time data will provide little information concerning the multicompartment pharmacokinetics of the parent drug or even concerning the metabolite itself. The slope of the terminal linear segment of a semilogarithmic plot of metabolite concentration versus time will probably be equal to either $-\lambda_n/2.303$ or $-\gamma_r/2.303$, whichever is smaller. Residual analysis will almost always result in hybrid constants that cannot be related to either the drug or the metabolite.

INTRAVENOUS INFUSION

Drug Concentrations in the Plasma

The disposition function for the central compartment following constant rate intravenous infusion of a drug that confers the pharmacokinetic characteristics of a multicompartment model on the body is identical to the disposition function for an intravenous bolus injection [Eq. (2.1)]:

$$d_{s,c} = \frac{\prod_{i=2}^{n} (s + E_i)}{\prod_{i=1}^{n} (s + \lambda_i)}$$

where all parameters are as defined previously. For intravenous infusion the input function in_s is given by

$$in_s = \frac{k_0(1 - e^{-Ts})}{s} \qquad (2.49)$$

where k_0 is the zero-order infusion rate in units of amount per time and T is the time when infusion ends. The Laplace transform for the amount of drug in the central compartment, $a_{s,c}$ is given by the product of the input and disposition function, (2.49) and (2.1), respectively. Hence

$$a_{s,c} = \frac{k_0(1 - e^{-Ts}) \prod\limits_{i=2}^{n} (s + E_i)}{s} \cdot \frac{1}{\prod\limits_{i=1}^{n} (s + \lambda_i)}$$

(2.50)

One may solve for X_c, the amount of drug in the central compartment, by taking the anti-Laplace of (2.50) (see Appendix B). The resulting equation is

$$X_c = k_0 \sum_{\ell=1}^{n} \frac{(1 - e^{\lambda_\ell T}) \prod\limits_{i=2}^{n} (E_i - \lambda_\ell)}{-\lambda_\ell \prod\limits_{\substack{i=1 \\ i \neq \ell}}^{n} (\lambda_i - \lambda_\ell)} e^{-\lambda_\ell t}$$

(2.51)

which can be written in concentration terms, employing the relationship $X_c = V_c C$ according to (2.5), as follows:

$$C = \frac{k_0}{V_c} \sum_{\ell=1}^{n} \frac{(1 - e^{\lambda_\ell T}) \prod\limits_{i=2}^{n} (E_i - \lambda_\ell)}{-\lambda_\ell \prod\limits_{\substack{i=1 \\ i \neq \ell}}^{n} (\lambda_i - \lambda_\ell)} e^{-\lambda_\ell t}$$

(2.52)

This equation describes the time course of drug in the plasma during infusion and after cessation of infusion. While infusion is continuing, $T = t$ and varies with time. When infusion ceases, T becomes a constant corresponding to the time infusion was stopped. Hence, by utilization of (2.52), the total plasma concentration-time curve during and following infusion can be fit with the aid of a digital computer. Consequently, it is not necessary to fit infusion curves by two discrete equations, one representing the infusion period and one representing the postinfusion period [5].

During infusion, $T = t$, and the term $(1 - e^{\lambda_\ell T})e^{-\lambda_\ell t}$ in (2.52) becomes $(e^{-\lambda_\ell t} - 1)$. Therefore,

$$C = \frac{k_0}{V_c} \sum_{\ell=1}^{n} \frac{\prod\limits_{i=2}^{n} (E_i - \lambda_\ell)}{-\lambda_\ell \prod\limits_{\substack{i=1 \\ i \neq \ell}}^{n} (\lambda_i - \lambda_\ell)} (e^{-\lambda_\ell t} - 1)$$

(2.53)

Expansion yields

$$
C = \frac{k_0}{V_c} \left[\sum_{\ell=1}^{n} \frac{\prod\limits_{i=2}^{n} (E_i - \lambda_\ell)}{\lambda_\ell \prod\limits_{\substack{i=1 \\ i \neq \ell}}^{n} (\lambda_i - \lambda_\ell)} - \sum_{\ell=1}^{n} \frac{\prod\limits_{i=2}^{n} (E_i - \lambda_\ell)}{\lambda_\ell \prod\limits_{\substack{i=1 \\ i \neq \ell}}^{n} (\lambda_i - \lambda_\ell)} e^{-\lambda_\ell t} \right]
$$

(2.54)

The first term in (2.54) can be simplified to give the following equation for C:

$$
C = \frac{k_0}{V_c} \left[\frac{\prod\limits_{i=2}^{n} E_i}{\prod\limits_{i=1}^{n} \lambda_i} - \sum_{\ell=1}^{n} \frac{\prod\limits_{i=2}^{n} (E_i - \lambda_\ell)}{\lambda_\ell \prod\limits_{\substack{i=1 \\ i \neq \ell}}^{n} (\lambda_i - \lambda_\ell)} e^{-\lambda_\ell t} \right]
$$

(2.55)

This equation describes the rise in drug concentration with time after the start of intravenous infusion. Plasma concentrations will increase with time until the rate of elimination equals the rate of infusion and then will remain constant. This plateau plasma drug concentration C_{ss} can be determined from (2.55) by setting time equal to infinity (i.e., by recognizing that the term $e^{-\lambda_\ell t}$ approaches zero with time). Thus

$$
C_{ss} = \frac{k_0 \prod\limits_{i=2}^{n} E_i}{V_c \prod\limits_{i=1}^{n} \lambda_i}
$$

(2.56)

It is evident that the plateau or steady-state concentration C_{ss} of drug is directly proportional to the rate of infusion. The term $\prod_{i=2}^{n} E_i /$ $V_c \prod_{i=1}^{n} \lambda_i$ can be expanded to $k_{21}k_{31} \cdots k_{n1}/V_c \lambda_1\lambda_2\lambda_3 \cdots \lambda_n$, which is equal to $1/V_c k_{10}$ or $1/Cl_s$ [see Eqs. (2.107), 2.169), and (2.215)]. Therefore, substitution of $1/Cl_s$ into (2.56) yields

$$
C_{ss} = \frac{k_0}{Cl_s}
$$

(2.57)

By knowing the clearance of a drug, the infusion rate required to maintain a certain plasma concentration of drug can be readily calculated employing the following rearrangement of (2.57):

$$k_0 = C_{ss} Cl_s \tag{2.58}$$

As is apparent from (2.57), the systemic clearance of a drug is readily calculated from the ratio of infusion rate to steady-state drug concentration in plasma:

$$Cl_s = \frac{k_0}{C_{ss}} \tag{2.59}$$

The terminal disposition rate constant, and hence half-life, of a drug may also be determined from data collected during infusion to steady state. Expansion of (2.55), substitution of C_{ss} for $k_0 \, \Pi_{i=2}^n E_i / V_c \, \Pi_{i=1}^n \lambda_i$ according to (2.56), and rearrangement gives

$$C_{ss} - C = \frac{k_0}{V_c} \sum_{\ell=1}^n \frac{\displaystyle\prod_{i=2}^n (E_i - \lambda_\ell)}{\lambda_\ell \displaystyle\prod_{\substack{i=1 \\ i \neq \ell}}^n (\lambda_i - \lambda_\ell)} e^{-\lambda_\ell t} \tag{2.60}$$

Based on this relationship, a plot of log $(C_{ss} - C)$ versus time will be nonlinear. However, since the values of λ_1 to λ_{n-1} are larger than λ_n, at some time during the infusion the terms $e^{-\lambda_1 t}$ to $e^{-\lambda_{n-1} t}$ will approach zero. At this time (2.60) will simplify to

$$C_{ss} - C = \frac{k_0 \displaystyle\prod_{i=2}^n (E_i - \lambda_n)}{V_c \lambda_n \displaystyle\prod_{\substack{i=1 \\ i \neq n}}^n (\lambda_i - \lambda_n)} e^{-\lambda_n t} \tag{2.61}$$

which in logarithmic terms becomes

$$\log (C_{ss} - C) = \log \frac{k_0 \displaystyle\prod_{i=2}^n (E_i - \lambda_n)}{V_c \lambda_n \displaystyle\prod_{\substack{i=1 \\ i \neq n}}^n (\lambda_i - \lambda_n)} - \frac{\lambda_n t}{2.303} \tag{2.62}$$

Therefore, a plot of log $(C_{ss} - C)$ versus t should eventually yield a linear segment with a slope of $-\lambda_n/2.303$ from which λ_n can be determined. Half-life $t_{1/2}$ can be determined either directly from the terminal linear segment of the resulting plot or from the relationship [Eq. (2.11)]

$$t_{1/2} = \frac{0.693}{\lambda_n}$$

The half-life and terminal disposition rate constant may also be determined from the declining drug concentration in the plasma versus time data collected following cessation of an intravenous infusion. Once infusion is stopped, T becomes a constant (i.e., the time at which infusion is ended). The term $(1 - e^{\lambda_\ell T})e^{-\lambda_\ell t}$ in (2.52) becomes $(1 - e^{\lambda_\ell T})e^{-\lambda_\ell(t'+T)}$ since

$$t = t' + T \tag{2.63}$$

where t' is the postinfusion time. Rearrangement of the term $(1 - e^{\lambda_\ell T})e^{-\lambda_\ell(t'+T)}$ yields $(e^{-\lambda_\ell T} - 1)e^{-\lambda_\ell t'}$. Therefore,

$$(1 - e^{\lambda_\ell T})e^{-\lambda_\ell t} = (e^{-\lambda_\ell T} - 1)e^{-\lambda_\ell t'} \tag{2.64}$$

in the postinfusion phase. Substitution of $(e^{-\lambda_\ell T} - 1)e^{-\lambda_\ell t'}$ for $(1 - e^{\lambda_\ell T})e^{-\lambda_\ell t}$ in (2.52) yields the following relationship between plasma concentration and time (t', postinfusion time) during the period after infusion [6]:

$$C = \frac{k_0}{V_c} \sum_{\ell=1}^{n} \frac{(e^{-\lambda_\ell T} - 1) \prod_{i=2}^{n} (E_i - \lambda_\ell)}{-\lambda_\ell \prod_{\substack{i=1 \\ i \neq \ell}}^{n} (\lambda_i - \lambda_\ell)} e^{-\lambda_\ell t'} \tag{2.65}$$

or

$$C = \sum_{\ell=1}^{n} R_\ell e^{-\lambda_\ell t'} \tag{2.66}$$

where

$$R_\ell = \frac{k_0}{V_c} \frac{(e^{-\lambda_\ell T} - 1) \prod_{i=2}^{n} (E_i - \lambda_\ell)}{-\lambda_\ell \prod_{\substack{i=1 \\ i \neq \ell}}^{n} (\lambda_i - \lambda_\ell)} \tag{2.67}$$

The coefficient R_ℓ can be related to A_ℓ, the zero-time intercept following intravenous injection. Rearrangement of (2.8) yields

$$\frac{A_\ell}{X_0} = \frac{\prod\limits_{\substack{i=2}}^{n} (E_i - \lambda_\ell)}{V_c \prod\limits_{\substack{i=1 \\ i \neq \ell}}^{n} (\lambda_i - \lambda_\ell)} \tag{2.68}$$

Substituting A_ℓ/X_0 for $\prod\limits_{i=2}^{n} (E_i - \lambda_\ell)/[V_c \prod\limits_{i=1, i \neq \ell}^{n} (\lambda_i - \lambda_\ell)]$ in (2.67) and solving for A_ℓ gives the relationship

$$A_\ell = \frac{R_\ell X_0 \lambda_\ell}{k_0 (1 - e^{-\lambda_\ell T})} \tag{2.69}$$

where X_0 is the administered dose and equals the product of the infusion rate and the infusion time (i.e., $k_0 T$).

From (2.66) it is readily apparent that upon stopping the infusion, drug concentrations in the plasma decline in a multiexponential manner when plotted semilogarithmically (Fig. 2.8). Determination of the constants λ_1 to λ_n and R_1 to R_n from postinfusion data may be carried out in the usual fashion (i.e., method of residuals, Appendix C, or computer curve-fitting, Appendix H). By knowing the duration of infusion and the infusion rate, A_1 to A_n can be calculated employing (2.69).

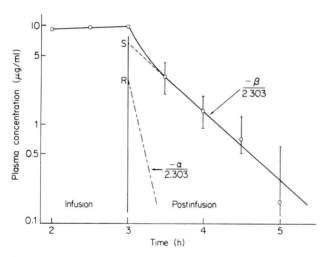

Fig. 2.8 Average oxacillin concentrations in plasma during and after constant rate intravenous infusion in four healthy volunteers. In the notation of the text, R, S, α, and β correspond to R_1, R_2, λ_1, and λ_2, respectively. (Data from Ref. 7.)

Equation (2.66), which describes the time course of drug following the cessation of infusion, is very useful since it is frequently
difficult or impossible to administer a drug by rapid intravenous
injection because of limited solubility of the drug (requiring a large
injection volume), or because of possible adverse pharmacologic effects. It may then become necessary to inject the drug slowly (i.e.,
as a short intravenous infusion).

If infusion is carried out until steady state is attained [i.e., the
infusion time T is sufficiently long so that the term $e^{-\lambda_\ell T}$ in (2.65)
approaches zero], the zero-time intercept R_ℓ, as defined by (2.67),
becomes

$$R_\ell = \frac{k_0}{V_c} \frac{\prod\limits_{i=2}^{n} (E_i - \lambda_\ell)}{\lambda_\ell \prod\limits_{\substack{i=1 \\ i \neq \ell}}^{n} (\lambda_i - \lambda_\ell)} \qquad (2.70)$$

Therefore, the decline of drug in the plasma after cessation of infusion to steady state is given by

$$C = \frac{k_0}{V_c} \sum_{\ell=1}^{n} \frac{\prod\limits_{i=2}^{n} (E_i - \lambda_\ell)}{\lambda_\ell \prod\limits_{\substack{i=1 \\ i \neq \ell}}^{n} (\lambda_i - \lambda_\ell)} e^{-\lambda_\ell t'} \qquad (2.71)$$

Equation (2.69) then reduces to

$$A_\ell = \frac{R_\ell X_0 \lambda_\ell}{k_0} \qquad (2.72)$$

where R_ℓ is as defined by (2.70). Once R_1 to R_n and λ_1 to λ_n are
estimated from postinfusion plasma concentration-time data, A_ℓ can
be calculated employing (2.72).

If a two-compartment system is considered (i.e., $n = 2$), the
larger the ratio of the zero-time intercepts A_1/A_2 following intravenous injection, the more readily one can discern the multicompartment characteristics of a drug. As A_1 approaches zero, the ratio
A_1/A_2 approaches zero and the plasma concentration-time curve becomes monoexponential (Fig. 2.9). On the other hand, if A_1 is exceedingly large relative to A_2, the plasma curve may again appear
to reflect a one-compartment model since, in this case, the plasma
levels during the distributive phase may decline in an apparent mono-

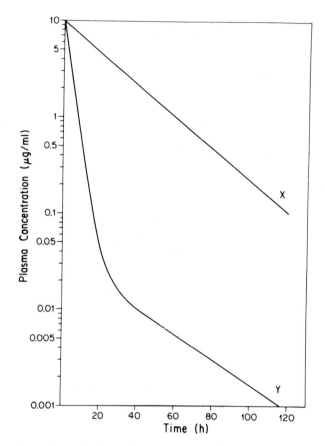

Fig. 2.9 Semilogarithmic plots of drug concentrations in plasma following intravenous injection of compounds X and Y. The disposition rate constants λ_1 and λ_2 are the same for both drugs, but the ratios of the coefficients (i.e., A_1/A_2) are markedly different, 0.3 for X and 300 for Y.

exponential fashion over several orders of magnitude of plasma drug concentration prior to reaching the terminal exponential phase (Fig. 2.9). This latter phase may not be observed, as the plasma concentration of drug may be well below the assay sensitivity for the drug in plasma.

For a drug that is administered by a bolus intravenous injection, the ratio of A_1 to A_2 is given by

$$\frac{A_1}{A_2} = \frac{\lambda_1 - E_2}{E_2 - \lambda_2} \qquad (2.73)$$

where A_1 and A_2 are obtained from (2.8). However, when a drug is infused to steady state, the analogous ratio R_1/R_2 is given by

$$\frac{R_1}{R_2} = \frac{\lambda_1 - E_2}{E_2 - \lambda_2} \frac{\lambda_2}{\lambda_1} \tag{2.74}$$

where R_1 and R_2 are obtained from (2.70). It follows that the ratio R_1/R_2 will always be less than the ratio A_1/A_2 since λ_2 is by definition smaller than λ_1. As a result, the ability to discern the multicompartment characteristics of a drug following infusion is

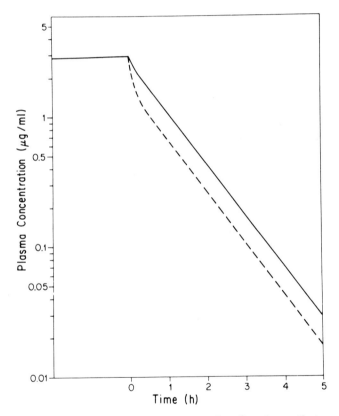

Fig. 2.10 Decline in plasma levels of a drug that confers two-compartment model characteristics on the body, following constant rate intravenous infusion to steady state (——) and following the rapid intravenous injection of a dose that gives an initial drug concentration equal to the steady-state concentration (-----). The biexponential characteristic of the drug is more evident following the bolus injection than after terminating the infusion.

usually decreased (Fig. 2.10). Hence the determination of the multicompartment model parameters following intravenous infusion may be
very difficult for drugs that do not display prominent multicompartment characteristics upon rapid intravenous injection. However, for
drugs with a very high A_1/A_2 ratio, infusion may be advantageous
from a pharmacokinetic analysis point of view since the multiexponential time course of a drug in the plasma may become more apparent. These general observations apply regardless of the number
of compartments required to describe the disposition characteristics
of a drug.

Simultaneous Rapid Intravenous Injection

The time required to obtain steady-state plasma levels C_{ss} by infusion will be quite long for a drug with a long half-life. It may be
convenient in such cases to administer an intravenous loading dose
to attain immediately the desired drug concentration and then attempt
to maintain this concentration by continuous infusion. The equation
describing the time course of the plasma concentration of drug following simultaneous injection of an intravenous loading dose and initiation of infusion is the sum of the two equations describing these two
processes individually, Eqs. (2.6) and (2.55), respectively. Thus

$$
C = \frac{X_0}{V_c} \sum_{\ell=1}^{n} \frac{\prod\limits_{\substack{i=2}}^{n} (E_i - \lambda_\ell)}{\prod\limits_{\substack{i=1 \\ i \neq \ell}}^{n} (\lambda_i - \lambda_\ell)} e^{-\lambda_\ell t}
$$

$$
+ \frac{k_0}{V_c} \left[\frac{\prod\limits_{i=2}^{n} E_i}{\prod\limits_{i=1}^{n} \lambda_i} - \sum_{\ell=1}^{n} \frac{\prod\limits_{i=2}^{n} (E_i - \lambda_\ell)}{\lambda_\ell \prod\limits_{\substack{i=1 \\ i \neq \ell}}^{n} (\lambda_i - \lambda_\ell)} e^{-\lambda_\ell t} \right] \qquad (2.75)
$$

Expanding (2.75), collecting the coefficients of the exponential terms,
and bringing these terms to a common denominator yields

$$
C = \frac{k_0}{V_c} \frac{\prod\limits_{i=2}^{n} E_i}{\prod\limits_{i=1}^{n} \lambda_i} + \sum_{\ell=1}^{n} \frac{X_0 \lambda_\ell - k_0}{V_c \lambda_\ell} \frac{\prod\limits_{i=2}^{n} (E_i - \lambda_\ell)}{\prod\limits_{\substack{i=1 \\ i \neq \ell}}^{n} (\lambda_i - \lambda_\ell)} e^{-\lambda_\ell t} \qquad (2.76)
$$

Since the variable, time, remains in (2.76), it is readily apparent that the plasma concentration following the intravenous injection and simultaneous intravenous infusion of a drug that distributes in the body according to a multicompartment model will not be constant. For the concentration of drug in plasma to be constant, the coefficient of the exponential term in (2.76) must equal zero. This will occur when either $X_0 \lambda_\ell - k_0$ and/or $E_i - \lambda_\ell$ in (2.76) are zero. This situation is not possible unless n = 1 (i.e., a one-compartment model).

The loading dose required to give an immediate plasma concentration of drug equal to the steady-state level C_{ss} would be $C_{ss}V_c$, since V_c relates the amount of drug in the body at time zero (i.e., the dose) to the plasma concentration at time zero. However, when a loading dose of $C_{ss}V_c$ is administered, and infusion is simultaneously initiated at a rate equal to $C_{ss}Cl_s$ [Eq. (2.58)], the plasma level will fall below the desired steady-state concentration, reach a minimum, then gradually increase until C_{ss} is obtained (Fig. 2.11). An alternative approach is to administer a loading dose equal to $C_{ss}V_\beta$ with infusion at a rate equal to $C_{ss}Cl_s$. V_β is the apparent volume of distribution of a drug that relates plasma concentration to the amount of drug in the body during the terminal exponential phase

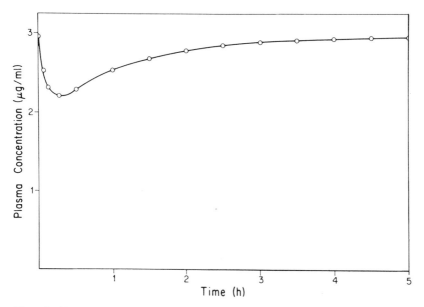

Fig. 2.11 Drug concentration in plasma on simultaneous rapid intravenous injection of a dose equal to $C_{ss}V_c$, and initiation and maintenance of an intravenous infusion at a rate equal to $C_{ss}Cl_s$. The drug in question displays multicompartment characteristics.

(i.e., $\ell = n$) of a plasma concentration versus time curve. This parameter is discussed in more detail later in the chapter. When a loading dose equal to $C_{ss}V_\beta$ is administered, the initial concentration of drug in the plasma will be higher than the desired steady-state level but will decrease with time to C_{ss} (Fig. 2.12). This alternative appears to be satisfactory for certain drugs (e.g., theophylline). However, with other drugs which also have a low therapeutic index (e.g., lidocaine), the initial levels may be sufficiently high as to produce toxicity. In practice a loading dose between the two extremes (i.e., between $V_c C_{ss}$ and $V_\beta C_{ss}$), although not ideal, would probably be the most satisfactory. This approach appears to have been successfully employed by Thomson et al. [9] and Rowland et al. [10] with lidocaine.

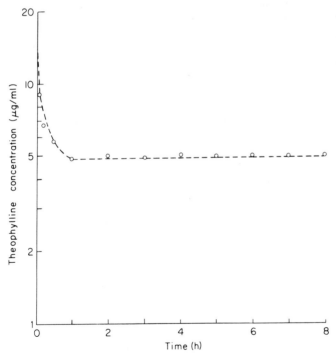

Fig. 2.12 Theophylline concentration in plasma on simultaneous rapid intravenous injection of a dose equal to $C_{ss}V_\beta$, and initiation and maintenance of an intravenous infusion at a rate equal to $C_{ss}Cl_s$. (From Ref. 8, subject F. S.; mean plateau concentration = 4.92 µg/ml).

Consecutive Constant Rate Intravenous Infusions

The administration of loading doses equal to $C_{ss}V_c$ or $C_{ss}V_\beta$, in conjunction with a zero-order infusion at a rate of $C_{ss}Cl_s$, presents disadvantages for drugs with pronounced multicompartment characteristics. The former may result in blood levels sufficiently below the desired drug concentration so that the patient is left unprotected for relatively long periods of time. The latter may produce untoward effects shortly after initiating therapy. An arbitrarily selected intermediate loading dose may still present one or the other problem. Interest in this issue has been considerable and several possible solutions have been considered.

Kruger-Thiemer [11] designed a dosing regimen for a drug with two-compartment characteristics that consists of an intravenous bolus dose equal to $C_{ss}V_c$ and a simultaneous intravenous infusion with an initial rate equal to $\lambda_1 C_{ss}V_c$ which decreases exponentially with time to a value of $C_{ss}Cl_s$. This approach is theoretically sound but presents formidable practical problems. Vaughan and Tucker [12], in an attempt to overcome the difficulties associated with administering a drug infusion at an exponentially declining rate, proposed approximating the exponential rate with a consecutive declining series of constant infusion rates.

A more realistic approach for the rapid achievement and maintenance of desired concentrations of drug in the plasma is the use of two consecutive constant rate intravenous infusions. The second or slower of the two infusions should be initiated immediately upon cessation of the first infusion, at a rate equal to $C_{ss}Cl_s$, where C_{ss} is equivalent to the desired drug concentration. Selection of the appropriate rate and appropriate infusion time for the first infusion is not as straightforward and requires consideration of several factors. Clearly, the initial infusion must be given at a sufficiently rapid rate to achieve desired drug concentrations shortly after initiating therapy. The first infusion must not be continued for too long a period; otherwise high blood levels associated with adverse effects may be reached. On the other hand, if the first infusion is discontinued too quickly, blood levels may fall below the desired range and remain there for an unacceptably long period of time.

The input function for the first infusion is given by Eq. (2.49):

$$in_{s1} = \frac{k_{01}(1 - e^{-Ts})}{s}$$

where k_{01} is the zero-order rate of the first infusion and T is the duration of this fast infusion. The input function for the second infusion, which is initiated at time T, is given by

$$in_{s2} = \frac{k_0(e^{-Ts} - e^{-T's})}{s} \tag{2.77}$$

where k_{02} is the zero-order rate of the second infusion and T' is the duration of this maintenance infusion. The disposition function $d_{s,c}$ for a multicompartment model has been described by Eq. (2.1).

The Laplace transform for the case where there are two consecutive infusions will be the sum of the two input functions in_{s1} and in_{s2} times the disposition function $d_{s,c}$. Therefore,

$$a_{s,c} = \left[\frac{k_{01}(1 - e^{-Ts})}{s} + \frac{k_{02}(e^{-Ts} - e^{-T's})}{s} \right] \frac{\prod\limits_{i=2}^{n} (s + E_i)}{\prod\limits_{i=1}^{n} (s + \lambda_i)} \tag{2.78}$$

The solution is (see Appendix B)

$$X_c = \sum_{\ell=1}^{n} \frac{k_{01}(1 - e^{\lambda_\ell T}) + k_{02}(e^{\lambda_\ell T} - e^{\lambda_\ell T'})}{-\lambda_\ell} \frac{\prod\limits_{i=2}^{n} (E_i - \lambda_\ell)}{\prod\limits_{\substack{i=1 \\ i \neq \ell}}^{n} (\lambda_i - \lambda_\ell)} e^{-\lambda_\ell t} \tag{2.79}$$

Equation (2.79) can be written in concentration terms as follows:

$$C = \sum_{\ell=1}^{n} \frac{k_{01}(1 - e^{\lambda_\ell T}) + k_{02}(e^{\lambda_\ell T} - e^{\lambda_\ell T'})}{-\lambda_\ell V_c} \frac{\prod\limits_{i=2}^{n} (E_i - \lambda_\ell)}{\prod\limits_{\substack{i=1 \\ i \neq \ell}}^{n} (\lambda_i - \lambda_\ell)} e^{-\lambda_\ell t} \tag{2.80}$$

When t is less than T, both T and T' are replaced by t and Eq. (2.80) reduces to Eq. (2.53). During the maintenance infusion (i.e., when $T < t < T'$), only T' is replaced by t and Eq. (2.80) may be written (on expansion) as

$$C = \sum_{\ell=1}^{n} \left[\frac{k_{01}(1 - e^{\lambda_\ell T}) \prod_{i=2}^{n}(E_i - \lambda_\ell)}{-\lambda_\ell V_c \prod_{\substack{i=1 \\ i \neq \ell}}^{n}(\lambda_i - \lambda_\ell)} e^{-\lambda_\ell t} \right.$$

$$+ \frac{k_{02}e^{\lambda_\ell T} \prod_{i=2}^{n}(E_i - \lambda_\ell)}{-\lambda_\ell V_c \prod_{\substack{i=1 \\ i \neq \ell}}^{n}(\lambda_i - \lambda_\ell)} e^{-\lambda_\ell t}$$

$$\left. + \frac{k_{02} \prod_{i=1}^{n}(E_i - \lambda_\ell)}{\lambda_\ell V_c \prod_{\substack{i=1 \\ i \neq \ell}}^{n}(\lambda_i - \lambda_\ell)} \right] \qquad (2.81)$$

Ultimately, as the maintenance infusion proceeds, steady state is achieved and drug concentration C_{ss} is equal to the summation of the third term on the right-hand side of Eq. (2.81). Substitution of C_{ss} for this term and rearrangement leads to an expression describing drug concentration at any time during the maintenance infusion compared to the steady-state drug concentration:

$$C - C_{ss} = \frac{1}{V_c} \sum_{\ell=1}^{n} [k_{01}(1 - e^{\lambda_\ell T}) + k_{02}e^{\lambda_\ell T}]$$

$$\left[\frac{1}{-\lambda_\ell} \frac{\prod_{i=2}^{n}(E_i - \lambda_\ell)}{\prod_{\substack{i=1 \\ i \neq \ell}}^{n}(\lambda_i - \lambda_\ell)} e^{-\lambda_\ell t} \right] \qquad (2.82)$$

Logically, the rate and duration of the loading infusion must be such that upon discontinuation (C_{max}, $t = T$) and initiation of the maintenance infusion, the drug concentration would exceed the desired drug concentration C_{ss}. Equation (2.82) tells us that under these conditions the time course of drug concentration may display one of two patterns: (1) blood levels will decline but may remain above the desired drug concentration and eventually approach C_{ss}; or (2) blood levels will decline but may fall below the desired drug concentration and then slowly rise to eventually approach C_{ss}.

Wagner [13] has devised a double infusion method (with drugs acting in the central compartment in mind) that results in blood levels, at all times during the second (maintenance) infusion, greater than or equal to C_{ss}. This requires that the term $C - C_{ss}$ in Eq. (2.82) be forbidden to take on a negative value. Since the second term of the summation in (2.82) will always be negative, the first term of the summation must be negative. This, in turn, requires that

$$k_{01} e^{\lambda_\ell T} \geq k_{01} + k_{02} e^{\lambda_\ell T} \tag{2.83}$$

or

$$k_{01} \geq \frac{k_{02}}{1 - e^{-\lambda_\ell T}} \tag{2.84}$$

for all values of ℓ. An infinite number of solutions for k_{01} will satisfy the requirement imposed by (2.84), but to avoid adverse effects we seek a minimum value of k_{01}. This is found when

$$k_{01} = \frac{k_{02}}{1 - e^{-\lambda_\ell T}} \tag{2.85}$$

As noted by Vaughan and Tucker [14], Eq. (2.85) has only one solution. This is readily seen by consecutively substituting Eq. (2.85) for k_{01} in the first summation term in Eq. (2.82) using $\ell = 1$, 2, 3, . . . , n. Since $\lambda_1 > \lambda_2 > \lambda_3 > \cdots > \lambda_n$, every value of ℓ other than $\ell = n$ will produce a positive rather than a negative value for the summation term. These outcomes violate the requirement established at the outset. Thus the appropriate rate for the loading infusion is given by

$$k_{01} = \frac{k_{02}}{1 - e^{-\lambda_n T}} \tag{2.86}$$

Under certain conditions Eq. (2.86) can be simplified to permit k_{01} to be estimated more easily. The series $e^{-x} = 1 - x + (x^2/2) - (x^3/6) + \cdots$ can be approximated accurately by $e^{-x} = 1 - x$, when $x \leq 0.1$. When this situation prevails, the denominator of (2.86) may be approximated by $\lambda_n T$ and the equation written as

$$k_{01} = \frac{k_{02}}{\lambda_n T} = \frac{1.44 k_{02} t_{1/2}}{T} \qquad (2.87)$$

This approach is illustrated by the data in Fig. 2.13.

Equation (2.87) tells us that the ratio of k_{01} to k_{02} is a function of the infusion time T for the first infusion. If T is short, the ratio of infusion rates is high and relatively high blood levels will be achieved. If we increase T, we decrease the ratio of infusion rates and decrease the maximum blood level (see Fig. 2.14). The blood level at the end of the first infusion, C_{max}, may be determined by replacing t and T' in Eq. (2.80) by T. Under these conditions Eq. (2.80) reduces to

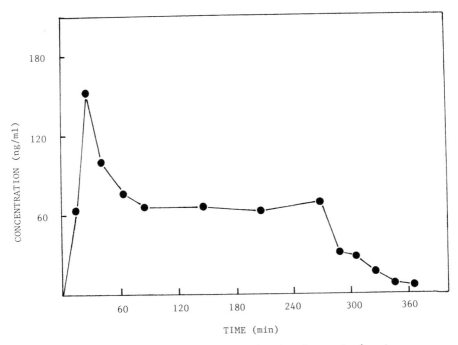

Fig. 2.13 Plot of propranolol concentration in plasma during two consecutive constant rate intravenous infusions in a representative cat. The second infusion was terminated at about 280 min. (From Ref. 15. © 1979 PJD Publications, Ltd.)

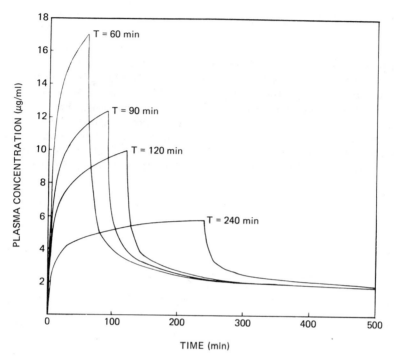

Fig. 2.14 Drug concentrations in plasma during two consecutive constant rate infusions. The maintenance infusion rate (k_{02}) was the same in each case. The loading infusion rate (k_{01}) was calculated according to Eq. (2.86), with infusion times (T) ranging from 60 to 240 min. (From Ref. 16.)

$$C_{max} = \sum_{\ell=1}^{n} \frac{k_{01}(1 - e^{\lambda_\ell T})}{-\lambda_\ell V_c} \frac{\prod_{i=2}^{n}(E_i - \lambda_\ell)}{\prod_{\substack{i=1 \\ i \neq \ell}}^{n}(\lambda_i - \lambda_\ell)} e^{-\lambda_\ell T} \tag{2.88}$$

which can be further simplified to yield

$$C_{max} = \frac{k_{01}}{V_c} \sum_{\ell=1}^{n} \frac{1 - e^{-\lambda_\ell T}}{\lambda_\ell} \frac{\prod_{i=1}^{n}(E_i - \lambda_\ell)}{\prod_{\substack{i=1 \\ i \neq \ell}}^{n}(\lambda_i - \lambda_\ell)} \tag{2.89}$$

Equation (2.89) provides a guideline for the estimation of T. After the initial selection of a desired infusion time, the maximum concentration it will produce may be determined by means of (2.89). If this value of C_{max} is inappropriately high and carries a risk of adverse effects, a longer infusion time must be considered and similarly evaluated.

FIRST-ORDER ABSORPTION

For a drug that enters the body by an apparent first-order absorption process (generally via the oral or intramuscular routes) and distributes in the body according to a multicompartment model, the disposition function for the central compartment is identical to the disposition function for an intravenous bolus injection given by (2.1):

$$d_{s,c} = \frac{\prod\limits_{i=2}^{n} (s + E_i)}{\prod\limits_{i=1}^{n} (s + \lambda_i)}$$

The following input function in_s is used to describe first-order absorption:

$$in_s = \frac{k_a FX_0}{s + k_a} \tag{2.90}$$

where k_a is the apparent first-order absorption rate constant and F is the fraction of the administered dose X_0 absorbed following drug administration. The Laplace transform for the amount of drug in the central compartment $a_{s,c}$ equals the product of the disposition and first-order input functions (i.e., $d_{s,c}$ and in_s), given by (2.1) and (2.90), respectively. Therefore,

$$a_{s,c} = \frac{k_a FX_0 \prod\limits_{i=2}^{n} (s + E_i)}{(s + k_a) \prod\limits_{i=1}^{n} (s + \lambda_i)} \tag{2.91}$$

Solving (2.91) for the amount of drug in the central compartment X_c by taking the anti-Laplace (see Appendix B) yields

$$X_c = k_a FX_0 \frac{\prod\limits_{i=2}^{n} (E_i - k_a)}{\prod\limits_{i=1}^{n} (\lambda_i - k_a)} e^{-k_a t}$$

$$+ k_a FX_0 \sum_{\ell=1}^{n} \frac{\prod\limits_{i=2}^{n} (E_i - \lambda_\ell)}{(k_a - \lambda_\ell) \prod\limits_{\substack{i=1 \\ i \neq \ell}}^{n} (\lambda_i - \lambda_\ell)} e^{-\lambda_\ell t} \qquad (2.92)$$

Expressing (2.92) in concentration terms employing the relationship $X_c = V_c C$ [according to (2.5)] results in the equation

$$C = \frac{k_a FX_0}{V_c} \frac{\prod\limits_{i=2}^{n} (E_i - k_a)}{\prod\limits_{i=1}^{n} (\lambda_i - k_a)} e^{-k_a t}$$

$$+ \frac{k_a FX_0}{V_0} \sum_{\ell=1}^{n} \frac{\prod\limits_{i=2}^{n} (E_i - \lambda_\ell)}{(k_a - \lambda_\ell) \prod\limits_{\substack{i=1 \\ i \neq \ell}}^{n} (\lambda_i - \lambda_\ell)} e^{-\lambda_\ell t} \qquad (2.93)$$

The absorption rate constant, for most drugs administered in readily available dosage forms, is probably significantly larger than the terminal disposition rate constant λ_n, and since by definition λ_1 to λ_{n-1} are larger than λ_n, at some time following administration the terms $e^{-k_a t}$ and $e^{-\lambda_1 t}$ to $e^{-\lambda_{n-1} t}$ approach zero and (2.93) reduces to

$$C = \frac{k_a FX_0}{V_c} \frac{\prod\limits_{i=2}^{n} (E_i - \lambda_n)}{(k_a - \lambda_n) \prod\limits_{\substack{i=1 \\ i \neq n}}^{n} (\lambda_i - \lambda_n)} e^{-\lambda_n t} \qquad (2.94)$$

Therefore, a plot of the logarithm of plasma concentration versus time following first-order input into a multicompartment model yields a multiexponential curve (Fig. 2.15), the terminal portion of which is

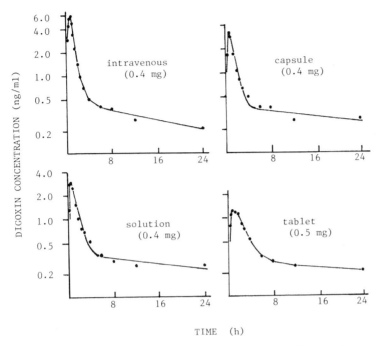

TIME   (h)

Fig. 2.15 Average digoxin concentrations in plasma after administration of an intravenous dose or an oral dose in one of three formulations
to 12 healthy volunteers. The multicompartment characteristics of
digoxin are evident after oral as well as after intravenous administration. (From Ref. 17.)

linear and described by (2.94). An estimate of the terminal disposition rate constant can be obtained from the slope, $\lambda_n/2.303$, of this
terminal linear segment.

Following oral administration of many drugs that display multicompartment characteristics after intravenous injection, we often fail
to observe a distributive phase. The plasma concentration-time
curves for such drugs appear biexponential rather than multiexponential (i.e., such curves behave as if the drug in question confers on
the body one-compartment rather than multicompartment characteristics). It has been illustrated through simulations, assuming a two-
compartment model (i.e., n = 2), that as k_a approaches λ_1, data will
still yield a curve consistent with a multicompartment system as illustrated in Fig. 2.15, even though the two exponentials are approximately equal to each other [18]. However, when k_a approaches E_2,
the data are best fit by a one-compartment model. Therefore, the
predominant distributive phase in Fig. 2.15 is characteristic of a multi-

compartment model where k_a is larger than E_2 and larger than or approaching λ_1.

Pharmacokinetic analysis of the blood level-time curve following an administration requiring first-order input (by the method of residuals, Appendix C, or nonlinear least-squares regression analysis, Appendix H), to obtain k_a and the disposition rate constants λ_1 to λ_n may not be possible without intravenous data, since such data are usually necessary for gaining an appreciation of the relative magnitudes of these rate constants. Assuming that the rate constant determined from the terminal slope is λ_n, λ_1 will be the rate constant calculated from the residual line if the data are best fit by a one-compartment model. When a one-compartment model adequately describes the data, k_a approaches E_2. As can be seen in (2.93), this causes the coefficient of the exponential term describing absorption to approach zero. If the data are multicompartmental in nature, it is not possible to predict whether the larger rate constant obtained from the residual lines should be assigned to k_a or to λ_1. As k_a approaches or becomes less than λ_n (i.e., a flip-flop model), the resulting plasma concentration versus time plot again defies analysis, since one cannot unambiguously assign the slow rate constant to either k_a or λ_n without intravenous data.

DETERMINATION OF PHARMACOKINETIC PARAMETERS

Calculation of k_{10}, k_{12}, k_{21}, and k'_e

Two-Compartment Model, Elimination Central. The disposition function $d_{s,c}$ for the central compartment of an n-compartment mammillary model [given by Eq. (2.1)] can also be written as follows (see Appendix B):

$$d_{s,c} = \frac{\prod\limits_{i=2}^{n} (s + E_i)}{\prod\limits_{i=1}^{n} (s + E_i) - \sum\limits_{j=2}^{n} [k_{1j} k_{j1} \prod\limits_{\substack{m=2 \\ m \neq j}}^{n} (s + E_m)]} \tag{2.95}$$

where k_{1j} and k_{j1} are first-order intercompartmental transfer rate constants, and E_i and E_m are the sum of the first-order exit rate constants out of compartment i or m. If the simplest case is considered (i.e., where a plasma concentration versus time curve is described by a biexponential equation), n will equal 2 (i.e., a two-compartment mammillary model; see Fig. 2.3) and (2.95) becomes

$$d_{s,c} = \frac{s + E_2}{(s + E_1)(s + E_2) - k_{12} k_{21}} \tag{2.96}$$

where $E_1 = k_{10} + k_{12}$ and $E_2 = k_{21}$. The constant k_{10} is the apparent first-order elimination rate constant from the central compartment, and k_{12} and k_{21} are the intercompartmental transfer rate constants (see Fig. 2.3). Expansion of the denominators of (2.96) and (2.1), when n = 2, yields

$$d_{s,c} = \frac{s + E_2}{s^2 + s(E_1 + E_2) + E_1 E_2 - k_{12}k_{21}} \qquad (2.97)$$

and

$$d_{s,c} = \frac{s + E_2}{s^2 + s(\lambda_1 + \lambda_2) + \lambda_1\lambda_2} \qquad (2.98)$$

respectively. By comparing (2.97) and (2.98) it can be shown that $\lambda_1 + \lambda_2 = E_1 + E_2$ and $\lambda_1\lambda_2 = E_1E_2 - k_{12}k_{21}$. Substitution of $k_{10} + k_{12}$ for E_1 and k_{21} for E_2 yields the following equations for λ_1 and λ_2:

$$\lambda_1 + \lambda_2 = k_{10} + k_{12} + k_{21} \qquad (2.99)$$

and

$$\lambda_1\lambda_2 = k_{10}k_{21} \qquad (2.100)$$

λ_1 is by definition greater than λ_2.

The specific equation that describes the biexponential decay in plasma concentrations following the intravenous bolus injection of a drug can be readily obtained by setting n = 2 in (2.7):

$$C = A_1 e^{-\lambda_1 t} + A_2 e^{-\lambda_2 t} \qquad (2.101)$$

where A_1 and A_2 are given by [see (2.8)]

$$A_1 = \frac{X_0(E_2 - \lambda_1)}{V_c(\lambda_2 - \lambda_1)} = \frac{X_0(k_{21} - \lambda_1)}{V_c(\lambda_2 - \lambda_1)} \qquad (2.102)$$

and

$$A_2 = \frac{X_0(E_2 - \lambda_2)}{V_c(\lambda_1 - \lambda_2)} = \frac{X_0(k_{21} - \lambda_2)}{V_c(\lambda_1 - \lambda_2)} \qquad (2.103)$$

The terms λ_1, λ_2, A_1, and A_2 are commonly referred to as α, β, A, and B in the literature.

As discussed previously in this chapter λ_1, λ_2, A_1, and A_2 are generally obtained from the nonlinear least-squares fit of plasma concentration versus time data to Eq. (2.101) (Appendix H). Once these parameters are determined, the constants k_{10}, k_{12}, and k_{21} can be calculated. The apparent volume of the central compartment, V_c, is given by (2.15) when $n = 2$:

$$V_c = \frac{X_0}{A_1 + A_2} \tag{2.104}$$

Substitution of $A_1 + A_2$ for X_0/V_c [obtained by rearrangement of (2.104)] in (2.103) yields

$$A_2 = \frac{(A_1 + A_2)(k_{21} - \lambda_2)}{\lambda_1 - \lambda_2} \tag{2.105}$$

which can be solved for k_{21}, since

$$k_{21} = \frac{A_1 \lambda_2 + A_2 \lambda_1}{A_1 + A_2} \tag{2.106}$$

The elimination rate constant from the central compartment can now be calculated since k_{21} is known (2.106) and $\lambda_1 \lambda_2 = k_{10} k_{21}$ (2.100). Hence

$$k_{10} = \frac{\lambda_1 \lambda_2}{k_{21}} \tag{2.107}$$

Recalling that $\lambda_1 + \lambda_2 = k_{10} + k_{12} + k_{21}$ (2.99), it follows that

$$k_{12} = \lambda_1 + \lambda_2 - k_{21} - k_{10} \tag{2.108}$$

All of these parameters, namely V_c, k_{10}, k_{12}, and k_{21}, can also be obtained from postinfusion data when the appropriate values of A_ℓ have been determined from the values of R_ℓ using Eqs. (2.69) and (2.72).

These constants may also be obtained from urinary excretion data. The following equation will describe the biexponential decline in an excretion rate versus time plot [set $n = 2$ in (2.23)]:

$$\frac{dX_u}{dt} = A_1' e^{-\lambda_1 t} + A_2' e^{-\lambda_2 t} \tag{2.109}$$

where

$$A_1' = k_e' X_0 \frac{E_2 - \lambda_1}{\lambda_2 - \lambda_1} = k_e' X_0 \frac{k_{21} - \lambda_1}{\lambda_2 - \lambda_1} \tag{2.110}$$

and

$$A_2' = k_e' X_0 \frac{E_2 - \lambda_2}{\lambda_1 - \lambda_2} = k_e' X_0 \frac{k_{21} - \lambda_2}{\lambda_1 - \lambda_2} \tag{2.111}$$

are obtained from (2.24). Rearrangement of (2.111) yields

$$k_{21} = \frac{A'_2 (\lambda_1 - \lambda_2)}{k'_e X_0} + \lambda_2 \qquad (2.112)$$

The parameter k'_e, the first-order urinary excretion rate constant, can be obtained for a two-compartment model from (2.27):

$$k'_e = \frac{A'_1 + A'_2}{X_0} \qquad (2.113)$$

Substitution for k'_e in (2.112) according to (2.113) gives

$$k_{21} = \frac{A'_2 (\lambda_1 - \lambda_2) X_0}{(A'_1 + A'_2) X_0} + \lambda_2 \qquad (2.114)$$

Canceling the X_0 terms and solving for a common denominator yields

$$k_{21} = \frac{A'_2 \lambda_1 - A'_2 \lambda_2 + A'_1 \lambda_2 + A'_2 \lambda_2}{A'_1 + A'_2} \qquad (2.115)$$

which when simplified becomes

$$k_{21} = \frac{A'_2 \lambda_1 + A'_1 \lambda_2}{A'_1 + A'_2} \qquad (2.116)$$

and is analogous to (2.106). The constants k_{10} and k_{12} can be solved for by employing the value of k_{21} from (2.114), and utilizing Eqs. (2.107) ($k_{10} = \lambda_1 \lambda_2 / k_{21}$) and (2.108) ($k_{12} = \lambda_1 + \lambda_2 - k_{21} - k_{10}$).

Amount unexcreted in the urine versus time data can also be used to determine k_{10}, k_{12}, and k_{21}. By setting $n = 2$ in (2.33), the following equation results:

$$X_u^\infty - X_u = A''_1 e^{-\lambda_1 t} + A''_2 e^{-\lambda_2 t} \qquad (2.117)$$

where

$$A''_1 = k'_e X_0 \frac{E_1 - \lambda_1}{\lambda_1 (\lambda_2 - \lambda_1)} = k'_e X_0 \frac{k_{21} - \lambda_1}{\lambda_1 (\lambda_2 - \lambda_1)} \qquad (2.118)$$

and

$$A''_2 = k'_e X_0 \frac{E_2 - \lambda_2}{\lambda_2 (\lambda_1 - \lambda_2)} = k'_e X_0 \frac{k_{21} - \lambda_2}{\lambda_2 (\lambda_1 - \lambda_2)} \qquad (2.119)$$

are obtained from (2.34) by setting $n = 2$. Setting $n = 2$ in (2.31) and solving for k_e' yields

$$k_e' = \frac{X_u^\infty \lambda_1 \lambda_2}{X_0 E_2} = \frac{X_u^\infty \lambda_1 \lambda_2}{X_0 k_{21}} \tag{2.120}$$

Substitution of $k_{10}k_{21}$ for $\lambda_1\lambda_2$ in (2.120) according to (2.100) and cancellation of common terms provides

$$k_e' = \frac{X_u^\infty k_{10}}{X_0} \tag{2.121}$$

Multiplying the numerator and denominator of (2.119) by λ_1 and expanding the numerator gives

$$A_2'' = k_e' X_0 \frac{\lambda_1 k_{21} - \lambda_1 \lambda_2}{\lambda_1 \lambda_2 (\lambda_1 - \lambda_2)} \tag{2.122}$$

The substitution of $k_{10}k_{21}$ for $\lambda_1\lambda_2$ in this equation followed by cancellation of the common parameter k_{21} yields

$$A_2'' = \frac{k_c' X_0 (\lambda_1 - k_{10})}{k_{10}(\lambda_1 - \lambda_2)} \tag{2.123}$$

X_u^∞ can be substituted for $k_e' X_0 / k_{10}$ in (2.123) based on a rearrangement of (2.121) to give

$$A_2'' = X_u^\infty \frac{\lambda_1 - k_{10}}{\lambda_1 - \lambda_2} \tag{2.124}$$

It can be readily shown from (2.117) that

$$X_u^\infty = A_1'' + A_2'' \tag{2.125}$$

Substituting $A_1'' + A_2''$ for X_u^∞ in (2.124) and solving for k_{10} yields

$$k_{10} = \frac{A_1'' \lambda_1 + A_2'' \lambda_2}{A_1'' + A_2''} \tag{2.126}$$

The constant k_{21} can be obtained by rearranging (2.100) to give

$$k_{21} = \frac{\lambda_1 \lambda_2}{k_{10}} \tag{2.127}$$

while Eq. (2.108) can be used to calculate k_{12}.

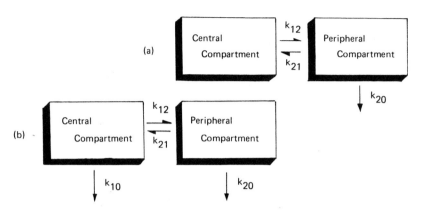

Fig. 2.16 Schematic representation of the body as a two-compartment
open model. In case (a), elimination is restricted to the peripheral
compartment; in case (b), elimination occurs from both compartments.

*Two-Compartment Model, Elimination Peripheral or Central and Periph-
eral.* Elimination in a two-compartment model may occur not only from
the central compartment but also from the peripheral compartment or
from both compartments simultaneously (Fig. 2.16). Although the
three two-compartment models are indistinguishable based solely on
plasma or urinary excretion data, additional information may be available that will require the use of one of the models in which elimination is not exclusive to the central compartment.

For the case where elimination occurs only from the peripheral
compartment, the following disposition function for the central compartment, $d_{s,c}$, may be written [see (2.95)]:

$$d_{s,c} = \frac{s + E_2}{(s + E_1)(s + E_2) - k_{12}k_{21}} \qquad (2.96)$$

However, $E_1 = k_{12}$ and $E_2 = k_{21} + k_{20}$ (see Fig. 2.16a), where k_{20} is
the apparent first-order elimination rate constant from the peripheral
compartment. The constants k_{12} and k_{21} are as defined previously.
Since there are two driving force compartments in the model, (2.96)
may also be written as

$$d_{s,c} = \frac{s + E_2}{(s + \lambda_1)(s + \lambda_2)} \qquad (2.128)$$

Expansion of (2.96) and (2.128) yields (2.97) and (2.98), respectively,
and $\lambda_1 + \lambda_2$ equals $E_1 + E_2$ and $\lambda_1\lambda_2$ equals $E_1E_2 - k_{12}k_{21}$. Substitution of k_{12} for E_1 and $k_{21} + k_{20}$ for E_2 yields the following expressions
for λ_1 and λ_2:

$$\lambda_1 + \lambda_2 = k_{12} + k_{21} + k_{20} \tag{2.129}$$

and

$$\lambda_1 \lambda_2 = k_{12} k_{20} \tag{2.130}$$

For intravenous administration the input function in_s equals X_0, the intravenous dose [Eq. (2.2)]. The Laplace transform for the amount of drug in the central compartment, $a_{s,c}$, is therefore

$$a_{s,c} = \frac{(s + E_2)X_0}{(s + \lambda_1)(s + \lambda_2)} \tag{2.131}$$

where $a_{s,c}$ equals the product of $d_{s,c}$ and in_s, E_2 equals $k_{21} + k_{20}$, and λ_1 and λ_2 are defined by (2.129) and (2.130). The anti-Laplace of this equation yields an expression for the amount of drug in the central compartment (X_c) as a function of time, which is

$$X_c = \frac{X_0(E_2 - \lambda_1)}{\lambda_2 - \lambda_1} e^{-\lambda_1 t} + \frac{X_0(E_2 - \lambda_2)}{\lambda_1 - \lambda_2} e^{-\lambda_2 t} \tag{2.132}$$

Substituting $k_{21} + k_{20}$ for E_2, converting to concentration terms employing Eq. (2.5) $(X_c = V_c C)$, and rearranging yields

$$C = \frac{X_0(\lambda_1 - k_{21} - k_{20})}{V_c(\lambda_1 - \lambda_2)} e^{-\lambda_1 t} + \frac{X_0(k_{21} + k_{20} - \lambda_2)}{V_c(\lambda_1 - \lambda_2)} e^{-\lambda_2 t} \tag{2.133}$$

or

$$C = A_1 e^{-\lambda_1 t} + A_2 e^{-\lambda_2 t}$$

which is identical to Eq. (2.101). However,

$$A_1 = \frac{X_0(\lambda_1 - k_{21} - k_{20})}{V_c(\lambda_1 - \lambda_2)} \tag{2.134}$$

and

$$A_2 = \frac{X_0(k_{21} + k_{20} - \lambda_2)}{V_c(\lambda_1 - \lambda_2)} \tag{2.135}$$

From a plot of log C versus time, estimates of A_1, A_2, λ_1, and λ_2 can be made (method of residuals, Appendix C; nonlinear regression analysis, Appendix H) from which V_c, k_{12}, k_{21}, and k_{20} can be determined.

The apparent volume of the central compartment can be estimated employing Eq. (2.104):

$$V_c = \frac{X_0}{A_1 + A_2}$$

where A_1 and A_2 are as defined by (2.134) and (2.135), respectively. Substitution of $A_1 + A_2$ for X_0/V_c [Eq. (2.104)] into (2.135) yields

$$A_1 = \frac{(A_1 + A_2)(k_{21} + k_{20} - \lambda_2)}{\lambda_1 - \lambda_2} \qquad (2.136)$$

Equation (2.99) can be rearranged to give

$$k_{21} + k_{20} - \lambda_2 = \lambda_1 - k_{12} \qquad (2.137)$$

Substituting $\lambda_1 - k_{12}$ for $k_{21} + k_{20} - \lambda_2$ into (2.136) and rearranging gives the following expression which can be employed to calculate k_{12}:

$$k_{12} = \frac{\lambda_1 A_1 + \lambda_2 A_2}{A_1 + A_2} \qquad (2.138)$$

The elimination rate constant from the peripheral compartment, k_{20}, can now be calculated since k_{12} is known [Eq. (2.138)] and since $\lambda_1 \lambda_2 = k_{12} k_{20}$ [Eq. (2.130)]. Rearranging (2.130) yields the following expression for k_{20}:

$$k_{20} = \frac{\lambda_1 \lambda_2}{k_{12}} \qquad (2.139)$$

The constant k_{21} can now be determined by rearrangement of (2.99) to yield

$$k_{21} = \lambda_1 + \lambda_2 - k_{12} - k_{20} \qquad (2.140)$$

The third type of two-compartment model, where elimination occurs from both the central and peripheral compartments (Fig. 2.16b), may be solved in a manner analogous to the other two-compartment models. A biexponential equation of the form $C = A_1 e^{-\lambda_1 t} + A_2 e^{-\lambda_2 t}$ will result. Relationships can be derived employing the methods and approaches developed above which relate the individual model constants k_{12}, k_{21}, k_{10}, and k_{20} to the hybrid constants λ_1, λ_2, A_1, and A_2. However, none of the model constants can be calculated independently, since in a mammillary disposition model, the maximum number of solvable rate constants Z is given by the following equation [5]:

$$Z = 2(n - 1) + 1 \qquad (2.141)$$

where n is the number of driving force compartments in the disposition model. There are two driving force compartments in any two-compartment model and therefore the maximum number of solvable rate constants is three. The model shown in Fig. 2.16b has four rate constants.

Three-Compartment Model. Triexponential equations may be required to describe adequately postintravenous injection data. In accordance with previous discussions, the simplest three-compartment model will be considered: that model where elimination occurs from a central compartment which is reversibly connected to a "shallow" and a "deep" peripheral compartment, compartments 2 and 3, respectively (Fig. 2.17).

The disposition function for the central compartment, $d_{s,c}$, may be obtained by setting n = 3 in (2.1) or (2.95). This will yield

$$d_{s,c} = \frac{(s + E_2)(s + E_3)}{(s + \lambda_1)(s + \lambda_2)(s + \lambda_3)} \tag{2.142}$$

and

$$d_{s,c} = \frac{(s + E_2)(s + E_3)}{(s + E_1)(s + E_2)(s + E_3) - k_{12}k_{21}(s + E_3) - k_{13}k_{31}(s + E_2)} \tag{2.143}$$

respectively, where $E_2 = k_{21}$, $E_3 = k_{31}$, and $E_1 = k_{12} + k_{13} + k_{10}$. The constants k_{12} and k_{21}, and k_{31} and k_{13} are the apparent first-order intercompartmental transfer rate constants between the shallow and central compartments, and deep and central compartments, respectively. The elimination rate constant from the central compartment is k_{10}. In (2.142) λ_1 is by definition greater than λ_2, which is in turn greater than λ_3.

Substituting k_{21} for E_2 and k_{31} for E_3 in (2.142) and (2.143) and $k_{12} + k_{13} + k_{10}$ for E_1 in (2.143) and expanding the denominators of (2.142) and (2.143) yields

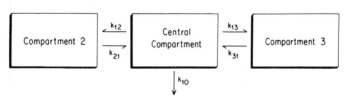

Fig. 2.17 Schematic representation of the body as a three-compartment open model with drug elimination from the central compartment.

$$d_{s,c} = \frac{(s + k_{21})(s + k_{31})}{s^3 + s^2(\lambda_1 + \lambda_2 + \lambda_3) + s(\lambda_1\lambda_2 + \lambda_1\lambda_3 + \lambda_2\lambda_3) + \lambda_1\lambda_2\lambda_3}$$

(2.144)

and

$$d_{s,c} = \frac{(s + k_{21})(s + k_{31})}{s^3 + s^2(k_{10} + k_{12} + k_{13} + k_{21} + k_{31})}$$
$$+ s(k_{10}k_{21} + k_{13}k_{21} + k_{10}k_{31} + k_{21}k_{31} + k_{31}k_{12}) + k_{21}k_{31}k_{10}$$

(2.145)

respectively. Comparing the coefficients in the denominators of (2.144) and (2.145), it is readily apparent that λ_1, λ_2, and λ_3 may be expressed in terms of the individual rate constants as

$$\lambda_1 + \lambda_2 + \lambda_3 = k_{10} + k_{12} + k_{13} + k_{21} + k_{31}$$

(2.146)

$$\lambda_1\lambda_2 + \lambda_1\lambda_3 + \lambda_2\lambda_3 = k_{10}k_{21} + k_{13}k_{21} + k_{10}k_{31} + k_{21}k_{31} + k_{31}k_{12}$$

(2.147)

and

$$\lambda_1\lambda_2\lambda_3 = k_{21}k_{31}k_{10}$$

(2.148)

The intravenous input function in_s is given by Eq. (2.2), that is, $in_s = X_0$, where X_0 is the intravenous dose. The Laplace transform for the amount of drug in the central compartment, $a_{s,c}$, which is the product of the input and disposition functions [given by (2.2) and (2.142), respectively], is

$$a_{s,c} = \frac{X_0(s + E_2)(s + E_3)}{(s + \lambda_1)(s + \lambda_2)(s + \lambda_3)}$$

(2.149)

Taking the anti-Laplace of (2.149) (Appendix B) yields the following expression for the amount of drug in the central compartment, X_c, as a function of time:

$$X_c = \frac{X_0(E_2 - \lambda_1)(E_3 - \lambda_1)}{(\lambda_2 - \lambda_1)(\lambda_3 - \lambda_1)}e^{-\lambda_1 t} + \frac{X_0(E_2 - \lambda_2)(E_3 - \lambda_2)}{(\lambda_1 - \lambda_2)(\lambda_3 - \lambda_2)}e^{-\lambda_2 t}$$
$$+ \frac{X_0(E_2 - \lambda_3)(E_3 - \lambda_3)}{(\lambda_1 - \lambda_3)(\lambda_2 - \lambda_3)}e^{-\lambda_3 t}$$

(2.150)

Substituting k_{31} for E_3, and k_{21} for E_2, rearranging, and expressing the equation in concentration terms by dividing by V_c according to (2.5) ($C = X_c/V_c$) yields

$$C = \frac{X_0(k_{21} - \lambda_1)(k_{31} - \lambda_1)}{V_c(\lambda_1 - \lambda_2)(\lambda_1 - \lambda_3)} e^{-\lambda_1 t} + \frac{X_0(k_{21} - \lambda_2)(\lambda_2 - k_{31})}{V_c(\lambda_1 - \lambda_2)(\lambda_2 - \lambda_3)} e^{-\lambda_2 t}$$

$$+ \frac{X_0(k_{21} - \lambda_3)(k_{31} - \lambda_3)}{V_c(\lambda_2 - \lambda_3)(\lambda_1 - \lambda_3)} e^{-\lambda_3 t} \tag{2.151}$$

or

$$C = A_1 e^{-\lambda_1 t} + A_2 e^{-\lambda_2 t} + A_3 e^{-\lambda_3 t} \tag{2.152}$$

where

$$A_1 = \frac{X_0(k_{21} - \lambda_1)(k_{31} - \lambda_1)}{V_c(\lambda_1 - \lambda_2)(\lambda_1 - \lambda_3)} \tag{2.153}$$

$$A_2 = \frac{X_0(k_{21} - \lambda_2)(\lambda_2 - k_{31})}{V_c(\lambda_1 - \lambda_2)(\lambda_2 - \lambda_3)} \tag{2.154}$$

and

$$A_3 = \frac{X_0(k_{21} - \lambda_3)(k_{31} - \lambda_3)}{V_c(\lambda_2 - \lambda_3)(\lambda_1 - \lambda_3)} \tag{2.155}$$

Therefore, from a plot of the logarithm of plasma concentration versus time after rapid intravenous injection, a triexponential curve should be obtained from which A_1, A_2, A_3, λ_1, λ_2, and λ_3 can be estimated (Fig. 2.18). Although such estimations can be made employing the method of residuals (Appendix C), the best method to determine these terms is to fit the curve by nonlinear least-squares regression analysis (Appendix H).

Once A_1, A_2, A_3, λ_1, λ_2, and λ_3 are known, the apparent volume of the central compartment V_c and the individual rate constants k_{12}, k_{21}, k_{13}, k_{31}, and k_{10} can be calculated. At time $t = 0$ the plasma concentration C_0 is given by the equation

$$C_0 = A_1 + A_2 + A_3 \tag{2.156}$$

Substitution for A_1, A_2, and A_3 according to (2.153), (2.154), and (2.155), respectively, in Eq. (2.156), bringing the resulting expression to a common denominator, expanding the numerator and denominator, and simplifying yields Eq. 2.14

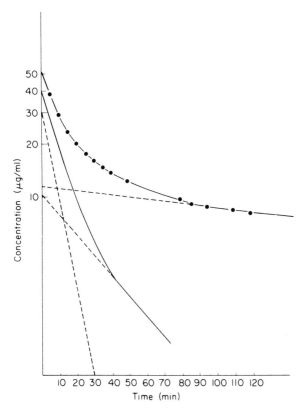

Fig. 2.18 Dacarbazine concentration in plasma following intravenous administration in the dog. Application of the method of residuals indicates that the data are described by the following triexponential equation: $C = 30.5 \exp(-0.117t) + 10.2 \exp(-0.028t) + 11.4 \exp(-0.003t)$, where t is expressed in minutes. (Data from Ref. 19.)

$$C_0 = \frac{X_0}{V_c}$$

Substitution of $A_1 + A_2 + A_3$ for C_0, according to (2.156), in (2.14) and rearrangement yields the following expression for V_c:

$$V_c = \frac{X_0}{A_1 + A_2 + A_3} \qquad (2.157)$$

By substituting $A_1 + A_2 + A_3$ for X_0/V_c in (2.154) and (2.155), and solving (2.154) for k_{21} and (2.155) for k_{31}, the following relationships are obtained:

$$k_{21} = \lambda_2 + \frac{A_2(\lambda_1 - \lambda_2)(\lambda_2 - \lambda_3)}{(A_1 + A_2 + A_3)(\lambda_2 - k_{31})} \tag{2.158}$$

and

$$k_{31} = \lambda_3 + \frac{A_3(\lambda_1 - \lambda_3)(\lambda_2 - \lambda_3)}{(A_1 + A_2 + A_3)(k_{21} - \lambda_3)} \tag{2.159}$$

respectively. Substitution of k_{21}, according to (2.158), in (2.159) and simplification yields the following quadratic equation:

$$k_{31}^2 - k_{31} \frac{\lambda_1 A_3 + \lambda_1 A_2 + \lambda_3 A_1 + \lambda_3 A_2 + \lambda_2 A_1 + \lambda_2 A_3}{A_1 + A_2 + A_3}$$

$$+ \frac{\lambda_1 \lambda_2 A_3 + \lambda_1 \lambda_3 A_2 + \lambda_2 \lambda_3 A_1}{A_1 + A_2 + A_3} = 0 \tag{2.160}$$

Similarly, substituting for k_{31}, according to (2.159), in (2.158) and simplifying yields a quadratic equation in k_{21} with identical coefficients:

$$k_{21}^2 - k_{21} \frac{\lambda_1 A_3 + \lambda_1 A_2 + \lambda_3 A_1 + \lambda_3 A_2 + \lambda_2 A_1 + \lambda_2 A_3}{A_1 + A_2 + A_3}$$

$$+ \frac{\lambda_1 \lambda_2 A_3 + \lambda_1 \lambda_3 A_2 + \lambda_2 \lambda_3 A_1}{A_1 + A_2 + A_3} = 0 \tag{2.161}$$

Equations (2.160) and (2.161) are of the form $ax^2 + bx + c = 0$, which may be solved by

$$x = \frac{-b \pm \sqrt{b^2 - 4ac}}{2a} \tag{2.162}$$

Therefore,

$$k_{21}, k_{31} = \frac{-b \pm \sqrt{b^2 - 4ac}}{2a} \tag{2.163}$$

where

$$a = 1 \tag{2.164}$$

$$b = - \frac{\lambda_1 A_3 + \lambda_1 A_2 + \lambda_3 A_1 + \lambda_3 A_2 + \lambda_2 A_1 + \lambda_2 A_3}{A_1 + A_2 + A_3} \tag{2.165}$$

and

$$c = \frac{\lambda_1 \lambda_2 A_3 + \lambda_1 \lambda_3 A_2 + \lambda_2 \lambda_3 A_1}{A_1 + A_2 + A_3} \tag{2.166}$$

Since k_{31} is the exit rate constant from the deep peripheral compartment, it will be smaller than k_{21}, the exit rate constant from the shallow peripheral compartment. Hence

$$k_{31} = \frac{1}{2}\left(-b - \sqrt{b^2 - 4c}\right) \tag{2.167}$$

and

$$k_{21} = \frac{1}{2}\left(-b + \sqrt{b^2 - 4c}\right) \tag{2.168}$$

Once k_{31} and k_{21} have been determined, the elimination rate constant from the central compartment k_{10} can be readily calculated from

$$k_{10} = \frac{\lambda_1 \lambda_2 \lambda_3}{k_{21} k_{31}} \tag{2.169}$$

which is obtained by rearrangement of (2.148).

Solving (2.146) and (2.147) for k_{13} yields

$$k_{13} = (\lambda_1 + \lambda_2 + \lambda_3) - (k_{10} + k_{21} + k_{31} + k_{12}) \tag{2.170}$$

and

$$k_{13} = \frac{(\lambda_1 \lambda_3 + \lambda_1 \lambda_2 + \lambda_1 \lambda_3) - (k_{10}k_{21} + k_{10}k_{31} + k_{21}k_{31} + k_{12}k_{31})}{k_{21}} \tag{2.171}$$

respectively. By subtracting (2.170) from (2.171) and solving for k_{12}, the following expression is obtained:

$$k_{12} = \frac{(\lambda_2 \lambda_3 + \lambda_1 \lambda_2 + \lambda_1 \lambda_3) - k_{21}(\lambda_1 + \lambda_2 + \lambda_3) - k_{10}k_{31} + k_{21}^2}{k_{31} - k_{21}} \tag{2.172}$$

Rearrangement of (2.146) yields

$$k_{13} = \lambda_1 + \lambda_2 + \lambda_3 - (k_{10} + k_{12} + k_{21} + k_{31}) \tag{2.173}$$

from which k_{13} can be calculated since the constants k_{10}, k_{12}, k_{21}, and k_{31} are known.

As with a two-compartment model, there are many types of three-compartment models where elimination may be assumed to occur from any one compartment or combination of compartments. These models

are indistinguishable based solely on plasma or urinary excretion
data. There are indications that a triexponential equation may be
necessary to characterize the pharmacokinetic profile of digoxin [20],
tubocurarine [21], 5-(dimethyltriazeno)imidazole-4-carboxamide [19],
and diazepam [22]. A three-compartment model involving peripheral
compartment elimination has been employed for bishydroxycoumarin
[23]. The derivation for this particular model is given therein.

Determination of the rate constants associated with multicompartment models may permit an assessment of the relative contribution of
distribution and elimination processes to the drug concentration versus
time profile of a drug. It may also aid in elucidating the mechanism of
drug interactions, and of the effects of disease, age, genetic influ-
ences, and other factors on drug disposition. However, it must be
kept in mind that these parameters are likely to be subject to considerable error. As pointed out by Westlake [24], these errors are
probably unimportant when the parameters are used to predict plasma
drug concentration. If the parameters are used to predict other features of the system (e.g., tissue drug concentrations), there may be
substantial errors in the predictions.

Relationship Between β and k_{10}. For multicompartment models a clear
distinction must be made between k_{10}, the elimination rate constant,
and the terminal disposition rate constant λ_n, which is frequently re-
ferred to as β in the literature. λ_n or β is equivalent to λ_2 or λ_3 in
the respective bi- or triexponential equations discussed above. The
difference between k_{10} and λ_n may be clearly illustrated employing the
simplest multiexponential equation, the biexponential equation. These
two constants may be related in the following manner. The fraction of
drug in the body that is in the central compartment, f_c, can be defined
as

$$f_c = \frac{X_c}{X} \qquad\qquad\qquad (2.174)$$

where X is the total amount of drug in the body and equals the sum of
the amounts of drug in the central and peripheral body compartments:

$$X = X_c + X_p \qquad\qquad\qquad (2.175)$$

Substitution of $X_c + X_p$ for X in (2.174) gives

$$f_c = \frac{X_c}{X_c + X_p} \qquad\qquad\qquad (2.176)$$

The appropriate values of X_c and X_p can be obtained from (2.4) and
(2.19), respectively. Setting n and j in these equations equal to 2,

which results in biexponential equations, then substituting these equations for X_c and X_p in (2.176), yields

$$f_c = \frac{X_0 \dfrac{E_2 - \lambda_1}{\lambda_2 - \lambda_1} e^{-\lambda_1 t} + X_0 \dfrac{E_2 - \lambda_2}{\lambda_1 - \lambda_2} e^{-\lambda_2 t}}{X_0 \dfrac{E_2 - \lambda_1}{\lambda_2 - \lambda_1} e^{-\lambda_1 t} + X_0 \dfrac{E_2 - \lambda_2}{\lambda_1 - \lambda_2} e^{-\lambda_2 t}}$$

$$+ X_0 \frac{k_{12}(E_2 - \lambda_1)}{(E_2 - \lambda_1)(\lambda_2 - \lambda_1)} e^{-\lambda_1 t} + X_0 \frac{k_{12}(E_2 - \lambda_2)}{(E_2 - \lambda_2)(\lambda_1 - \lambda_2)} e^{-\lambda_2 t}$$

$$(2.177)$$

Initial canceling of common terms and changing all coefficients to a common denominator, $\lambda_1 - \lambda_2$, which can then be canceled, gives

$$f_c = \frac{(\lambda_1 - E_2)e^{-\lambda_1 t} + (E_2 - \lambda_2)e^{-\lambda_2 t}}{(\lambda_1 - E_2)e^{-\lambda_1 t} + (E_2 - \lambda_2)e^{-\lambda_2 t} - k_{12}e^{-\lambda_1 t} + k_{12}e^{-\lambda_2 t}}$$

$$(2.178)$$

Substituting k_{21} for E_2 and collecting common terms in the denominator results in the following equation:

$$f_c = \frac{(\lambda_1 - k_{21})e^{-\lambda_1 t} + (k_{21} - \lambda_2)e^{-\lambda_2 t}}{(\lambda_1 - k_{21} - k_{12})e^{-\lambda_1 t} + (k_{21} - \lambda_2 + k_{12})e^{-\lambda_2 t}} \qquad (2.179)$$

In the postdistributive phase (i.e., as $e^{-\lambda_1 t}$ approaches zero),

$$f_c = f_c^* = \frac{(k_{21} - \lambda_2)e^{-\lambda_2 t}}{(k_{21} - \lambda_2 + k_{12})e^{-\lambda_2 t}} \qquad (2.180)$$

which readily reduces to

$$f_c^* = \frac{k_{21} - \lambda_2}{k_{21} + k_{12} - \lambda_2} \qquad (2.181)$$

Therefore, in the postdistributive phase the fraction of drug in the body that is in the central compartment is a constant, f_c^*.

The rate of change in the amount of drug in the body (dX/dt) equals the sum of the rates of change in the amounts of drug in the central and peripheral body compartments:

$$\frac{dX}{dt} = \frac{dX_c}{dt} + \frac{dX_p}{dt} \tag{2.182}$$

The differential equations for dX_c/dt and dXp/dt based on the model in Fig. 2.3 are

$$\frac{dX_c}{dt} = k_{21}X_p - k_{12}X_c - k_{10}X_c \tag{2.183}$$

and

$$\frac{dX_p}{dt} = k_{12}X_c - k_{21}X_p \tag{2.184}$$

respectively. Substitution for dX_c/dt and dX_p/dt, according to (2.183) and (2.184), respectively, in (2.182) yields

$$\frac{dX}{dt} = k_{21}X_p - k_{12}X_c - k_{10}X_c + k_{12}X_c - k_{21}X_p \tag{2.185}$$

which readily reduces to

$$\frac{dX}{dt} = -k_{10}X_c \tag{2.186}$$

By substituting for X_c, according to (2.4) with $n = 2$, in (2.186), the following equation is obtained:

$$\frac{dX}{dt} = -k_{10}\left[\frac{X_0(\lambda_1 - k_{21})}{\lambda_1 - \lambda_2} e^{-\lambda_1 t} + \frac{X_0(k_{21} - \lambda_2)}{\lambda_1 - \lambda_2} e^{-\lambda_2 t} \right] \tag{2.187}$$

Some time after administration $e^{-\lambda_1 t}$ approaches zero (i.e., during the postdistributive phase) and (2.187) reduces to

$$\frac{dX}{dt} = -k_{10} \frac{X_0(k_{21} - \lambda_2)}{\lambda_1 - \lambda_2} e^{-\lambda_2 t} \tag{2.188}$$

Rearrangement and expansion of (2.188) yields

$$\frac{dX}{dt} = -X_0 \frac{k_{10}k_{21} - k_{10}\lambda_2}{\lambda_1 - \lambda_2} e^{-\lambda_2 t} \tag{2.189}$$

Recognizing that $k_{10}k_{21} = \lambda_1\lambda_2$ [Eq. (2.100)], substituting $\lambda_1\lambda_2$ for $k_{10}k_{21}$ in (2.189), and rearranging the terms produces the relationship

$$\frac{dX}{dt} = -\lambda_2 \left[\frac{X_0(\lambda_1 - k_{10})}{\lambda_1 - \lambda_2} e^{-\lambda_2 t} \right] \tag{2.190}$$

It can now be shown that the term in brackets equals the amount of drug in the body during the postdistributive phase. The amount of drug in the body (X) is equal to $X_c + X_p$ [Eq. (2.175)] and is given by the denominator of (2.177):

$$X = X_0 \frac{E_2 - \lambda_1}{\lambda_2 - \lambda_1} e^{-\lambda_1 t} + X_0 \frac{E_2 - \lambda_2}{\lambda_1 - \lambda_2} e^{-\lambda_2 t}$$

$$+ X_0 \frac{k_{12}(E_2 - \lambda_1)}{(E_2 - \lambda_1)(\lambda_2 - \lambda_1)} e^{-\lambda_1 t} + X_0 \frac{k_{12}(E_2 - \lambda_2)}{(E_2 - \lambda_2)(\lambda_1 - \lambda_2)} e^{-\lambda_2 t} \tag{2.191}$$

Solving for X in the postdistributive phase (i.e., $e^{-\lambda_1 t} \to 0$), canceling the common term $E_2 - \lambda_2$, and substituting k_{21} for E_2 yields the following equation for the amount of drug in the body during the terminal exponential phase:

$$X = \frac{X_0(k_{21} - \lambda_2 + k_{12})}{\lambda_1 - \lambda_2} e^{-\lambda_2 t} \tag{2.192}$$

Rearrangement of (2.99) gives the expression

$$k_{21} - \lambda_2 + k_{12} = \lambda_1 - k_{10} \tag{2.193}$$

Therefore,

$$X = \frac{X_0(\lambda_1 - k_{10})}{\lambda_1 - \lambda_2} e^{-\lambda_2 t} \tag{2.194}$$

Substituting X for $X_0(\lambda_1 - k_{10})e^{-\lambda_2 t}/(\lambda_1 - \lambda_2)$, as given by (2.194), into (2.190) yields the following equation for the rate of change of drug levels in the body during the postdistributive phase:

$$\frac{dX}{dt} = -\lambda_2 X \tag{2.195}$$

Since $X_c = f_c X$ [Eq. (2.174)], (2.186) may be expressed as

$$\frac{dX}{dt} = -k_{10} f_c X \tag{2.196}$$

In the postdistributive phase,

$$\frac{dX}{dt} = -k_{10} f_c^* X \tag{2.197}$$

where f_c^* is given by (2.181). By comparing (2.196) and (2.197), one concludes that

$$\lambda_2 = f_c^* k_{10} \qquad (2.198)$$

It is clear from this equation that λ_2 is a function of both elimination (k_{10}) and distribution.

The dependence of λ_n or β on both distribution and elimination may be demonstrated in a different manner. It has been shown previously that $\lambda_1 + \lambda_2 = k_{12} + k_{21} + k_{10}$ [Eq. (2.99)] and $\lambda_1 \lambda_2 = k_{21} k_{10}$ [Eq. (2.100)]. Solving (2.100) for λ_1 yields

$$\lambda_1 = \frac{k_{21} k_{10}}{\lambda_2} \qquad (2.199)$$

Substituting this value for λ_1 into (2.99), multiplying each side of the equation by λ_2, and rearranging terms results in the quadratic equation

$$\lambda_2^2 - (k_{12} + k_{21} + k_{10}) \lambda_2 + k_{21} k_{10} = 0 \qquad (2.200)$$

which is of the form

$$ax^2 + bx + c = 0 \qquad (2.201)$$

The general solution of (2.201) is

$$x = \frac{-b \pm \sqrt{b^2 - 4ac}}{2a} \qquad (2.162)$$

Therefore,

$$\lambda_2 = \frac{1}{2} \left[(k_{12} + k_{21} + k_{10}) - \sqrt{(k_{12} + k_{21} + k_{10})^2 - 4 k_{21} k_{10}} \right]$$

$$\qquad (2.202)$$

The sign preceding the square root term is negative rather than positive since λ_1 has been assumed to be greater than λ_2. It can be readily demonstrated that the equation for λ_1 is identical to (2.202) except that a positive sign precedes the square root term.

The constant k_{10} is the elimination rate constant from the central compartment, and λ_2 reflects drug elimination from the body. The biologic half-life $t_{1/2}$ of a drug is calculated from λ_2 [Eq. (2.11)] rather than from k_{10}. Although λ_2 and half-life are hybrid parameters, they are among the most important functional pharmacokinetic parameters.

If, because of insufficient data, the plasma concentration of a drug with multicompartment characteristics after rapid intravenous injection show only the terminal exponential phase, what is actually the

λ_2 value will appear to be the elimination rate constant K in a one-compartment model.

Volume of Distribution and Clearance

The apparent volume of distribution is a useful pharmacokinetic parameter that relates the plasma or serum concentration of a drug to the total amount of drug in the body. Despite its name, this parameter usually has no direct physiologic meaning and does not refer to a real volume. However, it does provide some insight into the extent of extravascular distribution of a drug; that is, the greater the volume of distribution, the more extensive the extravascular distribution of a drug, and hence the lower the plasma or serum concentration of a drug for a given amount of drug in the body. For a drug with a plasma concentration versus time profile that can be adequately described by a single exponential following an intravenous bolus dose, there is only one volume of distribution parameter. There may be several volume parameters, however, for a drug whose disposition requires a multiexponential equation for its description. One volume term that has been mentioned in this chapter is V_c, the apparent volume of the central compartment. This parameter relates the drug concentration in the plasma to the amount of drug in the central compartment, and can be readily determined from the relationship given by (2.15)

$$V_c = \frac{X_0}{\sum_{\ell=1}^{n} A_\ell}$$

where X_0 is the intravenous dose and $\sum_{\ell=1}^{n} A_\ell$ is the sum of the n zero-time intercepts that would be obtained by applying the method of residuals to a plasma concentration-time curve after intravenous administration of a drug that requires n exponentials to characterize it. By assuming that a constant ratio of drug concentrations in the various tissues and fluids of the central compartment exists, V_c can be employed to estimate the amount of drug in the central compartment at any time regardless of the complexity of the model required to describe the time course of drug in the plasma.

An additional volume parameter in multicompartment systems is V_β. This parameter relates plasma concentration to amount of drug in the body during the terminal exponential phase of a plasma concentration versus time curve. The fraction of drug in the body which is in the central compartment during this terminal exponential phase, f_c^*, is given by

$$f_c^* = \frac{X_c}{X} \qquad (2.203)$$

$V_\beta C$ can be substituted for X in (2.203) since by definition $X = V_\beta C$ during the terminal phase. Therefore,

$$f_c^* = \frac{X_c}{V_\beta C} \tag{2.204}$$

Substitution of $V_c C$ for X_c, according to (2.5), in (2.204) and cancellation of the common term yields

$$f_c^* = \frac{V_c}{V_\beta} \tag{2.205}$$

Equation (2.198) can be rearranged to give

$$f_c^* = \frac{\lambda_2}{k_{10}} \tag{2.206}$$

where k_{10} is the first-order elimination rate constant and λ_2 is the disposition rate constant associated with the terminal exponential phase of a biexponential plasma concentration versus time curve. Although (2.198) was derived assuming that n = 2, a similar relationship would have resulted regardless of the number of exponentials required to describe a plasma concentration versus time curve provided that elimination is assumed to occur from the central compartment. Therefore, (2.206) can be written as

$$f_c^* = \frac{\lambda_n}{k_{10}} \tag{2.207}$$

By comparing (2.205) and (2.207), it becomes readily apparent that

$$\frac{V_c}{V_\beta} = \frac{\lambda_n}{k_{10}} \tag{2.208}$$

Rearrangement of (2.208) provides one approach for the determination of V_β:

$$V_\beta = \frac{V_c k_{10}}{\lambda_n} \tag{2.209}$$

Solving Eqs. (2.38) ($k_e' V_c = X_u^\infty / AUC$) and (2.121) ($k_e' = X_u^\infty k_{10} / X_0$) for X_u^∞ / k_e' yields

$$\frac{X_u^\infty}{k_e'} = V_c \cdot AUC \tag{2.210}$$

and

$$\frac{X_u^\infty}{k_e'} = \frac{X_0}{k_{10}} \tag{2.211}$$

Equating the right-hand sides of (2.210) and (2.211) and rearranging the resulting expression gives

$$V_c k_{10} = \frac{X_0}{AUC} \tag{2.212}$$

Substitution of this value of $V_c k_{10}$ for $V_c k_{10}$ in (2.209) results in the following general equation for the determination of V_β:

$$V_\beta = \frac{X_0}{\lambda_n \cdot AUC} \tag{2.213}$$

where AUC is the total area under the plasma concentration versus time curve. This method of calculating V_β is independent of the number of exponentials required to describe a plasma concentration versus time curve, and is analogous to the equation used to calculate volume of distribution in a one-compartment model: Eq. (1.35) ($V = X_0/K \cdot AUC$), where K is the first-order elimination rate constant of a drug. As mentioned previously, V_β, as determined by (2.213), can be used to determine the amount of drug in the body during the terminal exponential phase of a plasma concentration-time curve provided that elimination occurs only from the central compartment. Equation (2.213) can also be used to calculate V_β from intravenous infusion data. When infusion data are employed, X_0 is equal to the product of the infusion rate k_0 and infusion time T (i.e., $k_0 T$), and AUC is the total area under the plasma concentration versus time curve from the time of initiation of the infusion to time infinity after cessation of the infusion.

Methods for the calculation of the clearance Cl_s of a drug using both intravenous bolus and steady-state infusion data were presented earlier in the chapter. The relationships are

$$Cl_s = \frac{X_0}{AUC} \tag{2.43}$$

and

$$Cl_s = \frac{k_0}{C_{ss}} \tag{2.59}$$

where C_{ss} is the steady-state plasma concentration of a drug during an intravenous infusion. Equation (2.213) can be rearranged to yield

$$V_\beta \lambda_n = \frac{X_0}{AUC} \tag{2.214}$$

A comparison of (2.212), (2.214), and (2.43) reveals that

$$Cl_s = V_\beta \lambda_n = V_c k_{10} \tag{2.215}$$

Equation (2.215) can also be used to determine V_β once clearance is known since

$$V_\beta = \frac{Cl_s}{\lambda_n} \tag{2.216}$$

Substituting $0.693/t_{1/2}$ for λ_n [Eq. (2.11)] in (2.216) and solving for $t_{1/2}$ gives

$$t_{1/2} = 0.693 \frac{V_\beta}{Cl_s} \tag{2.217}$$

which again illustrates the dependence of $t_{1/2}$ on both the distribution and elimination characteristics of a drug.

An additional volume parameter and probably the most useful volume term to describe the apparent distribution space in a multicompartment system is V_{ss}, the apparent volume of distribution at steady state. This parameter was initially derived by Riggs [25], who equated it to the sum of the apparent volumes of the central and peripheral compartments. As its name implies, V_{ss} relates the amount of drug in the body to the drug concentration in the plasma at steady state during repetitive dosing or constant rate infusion:

$$X_{ss} = V_{ss} C_{ss} \tag{2.218}$$

and

$$\overline{X} = V_{ss} \overline{C} \tag{2.219}$$

where X_{ss} and C_{ss} are the amount of drug in the body and plasma concentration of drug at steady state, respectively, during constant rate infusion, and $\overline{X}$ and $\overline{C}$ are the "average" amount of drug in the body and plasma concentration of drug at steady state, respectively, during repetitive dosing.

Rearrangement of (2.219) yields the following relationship for V_{ss}:

$$V_{ss} = \frac{\overline{X}}{\overline{C}} \tag{2.220}$$

The amount of drug in the body at any time t after a single intravenous bolus dose in a multicompartment system is given by the difference between the administered dose X_0 and the amount eliminated up to that time, $(X_E)_0^t$:

$$X = X_0 - (X_E)_0^t \tag{2.221}$$

Solving (2.41) for dX_E/dt and integrating the resulting expression from time zero to t gives

$$(X_E)_0^t = Cl_s \int_0^t C \, dt \tag{2.222}$$

where Cl_s is clearance and $\int_0^t C \, dt$ is the area under the plasma concentration time curve described by (2.7). Substitution for $(X_E)_0^t$ in (2.221) according to (2.222) yields

$$X = X_0 - Cl_s \int_0^t C \, dt \tag{2.223}$$

Integrating (2.7) from time zero to t and substituting the resulting expression for $\int_0^t C \, dt$ in (2.223) gives

$$X = X_0 - Cl_s \sum_{\ell=1}^{n} \frac{A_\ell}{\lambda_\ell} (1 - e^{-\lambda_\ell t}) \tag{2.224}$$

The clearance of a drug is equal to the ratio of the intravenous dose to the total area under the drug concentration in the plasma versus time curve [i.e., $Cl_s = X_0/AUC$; Eq. (2.43)]. Substitution of $\sum_{\ell=1}^{n} A_\ell/\lambda_\ell$ for AUC, according to (2.40), in (2.43) yields

$$Cl_s = \frac{X_0}{\sum_{\ell=1}^{n} (A_\ell/\lambda_\ell)} \tag{2.225}$$

This value of Cl_s can then be substituted for Cl_s in (2.224) to give

$$X = X_0 - \frac{X_0 \sum_{\ell=1}^{n} [(A_\ell/\lambda_\ell)(1 - e^{-\lambda_\ell t})]}{\sum_{\ell=1}^{n} (A_\ell/\lambda_\ell)} \tag{2.226}$$

or

$$X = \frac{X_0 \left\{ \sum\limits_{\ell=1}^{n} (A_\ell/\lambda_\ell) - \sum\limits_{\ell=1}^{n} (A_\ell/\lambda_\ell) + \sum\limits_{\ell=1}^{n} [(A_\ell/\lambda_\ell)e^{-\lambda_\ell t}] \right\}}{\sum\limits_{\ell=1}^{n} (A_\ell/\lambda_\ell)}$$

(2.227)

On canceling common terms, the following results:

$$X = \frac{X_0 \sum\limits_{\ell=1}^{n} [(A_\ell/\lambda_\ell)e^{-\lambda_\ell t}]}{\sum\limits_{\ell=1}^{n} (A_\ell/\lambda_\ell)}$$

(2.228)

To convert the single-dose expression (2.228) to one describing the situation during a dosing interval at steady state, the exponential term in (2.228) is multiplied by $1/(1 - e^{-\lambda_\ell \tau})$, where τ is the dosing interval, which is obtained by setting k_i in the multiple-dosing function equal to λ_ℓ and recognizing that $e^{-N\lambda_\ell \tau}$ approaches zero at steady state (see Appendix B). Therefore,

$$X_{ss} = \frac{X_0 \sum\limits_{\ell=1}^{n} [A_\ell e^{-\lambda_\ell t}/\lambda_\ell (1 - e^{-\lambda_\ell \tau})]}{\sum\limits_{\ell=1}^{n} (A_\ell/\lambda_\ell)}$$

(2.229)

where X_{ss} is the amount of drug in the body during a dosing interval at steady state. The average amount of drug in the body at steady state $\overline{X}$ is defined as

$$\overline{X} = \frac{\int_0^\tau X_{ss}\, dt}{\tau}$$

(2.230)

Integration of the summation term in the numerator of (2.229) from $t = 0$ to $t = \tau$ yields

$$\int_0^\tau \sum\limits_{\ell=1}^{n} \frac{A_\ell e^{-\lambda_\ell t}}{\lambda_\ell (1 - e^{-\lambda_\ell \tau})} = \sum\limits_{\ell=1}^{n} \frac{-A_\ell e^{-\lambda_\ell t}}{\lambda_\ell^2 (1 - e^{-\lambda_\ell \tau})} \Bigg|_0^\tau = \sum\limits_{\ell=1}^{n} \frac{A_\ell}{\lambda_\ell^2}$$

(2.231)

It follows that

$$\bar{X} = \frac{X_0 \sum_{\ell=1}^{n} (A_\ell / \lambda_\ell^2)}{\tau \sum_{\ell=1}^{n} (A_\ell / \lambda_\ell)} \qquad (2.232)$$

The average concentration of drug in the plasma at steady state $\bar{C}$ is given by

$$\bar{C} = \frac{\int_0^\tau C_{ss} \, dt}{\tau} \qquad (3.25)$$

Substitution of $\sum_{\ell=1}^{n} A_\ell / \lambda_\ell$ for $\int_0^\tau C_{ss} \, dt$, according to (3.26), in (3.25) gives

$$\bar{C} = \frac{\sum_{\ell=1}^{n} (A_\ell / \lambda_\ell)}{\tau} \qquad (2.233)$$

The values of $\bar{X}$ and $\bar{C}$ as given by (2.232) and (2.233), respectively, can be substituted in (2.220) to yield

$$V_{ss} = \frac{X_0 \sum_{\ell=1}^{n} (A_\ell / \lambda_\ell^2)}{\left[\sum_{\ell=1}^{n} (A_\ell / \lambda_\ell) \right]^2} = \frac{X_0 \sum_{\ell=1}^{n} (A_\ell / \lambda_\ell^2)}{(AUC)^2} \qquad (2.234)$$

Therefore, once the estimates of A_ℓ and λ_ℓ are obtained from a fit of plasma concentration versus time data, V_{ss} can be readily estimated employing (2.234).

Although clearance and volume of distribution parameters have been discussed in this section, a more detailed presentation of their physiologic significance may be found in Chaps. 8 and 5, respectively.

REFERENCES

1. M. Rowland, S. Riegelman, and W. L. Epstein. Absorption kinetics of griseofulvin in man. *J. Pharm. Sci.* 57:984 (1968).
2. P. M. Bungay, R. L. Dedrick, and A. M. Guarino. Pharmacokinetic modeling of the dogfish shark (*Squalus acanthias*): Distribution and urinary and biliary excretion of phenol red and its glucuronide. *J. Pharmacokinet. Biopharm.* 4:377 (1976).

3. F. R. Sidell and W. A. Groff. Intramuscular and intravenous
    administration of small doses of 2-pyridinium aldoximine metho-
    chloride to man. *J. Pharm. Sci. 60*:1224 (1971).
4. W. J. Jusko, G. P. Lewis, and G. W. Schmitt. Ampicillin and
    hetacillin pharmacokinetics in normal and anephric subjects.
    Clin. Pharmacol. Ther. 14:90 (1973).
5. L. Z. Benet. General treatment of linear mammillary models
    with elimination from any compartment as used in pharmaco-
    kinetics. *J. Pharm. Sci. 61*:536 (1972).
6. J. C. K. Loo and S. Riegelman. Assessment of pharmacokinetic
    constants from postinfusion blood curves obtained after i.v.
    infusion. *J. Pharm. Sci. 59*:53 (1970).
7. M. Gibaldi. Estimation of the pharmacokinetic parameters of the
    two-compartment open model from post-infusion plasma concentra-
    tion data. *J. Pharm. Sci. 58*:1133 (1969).
8. P. A. Mitenko and R. I. Olgivie. Rapidly achieved plasma concen-
    tration plateaus, with observations on theophylline kinetics.
    Clin. Pharmacol. Ther. 13:329 (1972).
9. P. D. Thomson, K. L. Melmon, J. A. Richardson, K. Cohen,
    W. Steinbrunn, R. Cudihee, and M. Rowland. Lidocaine pharma-
    cokinetics in advanced heart failure, liver disease and renal
    failure in humans. *Ann. Intern. Med. 78*:499 (1973).
10. M. Rowland, P. D. Thomson, A. Guichard, and K. Melmon.
    Disposition kinetics of lidocaine in normal subjects. *Ann. N.Y.
    Acad. Sci. 179*:383 (1971).
11. E. Kruger-Thiemer. Continuous intravenous infusion and multi-
    compartment accumulation. *Eur. J. Pharmacol. 4*:317 (1968).
12. D. P. Vaughan and G. T. Tucker. General derivation of the
    ideal intravenous drug input required to achieve and maintain
    a constant plasma drug concentration. Theoretical application
    to lignocaine therapy. *Eur. J. Clin. Pharmacol. 10*:433 (1976).
13. J. G. Wagner. A safe method for rapidly achieving plasma con-
    centration plateaus. *Clin. Pharmacol. Ther. 16*:691 (1974).
14. D. P. Vaughan and G. T. Tucker. General theory for rapidly
    establishing steady state drug concentrations using two consec-
    utive constant rate intravenous infusions. *Eur. J. Clin.
    Pharmacol. 9*:235 (1975).
15. D. J. Weidler, N. S. Jallad, D. C. Garg, and J. G. Wagner.
    Pharmacokinetics of propranolol in the cat and comparisons with
    humans and three other species. *Res. Commun. Chem. Pathol.
    Pharmacol. 26*:105 (1979).
16. S. E. Tsuei, R. L. Nation, and J. Thomas. Design of infusion
    regimens to achieve and maintain a predetermined plasma drug
    level range. *Clin. Pharmacol. Ther. 28*:289 (1980).
17. B. L. Lloyd, D. J. Greenblatt, M. D. Allen, J. S. Harmatz,
    and T. W. Smith. Pharmacokinetics and bioavailability of digoxin

capsules, solution and tablets after single and multiple doses. *Am. J. Cardiol. 42*:129 (1978).

18. R. A. Ronfeld and L. Z. Benet. Interpretation of plasma concentration-time curves after oral dosing. *J. Pharm. Sci. 66*:178 (1977).

19. T. L. Loo, B. B. Tanner, G. E. Householder, and B. J. Shepard. Some pharmacokinetic aspects of 5-(dimethyltriazeno)-imidazole-4-carboxamide in the dog. *J. Pharm. Sci. 57*:2126 (1968).

20. J. E. Doherty, W. H. Perkins, and W. J. Flanigan. The distribution and concentration of tritiated digoxin in human tissues. *Ann. Intern. Med. 66*:116 (1976).

21. M. Gibaldi, G. Levy, and W. Hayton. Kinetics of the elimination and neuromuscular blocking effect of d-tubocurarine in man. *Anesthesiology 36*:213 (1972).

22. S. A. Kaplan, M. L. Jack, K. Alexander, and R. E. Weinfeld. Pharmacokinetic profile of diazepam in man following single intravenous and oral and chronic oral administrations. *J. Pharm. Sci. 62*:1789 (1973).

23. R. Nagashima, G. Levy, and R. A. O'Reilly. Comparative pharmacokinetics of coumarin anticoagulants: IV. Application of a three-compartment model to the analysis of the dose-dependent kinetics of bishydroxycoumarin elimination. *J. Pharm. Sci. 57*:1888 (1968).

24. W. J. Westlake. Problems associated with analysis of pharmacokinetic models. *J. Pharm. Sci. 60*:882 (1971).

25. D. S. Riggs. *The Mathematical Approach to Physiologic Problems.* Williams & Wilkins, Baltimore, Md., 1963, pp. 193—220.

3
Multiple Dosing

Some drugs, for example, analgesics, hypnotics, neuromuscular blocking agents, bronchodilators, and antiemetics, may be used effectively
as a single dose. More frequently, drugs are given on a continuous
basis. Moreover, most drugs are administered with sufficient frequency
that measurable and often pharmacologically significant levels of drug
persist in the body when a subsequent dose is administered. For
drugs administered in a fixed dose at a constant dosing interval (e.g.,
every 6 h or once a day), the peak plasma level following the second
and succeeding doses of a drug is almost always higher than the peak
level after the first dose, and therefore the drug accumulates in the
body relative to the initial dose. However, under these conditions
drug accumulation proceeds at a decreasing rate with increasing number of doses until a steady-state plasma level of drug is achieved. At
steady state, the plasma concentration of drug at any time during any
dosing interval should be identical to the concentration at the same time
during any other dosing interval. As will be demonstrated, the rate
and extent of accumulation of a drug is a function of the relative magnitudes of the dosing interval and the half-life of the drug. A model-
independent approach to multiple dosing (i.e., superposition) is discussed in Appendix E.

INTRAVENOUS ADMINISTRATION

The following general equation can be used to describe the plasma concentration versus time curve resulting from the intravenous injection
of a drug:

$$C = \sum_{\ell=1}^{n} A_\ell e^{-\lambda_\ell t} \tag{2.7}$$

where

$$A_\ell = \frac{X_0}{V_c} \frac{\prod\limits_{i=2}^{n} (E_i - \lambda_\ell)}{\prod\limits_{\substack{i=1 \\ i \neq \ell}}^{n} (\lambda_i - \lambda_\ell)} \qquad (2.8)$$

In these equations X_0 is the intravenous dose, V_c is the volume of the central compartment, E_i is the sum of the exit rate constants from the ith compartment, λ_i and λ_ℓ are disposition rate constant, and n is the number of exponentials required to describe the curve adequately. The maximum plasma concentration resulting from the intravenous administration of the first bolus dose of a drug, $(C_1)_{max}$, would occur at t = 0. Therefore,

$$(C_1)_{max} = \sum_{\ell=1}^{n} A_\ell \qquad (3.1)$$

The concentration of drug in the plasma at the end of the first dosing interval of length τ time units $(C_1)_{min}$ will be given by the relationship

$$(C_1)_{min} = \sum_{\ell=1}^{n} A_\ell e^{-\lambda_\ell \tau} \qquad (3.2)$$

which is obtained by setting t equal to τ in (2.7). Since there are usually measurable plasma concentrations of drug when a second dose is administered, administration of a second dose, equal in size to the first dose, will produce an immediate increase in plasma concentration of drug yielding a new maximum, $(C_2)_{max}$. This new maximum would be equal to the sum of the plasma concentration at the time of administration (i.e., at time t = τ) and the maximum concentration resulting from the first dose [i.e., $(C_1)_{max}$]. Therefore,

$$(C_2)_{max} = (C_1)_{max} + (C_1)_{min} \qquad (3.3)$$

Substitution for $(C_1)_{max}$ and $(C_1)_{min}$ according to (3.1) and (3.2), respectively, yields

$$(C_2)_{max} = \sum_{\ell=1}^{n} A_\ell + \sum_{\ell=1}^{n} A_\ell e^{-\lambda_\ell \tau} = \sum_{\ell=1}^{n} A_\ell (1 + e^{-\lambda_\ell \tau}) \qquad (3.4)$$

The minimum concentration of drug in the plasma after the second dose $(C_2)_{min}$ (assuming a constant dosing interval of τ) is given by

$$(C_2)_{min} = \sum_{\ell=1}^{n} A_\ell (1 + e^{-\lambda_\ell \tau}) e^{-\lambda_\ell \tau} \qquad (3.5)$$

which can be modified to yield

$$(C_2)_{min} = \sum_{\ell=1}^{n} A_\ell (e^{-\lambda_\ell \tau} + e^{-2\lambda_\ell \tau}) \qquad (3.6)$$

It follows that

$$(C_3)_{max} = \sum_{\ell=1}^{n} A_\ell + \sum_{\ell=1}^{n} A_\ell (e^{-\lambda_\ell \tau} + e^{-2\lambda_\ell \tau})$$

$$= \sum_{\ell=1}^{n} A_\ell (1 + e^{-\lambda_\ell \tau} + e^{-2\lambda_\ell \tau}) \qquad (3.7)$$

and

$$(C_3)_{min} = \sum_{\ell=1}^{n} A_\ell (1 + e^{-\lambda_\ell \tau} + e^{-2\lambda_\ell \tau}) e^{-\lambda_\ell \tau}$$

$$= \sum_{\ell=1}^{n} A_\ell (e^{-\lambda_\ell \tau} + e^{-2\lambda_\ell \tau} + e^{-3\lambda_\ell \tau}) \qquad (3.8)$$

where $(C_3)_{max}$ is the maximum plasma concentration following a third dose and $(C_3)_{min}$ is the minimum plasma concentration τ time units after the third dose.

On examination of (3.1), (3.4), and (3.7), it is readily apparent that a geometric series can be written for the maximum concentration of drug in the plasma following N doses, $(C_N)_{max}$:

$$(C_N)_{max} = \sum_{\ell=1}^{n} A_\ell (1 + e^{-\lambda_\ell \tau} + e^{-2\lambda_\ell \tau} + \cdots + e^{-(N-1)\lambda_\ell \tau})$$

$$(3.9)$$

If we let

$$r = 1 + e^{-\lambda_\ell \tau} + e^{-2\lambda_\ell \tau} + \cdots + e^{-(N-1)\lambda_\ell \tau} \qquad (3.10)$$

it follows that

$$(C_N)_{max} = \sum_{\ell=1}^{n} A_\ell r \qquad (3.11)$$

Multiplication of (3.10) by $e^{-\lambda_\ell \tau}$ yields

$$re^{-\lambda_\ell \tau} = e^{-\lambda_\ell \tau} + e^{-2\lambda_\ell \tau} + \cdots + e^{-(N-1)\lambda_\ell \tau} + e^{-N\lambda_\ell \tau} \qquad (3.12)$$

which when subtracted from (3.10) produces

$$r - re^{-\lambda_\ell \tau} = 1 - e^{-N\lambda_\ell \tau} \tag{3.13}$$

which can be solved for r to yield

$$r = \frac{1 - e^{-N\lambda_\ell \tau}}{1 - e^{-\lambda_\ell \tau}} \tag{3.14}$$

Substitution of this value of r in (3.11) yields the following general expression for the maximum concentration of drug in the plasma after intravenous administration of any number of doses:

$$(C_N)_{max} = \sum_{\ell=1}^{n} A_\ell \frac{1 - e^{-N\lambda_\ell \tau}}{1 - e^{-\lambda_\ell \tau}} \tag{3.15}$$

From a comparison of previous equations [i.e., (3.1) and (3.2), (3.4) and (3.5), and (3.7) and (3.8)] it is equally clear that

$$(C_N)_{min} = (C_N)_{max} e^{-\lambda_\ell \tau} \tag{3.16}$$

and, therefore,

$$(C_N)_{min} = \sum_{\ell=1}^{n} A_\ell \frac{1 - e^{-N\lambda_\ell \tau}}{1 - e^{-\lambda_\ell \tau}} e^{-\lambda_\ell \tau} \tag{3.17}$$

It is evident on examination of (3.15) and (3.17) that the concentration of drug in the plasma at any time during a dosing interval (i.e., C_N) is given by

$$C_N = \sum_{\ell=1}^{n} A_\ell \frac{1 - e^{-N\lambda_\ell \tau}}{1 - e^{-\lambda_\ell \tau}} e^{-\lambda_\ell t} \tag{3.18}$$

where t is the time elapsed since dose N was administered. Therefore, by knowing the zero-time intercepts and disposition rate constants, A_ℓ and λ_ℓ, respectively (both of which can be obtained following a single intravenous dose), the plasma concentration of a drug at any time during a dosing interval can be predicted provided that a fixed dose is administered every τ time units.

Equation (3.18) may also be obtained by a method that does not rely on a detailed derivation of the type presented above, and consequently is significantly more convenient (see Appendix B). Any equation that describes the time course of a drug in a driving force compartment after a single dose may be directly converted to a multiple-dose equation by multiplying each exponential term containing t by the function

$$\frac{1 - e^{-Nk_i\tau}}{1 - e^{-k_i\tau}}$$

where N and τ are as defined previously and k_i is the apparent first-order rate constant in each exponential term. Therefore, multiplication of (2.7), $C = \sum_{\ell=1}^{n} A_\ell e^{-\lambda_\ell t}$, by the multiple-dosing function, and setting k_i equal to λ_ℓ [since λ_ℓ is the rate constant in the exponential term of (2.7)] permits (2.7) to be directly converted to (3.18).

The drug concentration in the plasma, at any time during a dosing interval, will increase and then approach a constant value as the number of doses increases (see Fig. 3.1). The equation describing the time course of drug at the plateau or steady state can be obtained by setting N in (3.18) to infinity (i.e., by recognizing that the term $e^{-N\lambda_\ell\tau}$ approaches zero with increasing number of doses). Thus

$$C_{ss} = \sum_{\ell=1}^{n} A_\ell \frac{1}{1 - e^{-\lambda_\ell\tau}} e^{-\lambda_\ell t} \tag{3.19}$$

where C_{ss} is the plasma concentration of drug at any time during a dosing interval at steady state. Similarly, the equations for the maximum and minimum concentrations of drug in the plasma during a dosing interval at steady state, $(C_{ss})_{max}$ and $(C_{ss})_{min}$, respectively, can be written as

$$(C_{ss})_{max} = \sum_{\ell=1}^{n} A_\ell \frac{1}{1 - e^{-\lambda_\ell\tau}} \tag{3.20}$$

and

$$(C_{ss})_{min} = \sum_{\ell=1}^{n} A_\ell \frac{1}{1 - e^{-\lambda_\ell\tau}} e^{-\lambda_\ell\tau} \tag{3.21}$$

If the dosing interval τ is much greater than the half-life of a drug (where $t_{1/2} = 0.693/\lambda_n$), $(C_{ss})_{min}$ approaches zero. Under these conditions no accumulation will occur and the plasma concentration versus time profile will be the result of the administration of a series of single doses.

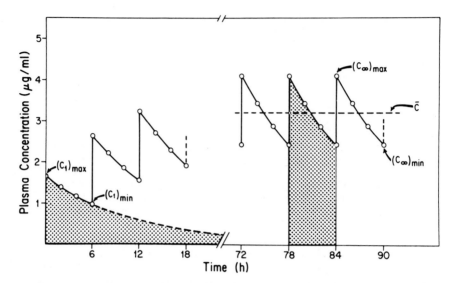

Fig. 3.1 Drug accumulation and attainment of steady state on multiple intravenous dosing of a fixed dose of drug every 6 h. Maximum and minimum drug concentrations after the first dose are denoted $(C_1)_{max}$ and $(C_1)_{min}$, respectively; those at steady state are denoted $(C_\infty)_{max}$ and $(C_\infty)_{min}$, respectively. The average drug concentration at steady state, $\bar{C}$, is also shown. The area under the drug concentration in plasma versus time curve during a dosing interval at steady state (shaded area) is the same as the total area under the curve after a single dose (shaded area bounded by solid and dashed lines).

As discussed in Chap. 2, one frequently finds in a two-compartment model that the larger the ratio of the zero-time intercepts A_1/A_2, the more readily one can discern the multicompartment characteristics of a drug. Equation (3.19) can be written as

$$C_{ss} = \sum_{\ell=1}^{n} U_\ell e^{-\lambda_\ell t} \tag{3.22}$$

where

$$U_\ell = A_\ell \frac{1}{1 - e^{-\lambda_\ell \tau}} \tag{3.23}$$

The ratio of U_1/U_2 would therefore be given by

$$\frac{U_1}{U_2} = \frac{A_1(1 - e^{-\lambda_2 \tau})}{A_2(1 - e^{-\lambda_1 \tau})} \qquad (3.24)$$

and will always be less than the ratio A_1/A_2. Since λ_1 is by definition greater than λ_2, the ratio $(1 - e^{-\lambda_2 \tau})/(1 - e^{-\lambda_1 \tau})$ will always be less than 1. Consequently, following multiple dosing the ability to discern the multicompartment characteristics of a drug is usually decreased. On the other hand, analytical limitations may prevent one from observing more than one exponential phase after a single intravenous administration of a drug that has an exceptionally large ratio of A_1 to A_2. In this case, multiple dosing makes the multicompartment characteristic of the drug more obvious. For a more detailed discussion of this phenomenon, see Chap. 2.

Average Steady-State Concentration

A parameter that is very useful in multiple dosing is the "average" concentration of drug in the plasma at steady state, $\bar{C}$. This parameter can be defined as

$$\bar{C} = \frac{\int_0^\tau C_{ss} dt}{\tau} \qquad (3.25)$$

where $\int_0^\tau C_{ss}\, dt$ is the area under the plasma concentration-time curve during a dosing interval at steady state (i.e., between time zero and τ) where τ is as defined previously. Integration of (3.19) from time zero to τ yields

$$\int_0^\tau C_{ss}\, dt = \sum_{\ell=1}^{n} \frac{A_\ell}{\lambda_\ell} \qquad (3.26)$$

This expression for the area under the plasma concentration-time curve from time zero to τ during a dosing interval at steady state is equivalent to (2.40), the equation for the area under the plasma concentration-time curve from time zero to infinity following a single intravenous dose (see Fig. 3.1). Therefore, the average plasma concentration of drug at steady state can be predicted from a single-dose study by employing the following relationship:

$$\bar{C} = \frac{\int_0^\infty C\, dt}{\tau} \qquad (3.27)$$

The area under the plasma concentration versus time curve, AUC or $\int_0^\infty C \, dt$, following a single intravenous dose, X_0, can be obtained by rearrangement of (2.214) to give

$$AUC = \frac{X_0}{V_\beta \lambda_n} \tag{3.28}$$

where V_β is the apparent volume of distribution and λ_n is the disposition rate constant associated with the terminal slope of a log plasma concentration-time curve and equals 0.693 divided by half-life (i.e., $0.693/t_{1/2}$) [Eq. (2.11)]. The relationship between these parameters and clearance Cl_s has also been presented previously:

$$Cl_s = V_\beta \lambda_n \tag{2.215}$$

Therefore, substituting $X_0/V_\beta \lambda_n$ for $\int_0^\infty C \, dt$ in (3.27) and setting $V_\beta \lambda_n$ equal to Cl_s yields

$$\overline{C} = \frac{X_0}{V_\beta \lambda_n \tau} = \frac{X_0}{Cl_s \tau} \tag{3.29}$$

which can also be written in terms of half-life, i.e.,

$$\overline{C} = \frac{1.44 X_0 t_{1/2}}{V_\beta \tau} \tag{3.30}$$

By knowing the AUC following a single dose, the clearance, or the half-life and volume of distribution of a drug, the average plasma concentration of a drug at steady state following the administration of a fixed dose X_0 at a constant time interval τ can be predicted. As can also be seen from (3.29) and (3.30), the size of the administered dose X_0 and the time interval at which this dose is administered, τ, can be adjusted to obtain a desired average steady-state plasma concentration. These equations assume that all parameters are constant over the entire dosing period.

The average plasma concentration of a drug at steady state as calculated employing (3.27), (3.29), or (3.30) is neither the arithmetic nor the geometric mean of $(C_{ss})_{max}$ and $(C_{ss})_{min}$. Rather, it is a plasma concentration value which when multiplied by τ equals the area under the plasma concentration-time curve over the time interval zero to τ at steady state. Therefore, from simple geometric considerations, $\overline{C}$ must represent a plasma concentration value between $(C_{ss})_{max}$ and $(C_{ss})_{min}$ (See Fig. 3.1). A limitation of the $\overline{C}$ approach is that it gives no information about the fluctuations in plasma levels [i.e., $\overline{C}$ gives no information as to the relative magnitudes of $(C_{ss})_{max}$ and $(C_{ss})_{min}$].

Accumulation

As discussed previously, the administration of a drug on a multiple-dose regimen will usually result in its accumulation in the body. The extent of accumulation of a given drug may be quantified in several ways. One approach is to determine the ratio of the minimum plasma concentration of drug at steady state $(C_{ss})_{min}$ to the minimum plasma concentration following the first dose $(C_1)_{min}$. This ratio can be defined as the accumulation factor R. Therefore,

$$R = \frac{(C_{ss})_{min}}{(C_1)_{min}} \tag{3.31}$$

Substitution for $(C_{ss})_{min}$ and $(C_1)_{min}$ in (3.31) according to (3.21) and (3.2), respectively, yields

$$R = \frac{\displaystyle\sum_{\ell=1}^{n} A_\ell \frac{1}{1 - e^{-\lambda_\ell \tau}} e^{-\lambda_\ell \tau}}{\displaystyle\sum_{\ell=1}^{n} A_\ell e^{-\lambda_\ell \tau}} \tag{3.32}$$

This relationship is rather complex. However, if all doses are administered in the postdistributive phase (i.e., $e^{-\lambda_1 \tau}$ to $e^{-\lambda_{n-1}\tau}$ approach zero) of a plasma concentration versus time curve, or if the plasma concentration versus time curve can be adequately described by a monoexponential equation [i.e., n = 1 in (3.32)], then (3.32) reduces to

$$R = \frac{1}{1 - e^{-\lambda_n \tau}} \tag{3.33}$$

Under these conditions the extent of accumulation can be predicted simply by knowing the terminal disposition rate constant of a drug, λ_n or K, or half-life $t_{1/2}$, since $t_{1/2} = 0.693/\lambda_n = 0.693/K$.

The ratio of $(C_{ss})_{max}$ to $(C_1)_{max}$ is also an appropriate expression of drug accumulation. According to Eqs. (3.20) and (3.1), this ratio is given by

$$\frac{(C_{ss})_{max}}{(C_1)_{max}} = \frac{\displaystyle\sum_{\ell=1}^{n} [A_\ell/(1 - e^{-\lambda_\ell \tau})]}{\displaystyle\sum_{\ell=1}^{n} A_\ell} \tag{3.34}$$

In the case of a drug that shows one-compartment model characteristics on intravenous administration, Eq. (3.34) may be simplified to
Eq. (3.33) where K replaces λ_n.

Another expression that has been used to characterize drug accumulation is the ratio of $\overline{C}$, the average drug concentration at steady
state, to $\overline{C}_1$, the average drug concentration during the first dosing
interval. Consider that the average drug concentration during any
dosing interval (i.e., $\overline{C}_N$) may be defined as

$$\overline{C}_N = \frac{\int_0^\tau C_N \, dt}{\tau} \tag{3.35}$$

where $\int_0^\tau C_N \, dt$ is the area under the plasma concentration-time
curve during the Nth dosing interval. Integration of (3.18) from
time zero to τ yields

$$\int_0^\tau C_N \, dt = \sum_{\ell=1}^{n} A_\ell \frac{1 - e^{-N\lambda_\ell \tau}}{\lambda_\ell} \tag{3.36}$$

Substitution of this value of $\int_0^\tau C_N \, dt$ in (3.34) and substitution for
$\int_0^\tau C_{ss} \, dt$ in (3.25) according to (3.26) yields

$$\overline{C}_N = \sum_{\ell=1}^{n} A_\ell \frac{1 - e^{-N\lambda_\ell \tau}}{\lambda_\ell \tau} \tag{3.37}$$

and at steady state

$$\overline{C} = \sum_{\ell=1}^{n} A_\ell \frac{1}{\lambda_\ell \tau} \tag{3.38}$$

respectively. Taking the ratio of $\overline{C}_N$ to $\overline{C}$ and canceling the common
term τ gives

$$\frac{\overline{C}_N}{\overline{C}} = \frac{\sum_{\ell=1}^{n} [A_\ell (1 - e^{-N\lambda_\ell \tau})/\lambda_\ell]}{\sum_{\ell=1}^{n} (A_\ell/\lambda_\ell)} \tag{3.39}$$

When N = 1, that is, for the first dose, (3.39) becomes

$$\frac{\overline{C}_1}{\overline{C}} = \frac{\sum_{\ell=1}^{n} [A_\ell (1 - e^{-\lambda_\ell \tau})/\lambda_\ell]}{\sum_{\ell=1}^{n} (A_\ell/\lambda_\ell)} \tag{3.40}$$

The inverse ratio $\overline{C}/\overline{C}_1$ may be used to express accumulation:

$$\frac{\overline{C}}{\overline{C}_1} = \frac{\sum\limits_{\ell=1}^{n} (A_\ell/\lambda_\ell)}{\sum\limits_{\ell=1}^{n} [A_\ell(1 - e^{-\lambda_\ell \tau})/\lambda_\ell]} \tag{3.41}$$

In the case of a drug that can be described by a one-compartment model on intravenous administration, Eq. (3.41) reduces to (3.33) where K replaces λ_n.

Equation (3.33) indicates that the larger the ratio of $t_{1/2}/\tau$, the greater will be the extent of accumulation. For example, consider a drug with a half-life of 24 h (i.e., $\lambda_n = 0.029\ h^{-1}$). If this drug is administered every 24 h (i.e., $\tau = 24$ h), according to Eq. (3.33) R equals 2.0. However, administration of the same dose every 6 h results in much greater accumulation (R = 6.3). Consequently, when τ is equal to or greater than the half-life of a drug, the extent of accumulation is relatively modest (≤ 2). If the ratio $t_{1/2}/\tau$ is large, however, the extent of accumulation may be substantial.

Time to Reach Steady State

The ratio $\overline{C}_N/\overline{C}$ as given by (3.39) can be employed to calculate the time required to reach a certain fraction of the ultimate steady-state level, where the fraction of the steady-state level, f_{ss}, is defined in terms of average plasma levels:

$$f_{ss} = \frac{\overline{C}_N}{\overline{C}} \tag{3.42}$$

Substitution for $\overline{C}_N/\overline{C}$ in (3.42) according to (3.39) gives

$$f_{ss} = \frac{\sum\limits_{\ell=1}^{n} [A_\ell(1 - e^{-N\lambda_\ell \tau})/\lambda_\ell]}{\sum\limits_{\ell=1}^{n} (A_\ell/\lambda_\ell)} \tag{3.43}$$

Equation (3.43) can be used to calculate the fraction of the ultimate steady state that is reached following the Nth dose. This equation cannot, however, be rearranged to obtain an expression for the time (i.e., $N\tau$) to reach a certain fraction of the steady-state level. The term $N\tau$ can only be estimated by numerical iteration. If the plasma concentration versus time profile of a drug can be adequately described by a monoexponential equation (i.e., n = 1), (3.43) reduces to

$$f_{ss} = 1 - e^{-NK\tau}$$ (3.44)

Rearrangement of (3.44) yields

$$e^{-NK\tau} = 1 - f_{ss}$$ (3.45)

the common logarithm of which is

$$-NK\tau = 2.303 \log (1 - f_{ss})$$ (3.46)

Equation (3.46) can be further rearranged to obtain an expression for $N\tau$. Thus

$$N\tau = - \frac{2.303}{K} \log (1 - f_{ss})$$ (3.47)

or

$$N\tau = -3.32 t_{1/2} \log (1 - f_{ss})$$ (3.48)

since K equals $0.693/t_{1/2}$ [Eq. (2.11)].

For a drug with one-compartment model characteristics the time required to reach a particular fraction of steady state is independent of the number of doses administered and the interval between administrations, but it is directly proportional to the half-life. From Eq. (3.48) it can be readily calculated that 3.32 and 6.64 half-lives would be required to reach 90 and 99%, respectively, of the steady-state plasma level of a drug. Since Eqs. (3.44) and (3.48) were derived based on a one-compartment system, they will be in error if used for a drug that demonstrates multicompartment characteristics.

A model-independent approach for the estimation of f_{ss} involves the use of areas under the plasma concentration versus time curve [1]. This approach is based on a simple extension of Eq. (3.43). Expansion of (3.43) yields

$$f_{ss} = \frac{\sum\limits_{\ell=1}^{n} (A_\ell / \lambda_\ell) - \sum\limits_{\ell=1}^{n} (A_\ell e^{-N\lambda_\ell \tau} / \lambda_\ell)}{\sum\limits_{\ell=1}^{n} (A_\ell / \lambda_\ell)}$$ (3.49)

The total area under a plasma concentration versus time curve, AUC, following the intravenous administration of a single dose of drug equals $\sum_{\ell=1}^{n} (A_\ell / \lambda_\ell)$ [Eq. (2.40)]. Substitution of AUC for $\sum_{\ell=1}^{n} (A_\ell / \lambda_\ell)$ in (3.49) gives

$$f_{ss} = \frac{AUC - \sum_{\ell=1}^{n} (A_\ell e^{-N\lambda_\ell \tau} / \lambda_\ell)}{AUC} \tag{3.50}$$

The integral of (2.7) $(C = \sum_{\ell=1}^{n} A_\ell e^{-\lambda_\ell t})$ from time t to ∞ provides
an expression for the area under a plasma concentration-time curve
following a single intravenous bolus dose from time t to ∞, AUC_t^∞:

$$AUC_t^\infty = \sum_{\ell=1}^{n} \frac{A_\ell e^{-\lambda_\ell t}}{\lambda_\ell} \tag{3.51}$$

Since $N\tau$ in (3.50) equals the time since the beginning of dosing (i.e.,
t), AUC_t^∞ can be substituted for $\sum_{\ell=1}^{n} (A_\ell e^{-N\lambda_\ell \tau} / \lambda_\ell)$ in (3.50) to yield

$$f_{ss} = \frac{AUC - AUC_t^\infty}{AUC} = \frac{AUC_0^t}{AUC} \tag{3.52}$$

Therefore, the fraction of steady state reached at time t after initiation of a multiple-dosing regimen can be determined by knowing the
areas, AUC and AUC_t^∞ or AUC_0^t obtained from a single bolus dose of
the drug. No model has to be assumed to permit the use of (3.52)
for determining f_{ss}.

Determination of a Loading Dose

As (3.48) indicates, a significant period of time may be required to
attain steady-state plasma concentrations for drugs with long half-
lives. A rational method to overcome the lapse in time before a steady-
state concentration is reached would be to administer an initial loading
dose. One approach to the calculation of a loading dose is as
follows. It is often desirable to maintain plasma concentrations of drug
greater than some minimum effective level. This level may be defined
as $(C_{ss})_{min}$. Therefore, the first dose (i.e., the loading dose X_0^*)
must be sufficiently high such that $(C_1)_{min}$ equals $(C_{ss})_{min}$, where
$(C_1)_{min}$ and $(C_{ss})_{min}$ are given by (3.21) and (3.2), respectively.
Substitution for A_ℓ according to (2.8), in (3.2) and (3.21), and substitution of X_0^* (the loading dose) for X_0 (the maintenance dose) in
(3.2) yields

$$(C_1)_{min} = \sum_{\ell=1}^{n} \frac{X_0^*}{V_c} \frac{\prod_{i=2}^{n} (E_i - \lambda_\ell)}{\prod_{\substack{i=1 \\ i \neq \ell}}^{n} (\lambda_i - \lambda_\ell)} e^{-\lambda_\ell \tau} \tag{3.53}$$

and

$$(C_{ss})_{min} = \sum_{\ell=1}^{n} \frac{X_0}{V_c} \frac{\prod\limits_{\substack{i=2}}^{n} (E_i - \lambda_\ell)}{\prod\limits_{\substack{i=1 \\ i \neq \ell}}^{n} (\lambda_i - \lambda_\ell)} \frac{1}{1 - e^{-\lambda_\ell \tau}} e^{-\lambda_\ell \tau} \tag{3.54}$$

respectively. Since $(C_1)_{min}$ as given by (3.53) must equal $(C_{ss})_{min}$,

$$\sum_{\ell=1}^{n} \frac{X_0^*}{V_c} \frac{\prod\limits_{\substack{i=2}}^{n} (E_i - \lambda_\ell)}{\prod\limits_{\substack{i=1 \\ i \neq \ell}}^{n} (\lambda_i - \lambda_\ell)} e^{-\lambda_\ell \tau} = \sum_{\ell=1}^{n} \frac{X_0}{V_c} \frac{\prod\limits_{\substack{i=2}}^{n} (E_i - \lambda_\ell)}{\prod\limits_{\substack{i=1 \\ i \neq \ell}}^{n} (\lambda_i - \lambda_\ell)} \frac{1}{1 - e^{-\lambda_\ell \tau}} e^{-\lambda_\ell \tau}$$

$$\tag{3.55}$$

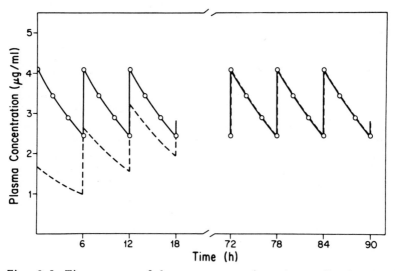

Fig. 3.2 Time course of drug concentration when a fixed dose of drug is given every 6 h (dashed line) and when the first dose of the regimen is replaced by an appropriately larger dose, a loading dose (solid line). Drug concentrations in plasma at steady state are identical, but steady state is attained much more quickly when a loading dose is used.

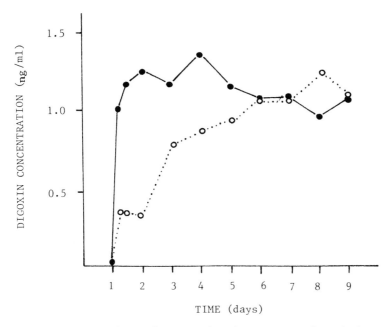

Fig. 3.3 Comparison of serum digoxin concentrations in human volunteers given a 2 mg loading dose followed by a 0.5 mg daily dose of the drug (●) and in those in whom the loading dose was omitted (○). (From Ref. 2.)

Solving (3.55) for X_0^* and canceling the common term V_c yields

$$X_0^* = X_0 \frac{\sum\limits_{\ell=1}^{n} \left\{ \left[\prod\limits_{\substack{i=2}}^{n} (E_i - \lambda_\ell) \middle/ \prod\limits_{\substack{i=1 \\ i\neq\ell}}^{n} (\lambda_i - \lambda_\ell) \right] [1/(1 - e^{-\lambda_\ell \tau})] e^{-\lambda_\ell \tau} \right\}}{\sum\limits_{\ell=1}^{n} \left\{ \left[\prod\limits_{\substack{i=2}}^{n} (E_i - \lambda_\ell) \middle/ \prod\limits_{\substack{i=1 \\ i\neq\ell}}^{n} (\lambda_i - \lambda_\ell) \right] e^{-\lambda_\ell \tau} \right\}}$$

$$(3.56)$$

In a one-compartment system (i.e., $n = 1$), or if all doses are administered in the postdistributive phase (i.e., $e^{-\lambda_1\tau}$ to $e^{-\lambda_{n-1}\tau}$ approach zero), (3.56) reduces to

$$X_0^* = X_0 \frac{1}{1 - e^{-\lambda_n \tau}} \tag{3.57}$$

Therefore, the loading dose is equal to the product of the maintenance dose and the accumulation factor. Administration of a loading dose X_0^* as calculated by (3.57) followed by a maintenance dose X_0 every τ time units in the postdistributive phase should produce an immediate minimum steady-state plasma concentration of drug (Figs. 3.2 and 3.3). For example, administration of a loading dose twice the size of the maintenance dose for a drug where the dosing interval τ equals the half-life will yield immediate minimum steady-state concentrations. If a loading dose were not given, approximately four half-lives would have been required to reach 90% of the ultimate steady state.

INTRAVENOUS INFUSION

Some drugs are administered as an intravenous infusion rather than an intravenous bolus injection. The relationship describing the rise in drug concentration in the plasma during infusion is

$$C = \frac{k_0}{V_c} \left[\frac{\prod\limits_{i=2}^{n} E_i}{\prod\limits_{i=1}^{n} \lambda_i} - \sum_{\ell=1}^{n} \frac{\prod\limits_{i=2}^{n} (E_i - \lambda_\ell)}{\lambda_\ell \prod\limits_{\substack{i=1 \\ i \neq \ell}}^{n} (\lambda_i - \lambda_\ell)} e^{-\lambda_\ell t} \right] \tag{2.55}$$

where k_0 is the zero-order infusion rate, and all other parameters are as defined previously. Administration of a second dose as an infusion, τ time units after administration of the first dose, where τ is in the postdistribution phase of the previous dose, would yield the following equation for plasma concentration (C_2) as a function of time

$$C_2 = (C_1)_{min} e^{-\lambda_n (t-\tau)} + \frac{k_0}{V_c} \left[\frac{\prod\limits_{i=2}^{n} E_i}{\prod\limits_{i=1}^{n} \lambda_i} - \sum_{\ell=1}^{n} \frac{\prod\limits_{i=2}^{n} (E_i - \lambda_\ell)}{\lambda_\ell \prod\limits_{\substack{i=1 \\ i \neq \ell}}^{n} (\lambda_i - \lambda_\ell)} e^{-\lambda_\ell (t-\tau)} \right] \tag{3.58}$$

If a third infusion is given τ time units after the second infusion, plasma concentrations resulting from this infusion would be given by the following equation:

$$C_3 = (C_2)_{min} e^{-\lambda_n(t-2\tau)} + \frac{k_0}{V_c} \left[\frac{\prod\limits_{i=2}^{n} E_i}{\prod\limits_{i=1}^{n} \lambda_i} - \sum_{\ell=1}^{n} \frac{\prod\limits_{i=2}^{n} (E_i - \lambda_\ell)}{\lambda_\ell \prod\limits_{\substack{i=1 \\ i \neq \ell}}^{n} (\lambda_i - \lambda_\ell)} e^{-\lambda_\ell(t-2\tau)} \right]$$

(3.59)

On examination of Eqs. (2.55), (3.58), and (3.59), it is readily apparent that a general equation can be written for the plasma concentration of drug following N doses, C_N, that is

$$C_N = (C_{N-1})_{min} e^{-\lambda_n(t-(N-1)\tau)}$$

$$+ \frac{k_0}{V_c} \left[\frac{\prod\limits_{i=2}^{n} E_i}{\prod\limits_{i=1}^{n} \lambda_i} - \sum_{\ell=1}^{n} \frac{\prod\limits_{i=2}^{n} (E_i - \lambda_\ell)}{\lambda_\ell \prod\limits_{\substack{i=1 \\ i \neq \ell}}^{n} (\lambda_i - \lambda_\ell)} e^{-\lambda_\ell(t-(N-1)\tau)} \right]$$

(3.60)

Since $t = (N - 1)\tau + t_i$ where t_i is some time during infusion (i.e., $0 \leq t_i \leq T$, where T is the infusion time), Eq. (3.60) can be written as follows:

$$C_N = (C_{N-1})_{min} e^{-\lambda_n t_i} + \frac{k_0}{V_c} \left[\frac{\prod\limits_{i=2}^{n} E_i}{\prod\limits_{i=1}^{n} \lambda_i} - \sum_{\ell=1}^{n} \frac{\prod\limits_{i=2}^{n} (E_i - \lambda_\ell)}{\lambda_\ell \prod\limits_{\substack{i=1 \\ i \neq \ell}}^{n} (\lambda_i - \lambda_\ell)} e^{-\lambda_\ell t_i} \right]$$

(3.61)

The maximum plasma concentration following the Nth infusion will occur when $t_i = T$ and is therefore given by the relationship

$$(C_N)_{max} = (C_{N-1})_{min} e^{-\lambda_n T} + \frac{k_0}{V_c} \left[\frac{\prod\limits_{i=2}^{n} E_i}{\prod\limits_{i=1}^{n} \lambda_i} - \sum_{\ell=1}^{n} \frac{\prod\limits_{i=2}^{n} (E_i - \lambda_\ell)}{\lambda_\ell \prod\limits_{\substack{i=1 \\ i \neq \ell}}^{n} (\lambda_i - \lambda_\ell)} e^{-\lambda_\ell T} \right]$$

(3.62)

The plasma concentration of a drug as a function of time following the cessation of infusion is given by

$$C = \sum_{\ell = 1}^{n} R_{\ell} e^{-\lambda_{\ell} t'} \tag{2.66}$$

where

$$R_{\ell} = \frac{k_0}{V_c} \frac{(e^{-\lambda_{\ell} T} - 1) \prod\limits_{i = 2}^{n} (E_i - \lambda_{\ell})}{-\lambda_{\ell} \prod\limits_{\substack{i = 1 \\ i \neq \ell}}^{n} (\lambda_i - \lambda_{\ell})} \tag{2.67}$$

and t' is the time postinfusion. Equation (2.66) can be readily converted to a multiple-dosing equation by multiplying it by the multiple-dosing function and setting k_i equal to λ_{ℓ}, yielding

$$C_N = \sum_{\ell = 1}^{n} R_{\ell} \frac{1 - e^{-N\lambda_{\ell} \tau}}{1 - e^{-\lambda_{\ell} \tau}} e^{-\lambda_{\ell} t'}$$

The minimum postinfusion concentration will occur when t' equals τ − T. If each dose is administered in the postdistribution phase of the previous dose, $\ell = n$. Therefore, $(C_{N-1})_{min}$, a value necessary to determine C_N and $(C_N)_{max}$ from Eqs. (3.61) and (3.62), is given by

$$(C_{N-1})_{min} = R_n \frac{1 - e^{-(N-1)\lambda_n \tau}}{1 - e^{-\lambda_n \tau}} e^{-\lambda_n (\tau - T)} \tag{3.63}$$

R_n is given by 2.67 when $\ell = n$.
At steady state, that is, when $e^{-(N-1)\lambda_n \tau}$ approaches zero

$$(C_{ss})_{min} = R_n \frac{1}{1 - e^{-\lambda_n \tau}} e^{-\lambda_n (\tau - T)} \tag{3.64}$$

The maximum concentration of drug at steady state, and the concentration of drug at steady state during infusion can be determined by setting $(C_{N-1})_{min}$ in Eqs. (3.61) and (3.62) equal to $(C_{ss})_{min}$; the latter is given by (3.64).

The average concentration of drug in the plasma at steady state, $\overline{C}$, resulting from multiple intravenous infusions can be determined from the same basic relationship used for the intravenous bolus case, namely $\overline{C} = \int_0^\tau C_{ss}\, dt/\tau$ [Eq. (3.25)]. It can be demonstrated that

$$\int_0^\tau C_{ss}\, dt = \int_0^\infty C\, dt \qquad (3.65)$$

Therefore,

$$\overline{C} = \frac{k_0 T}{V_c k_{10} \tau} \qquad (3.66)$$

since $\int_0^\infty C\, dt$ following an intravenous infusion equals $k_0 T/V_c k_{10}$ [see Eq. (2.212)]. The product $k_0 T$ equals the intravenous dose X_0, and $V_c k_{10} = V_\beta \lambda_n = Cl_s$ [Eq. (2.21)]. Therefore, the average plasma concentration of drug at steady state resulting from intravenous infusions can also be determined using Eqs. (3.27), (3.29), or (3.30).

Provided that the same underlying assumptions are met, an accumulation factor R, the time to reach a certain fraction of steady state Nτ, and a loading dose X_0^* can be determined for intravenous infusion data using the same relationships as used for intravenous bolus data:

$$R = \frac{1}{1 - e^{-\lambda_n \tau}} \qquad (3.33)$$

$$N\tau = -3.32 t_{1/2} \log(1 - f_{ss}) \qquad (3.48)$$

and

$$X_0^* = X_0 \frac{1}{1 - e^{-\lambda_n \tau}} \qquad (3.57)$$

respectively. Equation (3.48) applies only to a one-compartment model. In (3.57) X_0^* would equal the product of the loading infusion rate k_0^* and the loading infusion time T* for the loading dose, and X_0 would equal the product of the infusion rate k_0 and infusion time T for the maintenance dose. Therefore,

$$k_0^* T^* = k_0 T \frac{1}{1 - e^{-\lambda_n \tau}} \qquad (3.67)$$

Assuming that the infusion times for the loading and maintenance doses are the same (i.e., T* = T), (3.67) can be simplified to

$$k_0^* = k_0 \frac{1}{1 - e^{-\lambda_n \tau}} \qquad (3.68)$$

FIRST-ORDER ABSORPTION

The vast majority of drugs administered on a continuous basis are given orally. The equation describing the plasma concentration versus time curve following multiple dosing of a drug that is absorbed by an apparent first-order process can be arrived at directly. Multiplication of the exponential terms in (2.93), which describes the time course of drug in the plasma following first-order input, by the multiple-dosing function and setting k_i in each function equal to the rate constant in each exponential term (see Appendix B) yields

$$C_N = \frac{k_a F X_0}{V_c} \frac{\prod\limits_{i=2}^{n} (E_i - k_a)}{\prod\limits_{i=1}^{n} (\lambda_i - k_a)} \frac{1 - e^{-Nk_a \tau}}{1 - e^{-k_a \tau}} e^{-k_a t}$$

$$+ \frac{k_a F X_0}{V_c} \sum_{\ell=1}^{n} \frac{\prod\limits_{i=2}^{n} (E_i - \lambda_\ell)}{(k_a - \lambda_\ell) \prod\limits_{\substack{i=1 \\ i \neq \ell}}^{n} (\lambda_i - \lambda_\ell)} \frac{1 - e^{-N\lambda_\ell \tau}}{1 - e^{-\lambda_\ell \tau}} e^{-\lambda_\ell t}$$

$$(3.69)$$

where $0 \le t \le \tau$, k_a is an apparent first-order absorption rate constant, and F is the fraction of the orally administered drug that reaches the systemic circulation. All other parameters are as defined previously in this chapter. Equation (3.69) can be employed to predict the plasma concentration of drug at any time during any dosing interval. However, information that is often difficult to obtain, such as estimates of F/V_c and k_a, is required for such predictions. In such cases superposition (Appendix E) is an attractive alternative.

At steady state the time course of drug in the plasma during a dosing interval can be described by the equation

$$C_{ss} = \frac{k_a F X_0}{V_c} \frac{\prod\limits_{i=2}^{n} (E_i - k_a)}{\prod\limits_{i=1}^{n} (\lambda_i - k_a)} \frac{1}{1 - e^{-k_a \tau}} e^{-k_a t}$$

$$+ \frac{k_a F X_0}{V_c} \sum_{\ell=1}^{n} \frac{\prod_{i=2}^{n} (E_i - \lambda_\ell)}{(k_a - \lambda_\ell) \prod_{\substack{i=1 \\ i \neq \ell}}^{n} (\lambda_i - \lambda_\ell)} \frac{1}{1 - e^{-\lambda_\ell \tau}} e^{-\lambda_\ell t}$$

$$(3.70)$$

which is obtained by setting N equal to a sufficiently large number in (3.69) and realizing that the terms $e^{-Nk_a \tau}$ and $e^{-N\lambda_\ell \tau}$ then approach zero.

The average plasma concentration of drug at steady state, $\overline{C}$, as defined by (3.25) ($\overline{C} = \int_0^\tau C_{ss} \, dt/\tau$), can be calculated either by employing (3.25) directly, or by employing (3.27) ($\overline{C} = \int_0^\infty C \, dt/\tau$) or equations analogous to (3.29) ($\overline{C} = X_0/V_\beta \lambda_n \tau = X_0/Cl_s \tau$) or (3.30) ($\overline{C} = 1.44 X_0 t_{1/2}/V_\beta \tau$). Integration of (3.70) from time zero to τ yields

$$\int_0^\tau C_{ss} \, dt = \frac{k_a F X_0}{V_c} \frac{\prod_{i=2}^{n} (E_i - k_a)}{k_a \prod_{i=1}^{n} (\lambda_i - k_a)}$$

$$+ \frac{k_a F X_0}{V_c} \sum_{\ell=1}^{n} \frac{\prod_{i=2}^{n} (E_i - \lambda_\ell)}{\lambda_\ell (k_a - \lambda_\ell) \prod_{\substack{i=1 \\ i \neq \ell}}^{n} (\lambda_i - \lambda_\ell)} \qquad (3.71)$$

This equation can be further simplified to

$$\int_0^\tau C_{ss} \, dt = \frac{F X_0}{V_c} \left[\frac{\prod_{i=2}^{n} (E_i - k_a)}{\prod_{i=1}^{n} (\lambda_i - k_a)} + \sum_{\ell=1}^{n} \frac{k_a \prod_{i=2}^{n} (E_i - \lambda_\ell)}{\lambda_\ell (k_a - \lambda_\ell) \prod_{\substack{i=1 \\ i \neq \ell}}^{n} (\lambda_i - \lambda_\ell)} \right]$$

$$(3.72)$$

Expanding the term within the brackets for a given n, canceling common terms, and recognizing that $\prod_{i=2}^{n} E_i / \prod_{i=1}^{n} \lambda_i = 1/k_{10}$ [see (2.107) and (2.169)], where k_{10} is the first-order elimination rate constant from the central compartment, gives

$$\int_0^\tau C_{ss} \, dt = \frac{FX_0}{V_c k_{10}} \qquad (3.73)$$

Since

$$V_c k_{10} = V_\beta \lambda_n = Cl_s \qquad (2.215)$$

(3.73) can also be written as follows:

$$\int_0^\tau C_{ss} \, dt = \frac{FX_0}{V_\beta \lambda_n} = \frac{FX_0}{Cl_s} \qquad (3.74)$$

It can also be demonstrated that

$$\int_0^\tau C_{ss} \, dt = \int_0^\infty C \, dt \qquad (3.75)$$

where $\int_0^\infty C \, dt$ is the area under the plasma concentration-time curve from time zero to infinity following first-order input of a single dose.

Substituting $FX_0/V_\beta \lambda_n$ and/or FX_0/Cl_s for $\int_0^\tau C_{ss} \, dt$ in (3.25) and recognizing that $\lambda_n = 0.693/t_{1/2}$ [Eq. (2.11)] yields

$$\overline{C} = \frac{FX_0}{V_\beta \lambda_n \tau} = \frac{FX_0}{Cl_s \tau} = \frac{1.44 FX_0 t_{1/2}}{V_\beta \tau} \qquad (3.76)$$

As is evident from (3.76), $\overline{C}$ is dependent on the size of dose administered, the extent to which it is absorbed, and the dosing interval. However, $\overline{C}$ is independent of the rate of absorption and all other disposition rate constants, as evidenced by the absence of k_a and λ terms from (3.76). The same average plasma concentration of drug will be obtained whether the dose X_0 is administered as a single dose every τ time units, or is subdivided and administered at different times within τ time units; that is, 600 mg once a day is equivalent to 300 mg every 12 h, is equivalent to 150 mg every 6 h, and so on (see Figs. 3.4 and 3.5). However, upon subdividing the dose, the difference between the minimum and maximum plasma concentration will usually decrease.

Although Eq. (3.76) permits the estimation of average drug concentration at steady state based on the pharmacokinetic parameters of the drug, it is rarely used as such; a much simpler approach is available. Since $\overline{C} = \int_0^\tau C_{ss} \, dt/\tau$ and $\int_0^\tau C_{ss} \, dt = \int_0^\infty C \, dt$, $\overline{C}$ may be estimated directly from the ratio of total area under the drug concentration in plasma versus time curve after a single oral dose, to the dosing interval τ (see Fig. 3.6). This approach assumes that systemic availability and clearance are constants from dose to dose.

Accumulation can be determined by comparing the minimum plasma concentrations of drug at steady state and following the first dose,

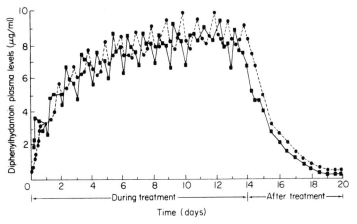

Fig. 3.4 Mean concentrations of phenytoin (diphenylhydantoin) in normal adult volunteers who received either 300 mg once a day (single-dose group: ■——■) or 100 mg three times a day (divided-dose group: ●---●). The average drug concentration at steady state is a function of the total daily dose (see Ref. 3).

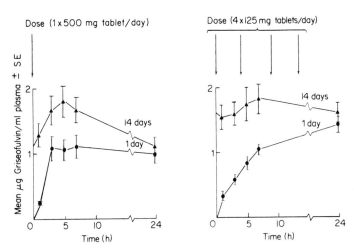

Fig. 3.5 Average concentrations of griseofulvin during the first and fourteenth day of drug administration in human volunteers who received 500 mg once a day or 125 mg four times a day. Theory predicts that the average drug concentration at steady state will be the same for both regimens but that the steady-state peak-to-trough ratio will be larger for the once-a-day regimen. (From Ref. 4.)

$R = (C_{ss})_{min}/(C_1)_{min}$ [Eq. (3.31)]. However, this method is relatively simple only when one is dealing with a situation in which each dose is administered in the postabsorptive-postdistributive phase of the preceding dose. This situation probably exists for a large number of drugs, although it may not be valid for sustained-release products and for drugs that are absorbed very slowly.

By setting N equal to 1 and t equal to τ in (3.69), an expression for the minimum plasma concentration following the first dose $(C_1)_{min}$ can be obtained:

$$
(C_1)_{min} = \frac{k_a FX_0}{V_c} \frac{\displaystyle\prod_{i=2}^{n}(E_i - k_a)}{\displaystyle\prod_{i=1}^{n}(\lambda_i - k_a)} e^{-k_a \tau}
$$

$$
+ \frac{k_a FX_0}{V_c} \sum_{\ell=1}^{n} \frac{\displaystyle\prod_{i=2}^{n}(E_i - \lambda_\ell)}{(k_a - \lambda_\ell) \displaystyle\prod_{\substack{i=1 \\ i \neq \ell}}^{n}(\lambda_i - \lambda_\ell)} e^{-\lambda_\ell \tau} \qquad (3.77)
$$

Similarly, by setting t equal to τ in (3.70), the following expression for the minimum plasma concentration at steady state $(C_{ss})_{min}$ results:

$$
(C_{ss})_{min} = \frac{k_a FX_0}{V_c} \frac{\displaystyle\prod_{i=2}^{n}(E_i - k_a)}{\displaystyle\prod_{i=1}^{n}(\lambda_i - k_a)} \frac{1}{1 - e^{-k_a \tau}} e^{-k_a \tau}
$$

$$
+ \frac{k_a FX_0}{V_c} \sum_{\ell=1}^{n} \frac{\displaystyle\prod_{i=2}^{n}(E_i - \lambda_\ell)}{(k_a - \lambda_\ell) \displaystyle\prod_{\substack{i=1 \\ i \neq \ell}}^{n}(\lambda_i - \lambda_\ell)} \frac{1}{1 - e^{-\lambda_\ell \tau}} e^{-\lambda_\ell \tau}
$$

$$(3.78)$$

Assuming that each dose is administered in the postabsorptive-postdistributive phase [i.e., as $e^{-k_a \tau}$ and $e^{-\lambda_1 \tau}$ to $e^{-\lambda_{n-1} \tau}$ approach zero], (3.77) and (3.78) become

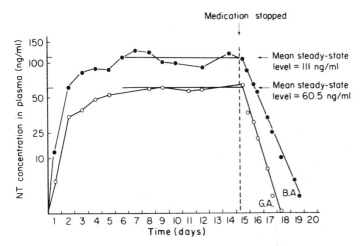

Fig. 3.6 Time course of plasma nortriptyline concentrations in two normal subjects, G. A. (O) and B. A. (●), who received 0.4 mg/kg three times a day for 2 weeks. The average drug concentrations predicted from the total area under the curve after a single dose were 53 and 116 ng/ml for G. A. and B. A., respectively. (From Ref. 5.)

$$(C_1)_{min} = \frac{k_a F X_0}{V_c} \frac{\prod\limits_{i=2}^{n} (E_i - \lambda_n)}{(k_a - \lambda_n) \prod\limits_{\substack{i=1 \\ i \neq \ell}}^{n} (\lambda_i - \lambda_n)} e^{-\lambda_n \tau} \qquad (3.79)$$

and

$$(C_{ss})_{min} = \frac{k_a F X_0}{V_c} \frac{\prod\limits_{i=2}^{n} (E_i - \lambda_n)}{(k_a - \lambda_n) \prod\limits_{\substack{i=1 \\ i \neq \ell}}^{n} (\lambda_i - \lambda_n)} \frac{1}{1 - e^{-\lambda_n \tau}} e^{-\lambda_n \tau} \qquad (3.80)$$

respectively. Therefore, the accumulation factor R, which is defined as $(C_{ss})_{min}/(C_1)_{min}$, equals $1/(1 - e^{-\lambda_n \tau})$ [Eq. (3.33)]. This expression can readily be employed to determine the extent of accumulation following first-order input every τ time units, since only an estimate of the terminal disposition rate constant is required. However, if each dose is not administered in the postabsorptive-postdistributive phase, a rather complex function would result for the accumulation factor. R would then be equal to the ratio of Eq. (3.78) to Eq. (3.77).

The time required to reach a certain fraction of the ultimate steady state following first-order input can also be estimated where the fraction of the steady-state concentration f_{ss} is as defined by (3.42), that is, $f_{ss} = \overline{C}_N/\overline{C}$, where $\overline{C}_N = \int_0^\tau C_N \, dt/\tau$ [Eq. (3.34)] and $\overline{C} = FX_0/Cl_s\tau = FX_0/V_\beta\lambda_n\tau$ [Eq. (3.76)]. Integration of (3.69) is relatively complex. However, the concentration-time profile following the oral administration of many if not most drugs can be adequately characterized by a one-compartment model with first-order input. Under these conditions, appropriate redefinition of the terms and integration of Eq. (3.69) from 0 to τ yields

$$\int_0^\tau C_N \, dt = \frac{k_a FX_0}{V(k_a - K)} \left(\frac{1 - e^{-Nk_a\tau}}{1 - e^{-k_a\tau}} \frac{e^{-k_a\tau}}{k_a} - \frac{1 - e^{-NK\tau}}{1 - e^{-K\tau}} \frac{e^{-K\tau}}{K} \right.$$

$$\left. + \frac{1 - e^{-NK\tau}}{1 - e^{-K\tau}} \frac{1}{K} - \frac{1 - e^{-Nk_a\tau}}{1 - e^{-k_a\tau}} \frac{1}{k_a} \right) \qquad (3.81)$$

which on rearrangement and simplification becomes

$$\int_0^\tau C_N \, dt = \frac{FX_0}{VK} \left(1 + \frac{Ke^{-Nk_a\tau}}{k_a - K} - \frac{k_a e^{-NK\tau}}{k_a - K} \right) \qquad (3.82)$$

Substitution of the value of $\int_0^\tau C_N \, dt$, as given in (3.82), into (3.34) yields the following expression for the average plasma concentration of drug during the Nth dosing interval:

$$\overline{C}_N = \frac{FX_0}{VK\tau} \left(1 + \frac{Ke^{-Nk_a\tau}}{k_a - K} - \frac{k_a e^{-NK\tau}}{k_a - K} \right) \qquad (3.83)$$

By substituting $\overline{C}$ for $FX_0/VK\tau$ according to (3.76) in (3.83) and dividing both sides of the equation by $\overline{C}$, one obtains

$$f_{ss} = \frac{\overline{C}_N}{\overline{C}} = 1 + \frac{Ke^{-Nk_a\tau}}{k_a - K} - \frac{k_a e^{-NK\tau}}{k_a - K} \qquad (3.84)$$

From (3.84) it is readily apparent that the time required to reach a certain fraction of the steady-state level is a complex function of the absorption and elimination rate constants. The larger the value of k_a relative to K, the less dependent on k_a is the time required to reach a given fraction of steady state [6]. At very large values of k_a relative to K (i.e., $k_a/K \geq 10$), Eq. (3.84) approaches

$$f_{ss} = 1 - e^{-NK\tau} \tag{3.44}$$

Therefore,

$$N\tau = -3.32 t_{1/2} \log (1 - f_{ss}) \tag{3.48}$$

Hence, when the absorption rate constant is significantly larger than the terminal disposition rate constant, the time required, $N\tau$, to reach a certain fraction of the steady-state level is a function only of the half-life of the drug. If this is not the case, then f_{ss} is also dependent on k_a. The smaller the value of k_a, the longer the time required to attain steady state or some fraction thereof.

Estimation of the time to steady state for a drug that shows multicompartment characteristics on oral administration is a task particularly well handled by the method of Chiou [1] [see Eq. (3.52)].

As discussed in the section on multiple dosing by intravenous administration, an initial loading dose may be desirable, since for drugs with long half-lives, a long period of time is required to reach steady state. The loading dose X_0^* required to achieve steady-state levels on the first dose may be determined by letting X_0 equal X_0^* in Eq. (3.77) [the equation for $(C_1)_{min}$] and setting this equal to the equation for $(C_{ss})min$ [Eq. (3.78)]:

$$\frac{k_a FX_0^*}{V_c} \frac{\prod_{i=2}^{n} (E_i - k_a)}{\prod_{i=1}^{n} (\lambda_i - k_a)} e^{-k_a \tau} + \frac{k_a FX_0^*}{V_c} \sum_{\ell=1}^{n} \frac{\prod_{i=2}^{n} (E_i - \lambda_\ell)}{(k_a - \lambda_\ell) \prod_{\substack{i=1 \\ i \neq \ell}}^{n} (\lambda_i - \lambda_\ell)} e^{-\lambda_\ell \tau}$$

$$= \frac{k_a FX_0}{V_c} \frac{\prod_{i=2}^{n} (E_i - k_a)}{\prod_{i=1}^{n} (\lambda_i - k_a)} \frac{1}{1 - e^{-k_a \tau}} e^{-k_a \tau}$$

$$+ \frac{k_a FX_0}{V_c} \sum_{\ell=1}^{n} \frac{\prod_{i=2}^{n} (E_i - \lambda_\ell)}{(k_a - \lambda_\ell) \prod_{\substack{i=1 \\ i \neq \ell}}^{n} (\lambda_i - \lambda_\ell)} \frac{1}{1 - e^{-\lambda_\ell \tau}} e^{-\lambda_\ell \tau} \tag{3.85}$$

Solving for X_0^* results in a relatively complex equation. However, by administration of the maintenance dose in the postabsorptive-post-distributive phase of the loading dose plasma concentration-time curve (i.e., $e^{-k_a \tau}$ and $e^{-\lambda_1 \tau}$ to $e^{-\lambda_{n-1} \tau}$ approach zero), the following equation is obtained for X_0^*:

$$X_0^* = X_0 \frac{1}{1 - e^{-\lambda_n \tau}} \qquad (3.57)$$

from which it is relatively simple to estimate a loading dose. This equation was employed to calculate a loading dose for drugs administered by the intravenous route. Irrespective of the size of the initial dose the steady-state plasma concentration of drug ultimately reached will be the same since the steady-state level is governed by the size of the maintenance dose (Fig. 3.7).

The drug concentration in plasma versus time curve after oral administration of many drugs can be adequately described by a one-compartment model. Setting n equal to 1 in (3.85) and canceling the common term $k_a F / V_c$ yields

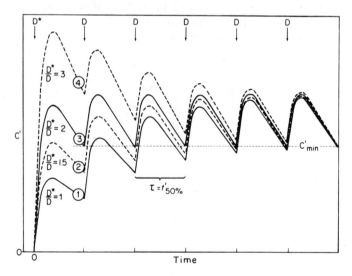

Fig. 3.7 Influence of the first dose of a multiple dose regimen on the time course of drug concentrations, C', in plasma. D* denotes the first dose (loading dose) and D denotes all subseqeunt doses (maintenance dose). The dosing interval was selected to equal the half-life of the drug (i.e., $\tau = t_{50\%}$). The ratio of D* to D varies from 1 to 3. (From Ref. 7.)

$$X_0^* \frac{e^{-k_a \tau}}{K - k_a} - X_0^* \frac{e^{-K\tau}}{K - k_a} = X^0 \frac{e^{-k_a \tau}}{(K - k_a)(1 - e^{-k_a \tau})}$$

$$- X^0 \frac{e^{-K\tau}}{(K - k_a)(1 - e^{-K\tau})} \tag{3.86}$$

By canceling the common term, $K - k_a$, bringing the right side of the equation to a common denominator, and solving for X_0^* gives

$$X_0^* = X^0 \frac{e^{-k_a \tau} - e^{-(k_a + K)\tau} - e^{-K\tau} + e^{-(k_a + K)\tau}}{(1 - e^{-k_a \tau})(1 - e^{-K\tau})(e^{-k_a \tau} - e^{-K\tau})} \tag{3.87}$$

Further simplification results in the following expression for X_0^*:

$$X_0^* = X^0 \frac{1}{(1 - e^{-k_a \tau})(1 - e^{-K\tau})} \tag{3.88}$$

If the maintenance dose is administered in the postabsorptive phase, (3.88) can be further simplified to yield (3.57) since the term $e^{-k_a \tau}$ approaches zero.

Assuming that the fraction F of each dose absorbed is constant during a multiple-dosing regimen, the time at which a maximum plasma concentration of drug at steady state occurs (t_{max}') may be arrived at by differentiating (3.70) with respect to time and setting the resultant equal to zero. Doing this and canceling the common term $k_a F X_0 / V_c$ yields

$$\frac{\prod\limits_{i=2}^{n} (E_i - k_a)}{\prod\limits_{i=1}^{n} (\lambda_i - k_a)} \frac{k_a}{1 - e^{-k_a \tau}} e^{-k_a t_{max}'}$$

$$= \sum\limits_{\ell=1}^{n} \frac{\prod\limits_{i=2}^{n} (E_i - \lambda_\ell)}{(\lambda_\ell - k_a) \prod\limits_{\substack{i=1 \\ i \neq \ell}}^{n} (\lambda_i - \lambda_\ell)} \frac{\lambda_\ell}{1 - e^{-\lambda_\ell \tau}} e^{-\lambda_\ell t_{max}'} \tag{3.89}$$

As is evident from examining (3.89) t_{max}' cannot be readily solved for. As discussed previously, plasma concentration versus time curves following oral drug administration can frequently be described by a one-compartment model. Under these conditions we may write that

$$\frac{1}{K - k_a} \frac{k_a}{1 - e^{-k_a \tau}} e^{-k_a t'_{max}} = \frac{1}{K - k_a} \frac{K}{1 - e^{-K\tau}} e^{-K t'_{max}} \qquad (3.90)$$

Canceling common terms and rearranging (3.90) gives

$$e^{(k_a - K)t'_{max}} = \frac{k_a (1 - e^{-K\tau})}{K(1 - e^{-k_a \tau})} \qquad (3.91)$$

By taking the common logarithm of both sides of (3.91) and dividing by $k_a - K$, the following expression is obtained for the time at which the maximum plasma concentration at steady state occurs:

$$t'_{max} = \frac{2.303}{k_a - K} \log \frac{k_a (1 - e^{-K\tau})}{K(1 - e^{-k_a \tau})} \qquad (3.92)$$

The time t_{max} at which a maximum plasma concentration occurs following a single dose is given by

$$t_{max} = \frac{2.303}{k_a - K} \log \frac{k_a}{K} \qquad (1.106)$$

Subtraction of (3.92) from (1.106) yields

$$t_{max} - t'_{max} = \frac{2.303}{k_a - K} \log \frac{1 - e^{-k_a \tau}}{1 - e^{-K\tau}} \qquad (3.93)$$

Since the right side of this equation is always positive, it is apparent that the maximum plasma concentration occurs at an earlier time at steady state than following a single dose. Frequently, the time at which the maximum plasma concentration is observed after the first dose, t_{max}, is the time at which the plasma is sampled after administration of subsequent doses to assess C_{max}. Based on mathematical principles this would not be a sound practice, since the time at which a maximum plasma concentration occurs is not constant until steady state is achieved.

DETERMINATION OF PHARMACOKINETIC PARAMETERS
FROM MULTIPLE-DOSING DATA

Estimates of all pharmacokinetic parameters can be made from steady-state intravenous plasma concentration-time data if τ is sufficiently large to permit an accurate determination of the intercept and disposition rate constant associated with the terminal phase of the concentration-time curve. Even if the dosing interval is too small to permit this, one can still estimate clearance Cl_S since only the area under the plasma concentration versus time curve at steady state, $\int_0^\tau C_{ss}$ dt or AUC, is required. Once AUC is known, Cl_S can be determined using (2.43) ($Cl_S = X_0/AUC$). Assuming that λ_n can be accurately determined, $t_{1/2}$ and V_β can be obtained employing (2.11) ($t_{1/2} = 0.693/\lambda_n$) and (2.216) ($V_\beta = Cl_S/\lambda_n$), respectively. Steady-state plasma concentrations can be described by

$$C_{ss} = \sum_{\ell=1}^{n} U_\ell e^{-\lambda_\ell t} \qquad (3.22)$$

The method of residuals (Appendix C) can be applied to the data, generating the coefficients and disposition rate constants, U_ℓ and λ_ℓ, respectively. Once these parameters are obtained, values of A_ℓ, the coefficients generated from intravenous single-dose data, can be calculated from

$$A_\ell = U_\ell (1 - e^{-\lambda_\ell \tau}) \qquad (3.94)$$

which is a rearrangement of (3.23). This then permits the volume of the central compartment V_c, and the steady-state volume of distribution V_{ss}, to be determined using (2.15) ($V_c = X_0/\sum_{\ell=1}^{n} A_\ell$), and (2.234) [$V_{ss} = X_0 \sum_{\ell=1}^{n} (A_\ell/\lambda_\ell^2)/\sum_{\ell=1}^{n} (A_\ell/\lambda_\ell)^2$]. The constants k_{10} [Eqs. (2.107) and (2.169)], k_{12} [Eqs. (2.108) and (2.172)], k_{21} [Eqs. (2.106) and (2.168)], k_{31} [Eq. (2.167)], and k_{13} [Eq. (2.173)] can also be determined from multiple-dose data once the values for A_ℓ and λ_ℓ are known.

REFERENCES

1. W. L. Chiou. Compartment-and model-independent linear plateau principle of drugs during a constant-rate absorption or intravenous infusion. J. Pharmacokinet. Biopharm. 8:311 (1980).
2. F. I. Marcus. Digitalis pharmacokinetics and metabolism. Am. J. Med. 58:452 (1975).

3. R. A. Buchanan, A. W. Kinkel, J. R. Goulet, and T. C. Smith. The metabolism of diphenylhydantoin (dilantin) following once-daily administration. *Neurology (N.Y.)* *22*:1809 (1972).

4. D. S. Platt. Plasma concentrations of griseofulvin in human volunteers. *Br. J. Dermatol.* *83*:382 (1970).

5. B. Alexanderson. Pharmacokinetics of nortriptyline in man after single and multiple oral doses: The predictability of steady-state plasma concentrations from single dose plasma-level data. *Eur. J. Clin. Pharamcol.* *4*:82 (1972).

6. J. M. Van Rossum and A. H. M. Tomey. Rate of accumulation and plateau plasma concentration of drugs after chronic medication. *J. Pharm. Pharmacol.* *20*:390 (1968).

7. E. Krüger-Thiemer and P. Bunger. The role of the therapeutic regimen in dosage design I. *Chemotherapy* *10*:61 (1965—66).

4

Absorption Kinetics and Bioavailability

Many pharmacokinetic studies are concerned principally with the *bio-availability* of the drug. Bioavailability, in simple terms, refers to the rate and extent of drug absorption. The rate at which a drug reaches the systemic circulation is an important consideration for drugs used to treat acute conditions, such as pain or insomnia, which can be ameliorated by a single dose. A drug that is absorbed slowly may not achieve sufficiently high concentrations at the site of action to elicit a desired effect or intensity of effect, even if the entire dose is absorbed. On the other hand, the extent of absorption is usually the more important factor for drugs that are administered repetitively for the treatment of subchronic or chronic conditions, such as infection, asthma, or epilepsy. The average drug concentration in plasma at steady state during repetitive administration is directly proportional to the amount absorbed from each dose but is independent of the rate of absorption. The rate of absorption does, however, influence the time course of drug concentration in plasma during a dosing interval at steady state. In some cases, very rapid absorption could produce transiently high drug concentrations in plasma that may be associated with adverse effects.

Comparative bioavailability refers to the relative bioavailability of a drug from two or more formulations. Comparative bioavailability studies are often carried out in place of clinical effect studies to determine whether two or more formulations containing the same active ingredients in the same amounts are therapeutically equivalent. It is assumed that two formulations that do not differ very much in the rate at which and extent to which they make the active ingredient available to the systemic circulation will not differ much in their therapeutic efficacy.

Pharmacokinetic theory is well developed and generally accepted for the determination of the extent or relative extent of absorption of a drug from a dosage form. Similar agreement does not exist with respect to characterizing the absorption rate of a drug. The results

of such analyses are usually dependent on the pharmacokinetic model
that is assumed and are usually descriptive rather than rigorous.
Characterization of absorption kinetics may be useful for determining
relative differences in absorption rates between formulations in comparative bioavailability studies.

ABSORPTION RATE

Curve-Fitting

The most common method of evaluating absorption kinetics is to assume that the drug concentration-time data can be described by one
of several pharmacokinetic compartment models and to fit the data to
an equation consistent with the assumed model by means of the method
of residuals (see Appendix C) or a nonlinear least-squares regression
program and a digital computer (see Appendix H). The most common
equations for a one-compartment model are

$$C = \frac{k_a F X_0}{V(k_a - K)} (e^{-Kt} - e^{-k_a t}) \tag{4.1}$$

which assumes first-order absorption and elimination,

$$C = \frac{k_a F X_0}{V(k_a - K)} [e^{-K(t-t_0)} - e^{-k_a(t-t_0)}] \tag{4.2}$$

which assumes a lag time t_0 before the onset of absorption,

$$C = \frac{k_0(e^{KT} - 1)e^{-Kt}}{VK} \tag{4.3}$$

which assumes zero-order absorption, where $T = t$ during the absorption period and T = absorption time (a constant) during the postabsorption period, and

$$\frac{dX_u}{dt} = \frac{k_e k_a F X_0}{k_a - K} (e^{-Kt} - e^{-k_a t}) \tag{4.4}$$

which uses urinary excretion data. The output of the computer
program contains estimates of the pharmacokinetic constants, including the absorption rate constant.

Ideally, one should have an independent estimate of K to differentiate the estimated rate constants and to avoid ambiguity in interpreting the results of such curve-fitting procedures. Serious problems
are encountered if the absorption is complex rather than a simple first-
or zero-order process. Sometimes most of the dose of a drug may be

relatively rapidly absorbed, but a small fraction of the dose is absorbed very slowly and absorption persists long after the time at which drug concentration in plasma reaches a maximum. In such cases the concentration-time curve may be apparently biexponential but the rate constant determined from the apparent postabsorption phase will be smaller than K. In this situation an independent estimate of K is needed. An example is shown in Fig. 4.1. Accurate estimates of k_a from urinary excretion data [see Eq. (4.4)] are possible only for drugs absorbed relatively slowly because urine collections cannot be made at very short intervals.

The absorption rate constants obtained by curve-fitting Eqs. (4.1) to (4.4) are at best estimates of the first-order loss of drug from the gastrointestinal tract, not of the first-order appearance of drug in the systemic circulation. If a drug undergoes simultaneous first-order absorption (rate constant k_{abs}) and first-order chemical or enzymatic degradation, k_d, in the gut, the apparent absorption

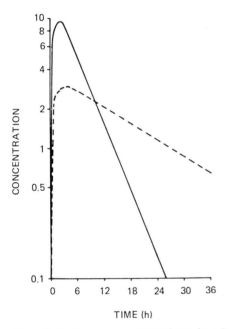

Fig. 4.1 Drug concentrations in plasma after oral administration of the same dose of drug as a conventional tablet (——) from which absorption is rapid and as a slowly dissolving tablet (---) from which absorption is slow. The half-life of the drug is 3.5 h, which is consistent with the value determined after giving the conventional tablet. The slow absorption found with the specialized dosage form results in an *apparent* half-life of 14 h.

rate constant, k_a, obtained on curve-fitting is actually the sum of k_{abs} and k_d [1]. Other factors that affect absorption, such as gastric emptying or gastrointestinal motility, can also distort the meaning of k_a [2,3]. In general, for any drug that is less than completely absorbed, it is unlikely that $k_a = k_{abs}$ [3].

Other problems in the estimation of k_a are encountered when curve-fitting concentration-time data to equations appropriate to a two-compartment model such as

$$C = Le^{-\lambda_1 t} + Me^{-\lambda_2 t} + Ne^{-k_a t}$$ (4.5)

[see Eq. (2.93)]. By definition $\lambda_1 > \lambda_2$ and it is likely for drugs that are rapidly absorbed that $k_a > \lambda_2$, but in all cases k_a may be smaller or larger than λ_1. There is no basis for assuming one or the other. Therefore, it is not possible to determine unambiguously k_a from drug concentration-time data obtained after oral administration. The dilemma may be resolved by independently estimating λ_1 and λ_2 after intravenous administration of the drug to the same subject. Some resolution may also be obtained by characterizing the pharmacokinetics of the drug after administration of a dosage form such as an oral solution, from which the drug is more rapidly absorbed. Most drug concentration in plasma-time data sets obtained after oral administration can be fitted with two exponential terms (i.e., a one-compartment model) rather than three exponential terms (i.e., a two-compartment model). However, intravenous administration of the same drug often suggests that the two-compartment model is more appropriate. Some reasons for this have been discussed in Chap. 2. Under these conditions, attempts to estimate the absorption rate constant from data obtained after oral administration can result in substantial error. It has been shown that if such data are fitted to Eq. (4.1), the larger of the two rate constants would not be equal to the absorption rate constant but, under certain conditions, may be equal to λ_1 [4]. Since for virtually all drugs the time course of concentration in plasma after intravenous administration shows multicompartment characteristics, and for most drugs a two- or three-compartment model is most appropriate, it follows that the estimate of an absorption rate constant from data obtained after oral administration of any drug, by assuming a one-compartment model, will be incorrect even if the drug were truly absorbed by apparent first-order kinetics.

Wagner [5] has proposed that although the absorption rate constant determined from a one-compartment fit of concentration-time data after oral administration of a drug that shows two-compartment characteristics after intravenous administration is incorrect, the ratio of the absorption rate constants calculated for two dosage forms using one-compartment analyses would be a good approximation of the actual ratio of the absorption rate constants. Ronfeld and Benet [4] examined the same question and concluded that the approximation error could be substantially larger than suggested by Wagner [5], but that a qualitative evaluation of the relative merits of different dosage forms could be accurately made with one-compartment fits.

Percent Absorbed-Time Plots

The problems associated with the characterization of absorption kinetics by curve-fitting have prompted many investigators to seek better methods of analysis. One of the most important of these alternative methods is based on the construction and evaluation of percent absorbed-time plots [6, 7], which do not require the assumption of zero- or first-order absorption.

One-Compartment Model (Wagner-Nelson Method). The amount of drug that has been absorbed into the systemic circulation, X_A, at any time after administration will equal the sum of the amount of drug in the body, X, and the cumulative amount of drug eliminated, X_E, by urinary excretion, by metabolism, and by all other routes at that time. Thus

$$X_A = X + X_E \qquad (4.6)$$

which when differentiated with respect to time becomes

$$\frac{dX_A}{dt} = \frac{dX}{dt} + \frac{dX_E}{dt} \qquad (4.7)$$

The term dX_E/dt (elimination rate of drug) is by definition equal to the product of the amount of drug in the body X and the apparent first-order elimination rate constant of drug from the body;

$$\frac{dX_E}{dt} = KX \qquad (4.8)$$

Substitution of KX for dX_E/dt in Eq. (4.7) yields

$$\frac{dX_A}{dt} = \frac{dX}{dt} + KX \qquad (4.9)$$

Since X equals VC, where V and C are the apparent volume of distribution and plasma concentration of drug, respectively, Eq. (4.9) may be written as

$$\frac{dX_A}{dt} = V\frac{dC}{dt} + KVC \qquad (4.10)$$

Integration of Eq. (4.10) from time zero to T yields the following expression for the amount of drug absorbed to time T, $(X_A)_T$:

$$(X_A)_T = VC_T + KV \int_0^T C \, dt \qquad (4.11)$$

where C_T is the plasma concentration of drug at time T and $\int_0^T C \, dt$ is the area under the plasma concentration versus time curve from time zero to T. An equation for the amount of drug ultimately absorbed, $(X_A)_\infty$, can be obtained by integrating (4.10) from time zero to infinity and recognizing that C equals zero at both times zero and infinity. Thus

$$(X_A)_\infty = KV \int_0^\infty C \, dt \qquad (4.12)$$

where $\int_0^\infty C \, dt$ is the total area under the plasma concentration versus time curve. Dividing (4.11) by (4.12) and canceling common terms yields the expression for the fraction absorbed to time T:

$$\frac{(X_A)_T}{(X_A)_\infty} = \frac{C_T + K \int_0^T C \, dt}{K \int_0^\infty C \, dt} \qquad (4.13)$$

Equation (4.13) relates the cumulative amount of drug absorbed after a certain time to the amount of drug ultimately absorbed, rather than to the dose administered. By collecting blood after a single oral dose and determining drug concentrations in plasma and the elimination rate constant, one can calculate the fraction absorbed for various times after administration. The calculations required to construct a percent absorbed-time plot are outlined in Table 4.1 and are based on the concentration-time data in columns 1 and 2. A plot of $C_T + K \int_0^T C \, dt$ versus time, as shown in Fig. 4.2, indicates that the curve is asymptotic and approaches the value of $K \int_0^\infty C \, dt$. After about 18 h $C_T + K \int_0^T C \, dt$ is independent of time and closely approximates $K \int_0^\infty C \, dt$, indicative of the fact that absorption is negligible and $(X_A)_T \backsim (X_A)_\infty$. The percent absorbed-time plot is shown in Fig. 4.3. The data suggest that absorption is relatively slow since at 2 h only about half of the absorption has taken place.

It is important to remember that percent absorbed-time plots tell us nothing about the extent of absorption. In principle one can obtain similar plots for two formulations of a drug that differ substantially in terms of how much of the drug is eventually absorbed. This difference will be reflected in the $C_T + K \int_0^T C \, dt$ versus time plots.

An important characteristic of the Wagner-Nelson method for evaluating absorption data is that no model is assumed for the absorption process. One often finds, however, that a plot of percent unabsorbed (i.e., $100\{1 - [(X_A)_T/(X_A)_\infty]\}$) versus time on semi-

Table 4.1 Calculation of Absorption Data Using the Wagner-Nelson Method

Time (h)	Drug Concentration (μg/ml)	$\int_0^T C\,dt$	$K\int_0^T C\,dt$	$C_T + K\int_0^T C\,dt$	Fraction Absorbed
0	0	0	0	0	0
1	1.88	0.94	0.08	1.96	0.29
2	3.05	3.41	0.29	3.34	0.49
3	3.74	6.80	0.59	4.33	0.64
5	4.21	14.75	1.27	5.48	0.81
7	4.08	23.04	1.98	6.06	0.90
9	3.70	30.82	2.65	6.35	
12	3.02	40.90	3.52	6.54	
18	1.86	55.54	4.78	6.64	
24	1.12	64.48	5.55	6.67	
36	0.40	73.60	6.33	6.73	
48	0.14	76.84	6.61	6.75	
60	0.05	77.98	6.71	6.76	
72	0.02	78.38	6.74	6.76	
	0	78.60	6.76	6.76	

Notes: The example concerns a drug absorbed and eliminated by first-order processes; a one-compartment model is assumed. The drug is eliminated with a half-life of 8 h ($K = 0.086\ h^{-1}$).

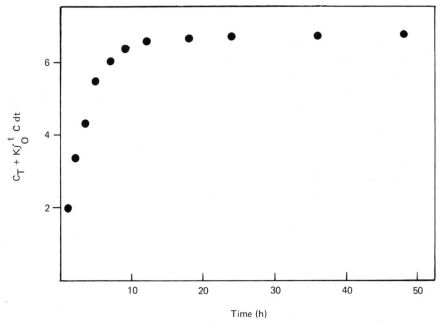

Fig. 4.2 Plot of the numerator of Eq. (4.13) (i.e., $C_T + K \int_0^t C \, dt$) versus time, based on the data in Table 4.1. Drug absorption is essentially complete after about 18 h. Thereafter, the value of $C_T + K \int_0^t C \, dt$ is a constant equal to $K \int_0^\infty C \, dt$ [i.e., the denominator of Eq. (4.13)].

logarithmic coordinates approximates a straight line. This suggests apparent first-order absorption and the apparent absorption rate constant may be estimated from the slope, which is equal to $-k_a/2.303$. A linear relationship between percent unabsorbed and time on rectilinear coordinates suggests apparent zero-order absorption. If sufficient data are available, one may be able to characterize more complex absorption kinetics (see Fig. 4.4).

Urinary excretion data can also be employed to construct percent absorbed-time plots. The excretion rate of intact drug in the urine, dX_u/dt, is given by

$$\frac{dX_u}{dt} = k_e X \qquad (4.14)$$

where k_e is the apparent first-order excretion rate constant and X is the amount of drug in the body. Since X equals VC, it follows that

$$\frac{dX_u}{dt} = k_e VC \qquad (4.15)$$

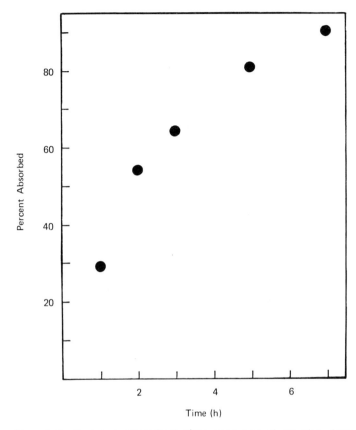

Fig. 4.3 Percent absorbed-time plot based on the data in Table 4.1. A plot of percent unabsorbed versus time on semilogarithmic coordinates would reveal apparent first-order absorption.

Rearranging terms yields

$$C = \frac{dX_u/dt}{k_e V} \tag{4.16}$$

Substituting this value of C in (4.10) and canceling common terms gives

$$\frac{dX_A}{dt} = \frac{1}{k_e} \frac{d(dX_u/dt)}{dt} + \frac{K}{k_e} \frac{dX_u}{dt} \tag{4.17}$$

which when integrated from time zero to T becomes

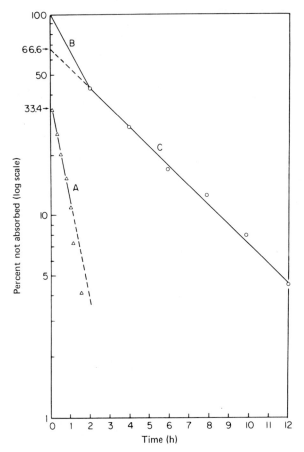

Fig. 4.4 Plot of percent sulfaethidole remaining to be absorbed (log scale) versus time after oral administration of a sustained-release suspension of the drug (see Ref. 6). The data show two components in the absorption phase and suggest that, under these conditions, drug absorption can be described by two parallel first-order processes.

$$(X_A)_T = \frac{1}{k_e}\left(\frac{dX_u}{dt}\right)_T + \frac{K}{k_e}(X_u)_T \qquad (4.18)$$

where $(dX_u/dt)_T$ is the excretion rate of intact drug in the urine at time T and $(X_u)_T$ is the cumulative amount of intact drug eliminated in the urine to time T. An equation for the total amount of drug ultimately absorbed, $(X_A)_\infty$, can be obtained by setting T equal to infinity in Eq. (4.18) and recognizing that dX_u/dt equals zero at time infinity. Thus,

$$(X_A)_\infty = \frac{K}{k_e} X_u^\infty \qquad (4.19)$$

where X_u^∞ is the total amount of unchanged drug eliminated in the urine. The fraction absorbed at any time T, $(X_A)_T/(X_A)_\infty$, is determined by dividing (4.18) by (4.19) and canceling common terms:

$$\frac{(X_A)_T}{(X_A)_\infty} = \frac{(dX_u/dt)_T + K(X_u)_T}{KX_u^\infty} \qquad (4.20)$$

Equation (4.20) indicates that, in principle, percent absorbed-time plots can be constructed based solely on urinary excretion data. Urine must be collected long enough to estimate K accurately but need not be collected to time infinity. A plot of $(dX_u/dt)_T + K(X_u)_T$ versus time is asymptotic, approximating KX_u^∞ when absorption is negligible.

In theory, percent absorbed-time plots may also be constructed from metabolite concentration in plasma versus time data or from urinary excretion rates of metabolite [8, 9], but the required assumptions make these methods of limited value.

The most serious limitation of the Wagner-Nelson method is that it applies rigorously only to drugs with one-compartment characteristics. In all other cases it is an approximation. It has been shown that the application of the Wagner-Nelson method to assess the absorption of drugs with multicompartment characteristics results in an underestimation of the time at which absorption ceases and an overestimation of the absorption rate [7]. The extent of error for a drug with two-compartment characteristics depends on the ratio of k_{10} or k_{el} to λ_2 [10]. If λ_2/k_{10} is ≥ 0.8, then in all likelihood the Wagner-Nelson method provides a reasonable approximation of the time course of absorption. Clearly, the Wagner-Nelson method should not be applied if drug concentration-time data after oral administration indicate multicompartment characteristics (see Fig. 2.15). A dilemma is encountered, however, when the concentration-time curve after oral administration of a drug that shows multicompartment characteristics on intravenous injection suggests a one-compartment model. Analysis of these data by the Wagner-Nelson method may produce incorrect results. One way of resolving this dilemma is to construct the percent absorbed-time plot using the Loo-Riegelman method, described in the next section. Unfortunately, this method requires concentration-time data obtained after both intravenous and oral administration and can be used in few instances. For this reason, the Wagner-Nelson method is likely to be applied in bioavailability studies for some time to come, despite the uncertainties.

Multicompartment Models (Loo-Riegelman Method). The Loo-Riegelman method requires drug concentration-time data after both oral and in-

travenous administration of the drug to the same subject. It can be
applied generally to linear multicompartment pharmacokinetic models.
The derivation that follows is based on a drug with two-compartment
characteristics. The amount of drug absorbed into the systemic circulation at any time is given by

$$X_A = X_c + X_E + X_p \tag{4.21}$$

where X_E is the cumulative amount of drug eliminated by all pathways and X_c and X_p are the amounts of drug in the central and
peripheral compartments, respectively. Differentiation of (4.21)
with respect to time yields

$$\frac{dX_A}{dt} = \frac{dX_c}{dt} + \frac{dX_E}{dt} + \frac{dX_p}{dt} \tag{4.22}$$

The rate of elimination of drug, dX_E/dt, assuming first-order
kinetics, is by definition

$$\frac{dX_E}{dt} = k_{10}X_c \tag{4.23}$$

where k_{10} is the apparent first-order elimination rate constant of
drug from the central compartment. By substituting $k_{10}X_c$ for
dX_E/dt in (4.22) and dividing both sides of the equation by the apparent volume of the central compartment, V_c, one obtains

$$\frac{1}{V_c}\frac{dX_A}{dt} = \frac{1}{V_c}\frac{dX_c}{dt} + \frac{1}{V_c}k_{10}X_c + \frac{1}{V_c}\frac{dX_p}{dt} \tag{4.24}$$

Since X_c/V_c equals the drug concentration in plasma, C, Eq. (4.24)
can be written

$$\frac{1}{V_c}\frac{dX_A}{dt} = \frac{dC}{dt} + k_{10}C + \frac{1}{V_c}\frac{dX_p}{dt} \tag{4.25}$$

Integration of (4.25) from time zero to T yields the following expression for the amount of drug absorbed to time T:

$$\frac{(X_A)_T}{V_c} = C_T + k_{10}\int_0^T C\ dt + \frac{(X_p)_T}{V_c} \tag{4.26}$$

where $\int_0^T C\ dt$ is as defined previously in this chapter and C_T and
$(X_p)_T$ are the plasma concentration and amount of drug in the peripheral compartment at time T, respectively. The expression for the
amount of drug ultimately absorbed, $(X_A)_\infty$, is obtained by integrating (4.25) from time zero to infinity, which yields

$$\frac{(X_A)_\infty}{V_c} = k_{10} \int_0^\infty C \, dt \tag{4.27}$$

where $\int_0^\infty C \, dt$ is as defined previously. The fraction absorbed at any time T, $(X_A)_T / (X_A)_\infty$, is given by

$$\frac{(X_A)_T}{(X_A)_\infty} = \frac{C_T + k_{10} \int_0^T C \, dt + (X_p)_T / V_c}{k_{10} \int_0^\infty C \, dt} \tag{4.28}$$

Values for C_T, $\int_0^T C \, dt$, and $\int_0^\infty C \, dt$ are obtained from the oral absorption study. The rate constant k_{10} is estimated from a previous or subsequent intravenous study of the same subject. The amount of drug in the peripheral compartment as a function of time after oral administration divided by the volume of the central compartment can be estimated by a rather complicated approximation procedure requiring both oral and intravenous data.

The differential equation for the rate of change in the amount of drug in the peripheral compartment with time is given by

$$\frac{dX_p}{dt} = k_{12}X_c - k_{21}X_p \tag{4.29}$$

where k_{12} and k_{21} are apparent first-order intercompartmental transfer rate constants. If one assumes that the amount of drug in the central compartment between two consecutive sampling periods can be approximated by a straight line, then

$$X_c = (X_c)_0 + \frac{\Delta X_c}{\Delta t} t \tag{4.30}$$

where $(X_c)_0$ and X_c are the amounts of drug in the central compartment at the time of the first of any two consecutive sampling periods (i.e., time t_0) and at time t, respectively; $(\Delta X_c / \Delta t)$ is the slope of this line; and t is any time within the sampling period and varies from 0 to Δt. Substitution for X_c in Eq. (4.29) yields

$$\frac{dX_p}{dt} = k_{12}(X_c)_0 + k_{12}\frac{\Delta X_c}{\Delta t} t - k_{21}X_p \tag{4.31}$$

the Laplace transform of which is

$$s\overline{X}_p - (X_p)_0 = \frac{k_{12}(X_c)_0}{s} + \frac{k_{12}(\Delta X_c / \Delta t)}{s^2} - k_{21}\overline{X}_p \tag{4.32}$$

where $(X_p)_0$ is the amount of drug in the peripheral compartment at time t_0 and s is the Laplace operator. Solving (4.32) for $\overline{X}_p$ yields

$$\overline{X}_p = \frac{(X_p)_0}{s + k_{21}} + \frac{k_{12}(X_c)_0}{s(s + k_{21})} + \frac{k_{12}(\Delta X_c / \Delta t)}{s^2(s + k_{21})} \tag{4.33}$$

By taking the anti-Laplace of this equation (see Appendix A), an expression for the amount of drug in the peripheral compartment as a function of time can be obtained. That is,

$$X_p = (X_p)_0 e^{-k_{21}t} + \frac{k_{12}(X_c)_0}{k_{21}}(1 - e^{-k_{21}t}) + \frac{k_{12}(\Delta X_c / \Delta t)}{k_{21}} t$$

$$- \frac{k_{12}(\Delta X_c / \Delta t)}{k_{21}^2}(1 - e^{-k_{21}t}) \tag{4.34}$$

which may be simplified to

$$X_p = (X_p)_0 e^{-k_{21}t} + \frac{k_{12}(X_c)_0}{k_{21}}(1 - e^{-k_{21}t})$$

$$+ \frac{k_{12}(\Delta X_c / \Delta t)}{k_{21}^2}(e^{-k_{21}t} + k_{21}t - 1) \tag{4.35}$$

Dividing Eq. (4.35) by V_c and setting time equal to the time between any two consecutive sampling periods, Δt, yields

$$\frac{(X_p)_T}{V_c} = \frac{(X_p)_0}{V_c} e^{-k_{21}\Delta t} + \frac{k_{12}C_0}{k_{21}}(1 - e^{-k_{21}\Delta t})$$

$$+ \frac{k_{12}(\Delta C / \Delta t)}{k_{21}^2}(e^{-k_{21}\Delta t} + k_{21}\Delta t - 1) \tag{4.36}$$

If the sampling period is relatively short so that $k_{21}t \leq 0.5$ [11], the third term of Eq. (4.36) may be reduced by expressing the exponential term $e^{-k_{21}\Delta t}$ as a two-term Taylor expansion (i.e., $e^{-x} = 1 - x + x^2/2$). Equation (4.36) then simplifies to

$$\frac{(X_p)_T}{V_c} = \frac{(X_p)_0}{V_c} e^{-k_{21}\Delta t} + \frac{k_{12}C_0}{k_{21}}(1 - e^{-k_{21}\Delta t}) + \frac{k_{12}(\Delta C / \Delta t)(\Delta t)^2}{2} \tag{4.37}$$

The calculations involved in estimating values of $(X_p)_T/V_c$ as a function of time based on concentration-time data obtained after oral administration and estimates of k_{12} and k_{21} obtained after an intravenous study are shown in Table 4.2. The values can then be used in Eq. (4.28) to generate percent absorbed-time data as shown in Table 4.3.

The Loo-Riegelman method can also be applied to urinary excretion data. In this case the equation analogous to Eq. (4.28) is

$$\frac{(X_A)_T}{(X_A)_\infty} = \frac{(dX_u/dt)_T + k_{10}(X_u)_T + k_e'(X_p)_T}{k_{10}X_u^\infty} \tag{4.38}$$

where

$$k_e'(X_p)_T = k_e'(X_p)_0 e^{-k_{21}\Delta t} + \frac{k_{12}(dX_u/dt)_0}{k_{21}}(1 - e^{-k_{21}\Delta t})$$

$$+ \frac{k_{12}[\Delta(dX_u/dt)/\Delta t]}{k_{21}^2}(e^{-k_{21}\Delta t} + k_{21}\Delta t - 1) \tag{4.39}$$

Equation (4.39) is analogous to Eq. (4.36) and may be simplified by applying the two-term Taylor expansion if appropriate.

Although the application of the Loo-Riegelman method is limited because of the requirement for concentration-time data obtained after both oral and intravenous administration, it is a very useful and rigorous approach for the evaluation of absorption kinetics. The method can be used for drugs that distribute in any number of pharmacokinetic compartments. For example, the fraction absorbed equation for a drug that can be described after intravenous injection by a three-compartment model with linear elimination from the central compartment (see Fig. 2.17) is

$$\frac{(X_A)_T}{(X_A)_\infty} = \frac{C_T + k_{10}\int_0^T C\,dt + (X_2)_T/V_c + (X_3)_T/V_c}{k_{10}\int_0^\infty C\,dt} \tag{4.40}$$

where X_2 and X_3 are the amounts of drug in each peripheral compartment. Individual equations analogous to Eq. (4.36) must be written for the amount of drug in each peripheral compartment. For example,

$$\frac{(X_3)_T}{V_c} = \frac{(X_3)_0}{V_c}e^{-k_{21}\Delta t} + \frac{k_{13}C_0}{k_{31}}(1 - e^{-k_{31}\Delta t})$$

$$+ \frac{k_{13}(\Delta C/\Delta t)}{k_{31}^2}(e^{-k_{31}\Delta t} + k_{31}\Delta t - 1) \tag{4.41}$$

Pharmacokinetics

Table 4.2 Calculation of Absorption Data Using
the Loo-Riegelman Method

Time T	Drug Concentration in Plasma, C_T	ΔC	Δt	C_0	$(X_p)_0/V_c$
0	0.00	—	—	—	—
0.5	3.00	3.0	0.5	0.00	0.000
1.0	5.20	2.2	0.5	3.00	0.218
1.5	6.50	1.3	0.5	5.20	0.749
2.0	7.30	0.8	0.5	6.50	1.433
2.5	7.60	0.3	0.5	7.30	2.157
3.0	7.75	0.15	0.5	7.60	2.849
3.5	7.70	−0.05	0.5	7.75	3.471
4.0	7.60	−0.1	0.5	7.70	4.019
5.0	7.10	−0.5	1.0	7.60	4.469
6.0	6.60	−0.5	1.0	7.10	5.103
7.0	6.00	−0.6	1.0	6.60	5.442
9.0	5.10	−0.9	2.0	6.00	5.552
11.0	4.40	−0.7	2.0	5.10	5.318
15.0	3.30	−1.1	4.0	4.40	4.861

Notes: The estimation of $(X_p)_T/V_c$ following oral administration is
based on Eq. (4.37). A two-compartment model and first-order disposition are assumed: $k_{12} = 0.29$, $k_{21} = 0.31$, and $k_{10} = 0.16$.

Although the Loo-Riegelman method was developed based on multicompartment models in which elimination takes place only from the central compartment, Wagner [12] has shown that the method is equally valid whether elimination occurs from the central compartment alone, from the peripheral compartment(s) alone, or from both (all) compartments.

An inherent limitation of the Loo-Riegelman method is the intrasubject variability in pharmacokinetic parameters such as k_{10}, k_{12}, and k_{21} between the intravenous and oral studies. The assumption must be made that the kinetics of drug distribution and elimination remain unchanged in the interval between doses. A method that eliminates intrasubject variability is the simultaneous administration

$\dfrac{(X_p)_0}{V_c} e^{-k_{21}\Delta t}$	$\dfrac{k_{12}(C)_0}{k_{21}}(1 - e^{-k_{21}\Delta t})$	$\left(\dfrac{k_{12}(\Delta t)^2}{2}\right)\dfrac{\Delta C}{\Delta t}$	$(X_p)_T/V_c$
—	—	—	0.000
0.000	0.000	0.218	0.218
0.187	0.402	0.160	0.749
0.642	0.697	0.094	1.433
1.228	0.871	0.058	2.157
1.849	0.978	0.022	2.849
2.442	1.018	0.011	3.471
2.976	1.039	−0.004	4.019
3.444	1.032	−0.007	4.469
3.276	1.900	−0.073	5.103
3.740	1.775	−0.073	5.442
3.989	1.650	−0.087	5.552
2.987	2.592	−0.261	5.318
2.861	2.203	−0.203	4.861
1.361	3.168	−0.638	3.891

of the oral and intravenous doses. The oral dose would consist of
drug in the formulation to be evaluated and the intravenous dose
would be a solution containing labeled drug (i.e., either a radioactive
or a stable isotope) [13, 14]. The concentration of labeled drug in
plasma must be determined by methods specific for unchanged drug.

Deconvolution Method

Deconvolution is a model-independent method for determining absorption rates. Our discussion will be limited to the application of, rather
than the mathematical basis for, the method. It was introduced by
Rescigno and Segre [15] in 1966, but its use has been limited. The

Table 4.3 Calculation of Absorption Data Using the Loo-Riegelman Method [see Eq. (4.28)]

T	C_T	$k_{10}\int_0^T C\,dt$	$(X_p)_T/V_c$	$(X_A)_T/(X_A)_\infty$	Percent Unabsorbed
0.5	3.00	0.12	0.22	0.165	83.5
1.0	5.20	0.45	0.75	0.316	68.4
1.5	6.50	0.92	1.43	0.437	56.3
2.0	7.30	1.47	2.16	0.540	46.0
2.5	7.60	2.06	2.85	0.618	38.2
3.0	7.75	2.68	3.47	0.687	31.3
3.5	7.70	3.30	4.02	0.742	25.8
4.0	7.60	3.91	4.47	0.790	21.0
5.0	7.10	5.08	5.10	0.854	14.6
6.0	6.60	6.18	5.44	0.901	9.9
7.0	6.00	7.19	5.55	0.926	7.4
9.0	5.10	8.96	5.32	0.958	4.2
11.0	4.40	10.48	4.86	0.976	2.4
15.0	3.30	12.95	3.89	0.996	0.4

Notes: A two-compartment open model and first-order disposition are assumed: $k_{10} = 0.16$. Values for $(X_p)_T/V_c$ are taken from Table 4.2, $\int_0^\infty C\,dt = 126.44$.

deconvolution method requires no assumptions regarding the number of compartments in the model or the kinetics of absorption. Linear distribution and elimination are assumed. Like the Loo-Riegelman method, deconvolution requires data obtained after both oral and intravenous administration in the same subject and assumes no differences in the pharmacokinetics of drug distribution and elimination from one study to the other. Drug concentrations must be measured at the same times following both oral and intravenous administration during the time that drug is absorbed after oral administration [16]. However, the deconvolution method does not require the determination of drug concentrations in plasma at equally spaced intervals during or after the absorption phase [17]. The accuracy of the method depends on the size of the sampling interval. The same applies to the Loo-Riegelman method [12].

Under these conditions the fraction unabsorbed or the fraction remaining FR in the gastrointestinal tract after a certain time, expressed in terms of the sampling interval, is given by [16]

$$(FR)_{n\Delta t} = \frac{H_{(n+1)\Delta t}}{H_{\Delta t}} - \sum_{\substack{i=2 \\ j=n}}^{\substack{j=1 \\ i=n+1}} \frac{F_i \Delta t}{F_{\Delta t}} [FR]_{(j-1)\Delta t} \qquad (4.42)$$

where

$$(FR)_{n\Delta t} = 1 - \frac{(X_A)_T}{(X_A)_\infty} = 1 - \frac{(X_A)_{n\Delta t}}{(X_A)_\infty} \qquad (4.43)$$

and $n \Delta t$ is the time after n sampling intervals equal to Δt. H is a function describing the drug concentration-time curve following oral administration and F is a function describing the drug concentration-time curve following intravenous bolus administration. $F_{n\Delta t}$ may be given by the drug concentration in plasma at $n \Delta t$ or the area under the drug concentration-time curve between $n \Delta t$ and $(n - 1) \Delta t$. $H_{n\Delta t}$ can only be expressed in terms of concentration. When both H and F are expressed in terms of drug concentrations in plasma, the method is termed point-point.

Consider a situation where drug is administered intravenously and orally on two occasions and blood samples are obtained every 15 min (i.e., $\Delta t = 15$). Using the point-point method, the fraction remaining unabsorbed 15 min after oral administration is given by Eq. (4.42) as follows:

$$(FR)_{\Delta t} = \frac{C_{2\Delta t}^{oral}}{C_{\Delta t}^{oral}} - \frac{C_{2\Delta t}^{i.v.}}{C_{\Delta t}^{i.v.}} (FR)_0 \qquad (4.44)$$

where $(FR)_{\Delta t}$ is the fraction unabsorbed 15 min after oral administration; $(FR)_0$ is the fraction unabsorbed at $t = 0$ and is equal to 1.0; $C^{oral}_{2\Delta t}$ and $C^{oral}_{\Delta t}$ are the drug concentrations in plasma 30 and 15 min, respectively, after oral administration; and $C^{i.v.}_{2\Delta t}$ and $C^{i.v.}_{\Delta t}$ are the drug concentrations in plasma 30 and 15 min, respectively, after intravenous bolus administration. The fraction remaining unabsorbed 30 min after oral administration is given by

$$(FR)_{2\Delta t} = \frac{C^{oral}_{3\Delta t}}{C^{oral}_{\Delta t}} - \frac{C^{i.v.}_{2\Delta t}}{C^{i.v.}_{\Delta t}} (FR)_{\Delta t} - \frac{C^{i.v.}_{3\Delta t}}{C^{i.v.}_{\Delta t}} (FR)_0 \qquad (4.45)$$

where $(FR)_{\Delta t}$ is obtained by first solving Eq. (4.44). Table 4.4 provides a numerical illustration of how the fraction remaining unabsorbed can be calculated by deconvolution using the point-point method.

For a one-compartment model with first-order absorption and first-order elimination, $(FR)_{n\Delta t}$ should be equal to $e^{-nk_a \Delta t}$. This is readily demonstrated by substituting the appropriate equations in Eq. (4.42). Under these conditions $(FR)_{\Delta t}$ is given by

Table 4.4 Calculation of Absorption Data Using Deconvolution (Point-Point Method) (see Ref. 16)

Time	$C^{i.v.}$	C^{oral}	FR^a
0	100.0	0.0	1.00
1	84.0	58.6	0.35
2	70.6	69.9	0.12
3	59.9	65.9	0.05
4	49.4	57.9	
5	41.5	49.6	

[a]FR denotes the fraction remaining unabsorbed:

$$FR_1 = \frac{69.9}{58.6} - \frac{70.6}{84.0} (1.00) \qquad (Eq.\ 4.44)$$

$$FR_2 = \frac{65.9}{58.6} - \frac{70.6}{84.0} (0.35) - \frac{59.9}{84.0} (1.00) \qquad (Eq.\ 4.45)$$

$$FR_3 = \frac{57.9}{58.6} - \frac{70.6}{84.0} (0.12) - \frac{59.9}{84.0} (0.35) - \frac{49.4}{84.0} (1.00)$$

$$(FR)_{\Delta t} = \frac{A(e^{-2K\Delta t} - e^{-2k_a\Delta t})}{A(e^{-K\Delta t} - e^{-k_a\Delta t})} - \frac{Be^{-2K\Delta t}}{Be^{-K\Delta t}} \qquad (4.46)$$

where $A = k_a FX_0/V(k_a - K)$ and $B = X_0/V$. Canceling common terms and rearranging terms yields

$$(FR)_{\Delta t} = \frac{e^{-2K\Delta t} - e^{-2k_a\Delta t} - e^{-K\Delta t}(e^{-K\Delta t} - e^{-k_a\Delta t})}{e^{-K\Delta t} - e^{-k_a\Delta t}} \qquad (4.47)$$

which may be simplified to yield

$$(FR)_{\Delta t} = \frac{e^{-k_a\Delta t}(e^{-K\Delta t} - e^{-k_a\Delta t})}{e^{-K\Delta t} - e^{-k_a\Delta t}} = e^{-k_a\Delta t} \qquad (4.48)$$

Benet and Chiang [18] recommend the use of the point-area method rather than the point-point method. In the point-area method, H is

Table 4.5 Calculation of Absorption Data Using Deconvolution (Point-Area Method) (see Ref. 16)

Time	$\int_0^t C^{i.v.} dt$	$\int_{t_1}^{t_2} C^{i.v.} dt$	C^{oral}	FR^a
0	0.0	91.8	0.0	1.00
1	91.8	77.1	58.6	0.35
2	169.9	64.8	69.9	0.125
3	233.7	54.4	65.9	0.04
4	288.1	45.7	57.9	
5	333.8		49.6	

^{a}FR denotes fraction remaining unabsorbed:

$$FR_1 = \frac{69.9}{58.6} - \frac{77.1}{91.8}(1.00)$$

$$FR_2 = \frac{65.9}{58.6} - \frac{77.1}{91.8}(0.35) - \frac{64.8}{91.8}(1.00)$$

$$FR_3 = \frac{57.9}{58.6} - \frac{77.1}{91.8}(0.125) - \frac{64.8}{91.8}(0.35) - \frac{54.4}{91.8}(1.00)$$

given by the drug concentration in plasma at time n Δt after oral administration and F is given by the area under the drug concentration versus time curve over the sampling interval after intravenous administration. The use of the point-area method to evaluate the time course of absorption is illustrated in Table 4.5.

Intercept Method

Vaughan [19] has proposed a method for evaluating the in vivo release rate constant of a drug from its oral formulations. The method is model independent but requires data after oral administration of both the formulation and a solution of the drug and assumes that absorption as well as distribution and elimination are first-order processes.

The drug concentration in plasma after a single oral dose D_s in solution can usually be described by a summation of exponential terms:

$$C_s = D_s \sum_{i=1}^{N} A_i e^{-\alpha_i t} \qquad (4.49)$$

where A_i and α_i are constants and $\alpha_i > \alpha_{i+1}$. If after oral administration of the formulation containing a dose D_f, the drug is released from the formulation in a first-order fashion prior to absorption, drug concentrations in plasma are given by [19]

$$C_f = fD_f k_r \left(\sum_{i=1}^{N} \frac{A_i}{\alpha_i - k_r} \right) e^{-k_r t} + \sum_{i=1}^{N} \frac{fD_f k_r A_i e^{-\alpha_i t}}{k_r - \alpha_i} \qquad (4.50)$$

where f is the fraction of the dose D_f that is absorbed relative to the amount absorbed after the solution and k_r is the first-order release rate constant from the formulation. Provided that $k_r > \alpha_N$ both C_s and C_f will, at some time after administration, be described by single exponential functions:

$$C_s = D_s A_N e^{-\alpha_N t} \qquad (4.51)$$

and

$$C_f = \frac{fD_f k_r A_N e^{-\alpha_N t}}{k_r - \alpha_N} \qquad (4.52)$$

where α_N is equal to λ_n for a multicompartment system or to K for a one-compartment system. The intercepts I of the extrapolations of the final exponential regressions of log C_s versus time and log C_f

versus time, with the concentration axis, are given by the coefficients of the terms on the right-hand side of Eqs. (4.51) and (4.52):

$$I_s = D_s A_N \qquad (4.53)$$

and

$$I_f = \frac{fD_f k_r A_N}{k_r - \alpha_N} \qquad (4.54)$$

Dividing Eq. (4.53) by (4.54), canceling common terms, and rearranging the resulting equation yields an expression for k_r:

$$k_r = \frac{\alpha_N}{1 - fD_f I_s / D_s I_f} \qquad (4.55)$$

Hence k_r may be calculated from drug concentration-time data obtained after oral administration of a solution and a formulation. In principle, Eq. (4.55) may also be used with urinary excretion rate data. Vaughan [19] has provided an example based on urinary excretion rate data to illustrate the use of Eq. (4.55). A 15 mg dose of methylamphetamine was given as an aqueous solution and as a tablet formulation. The cumulative urinary excretion of unchanged drug was 50.4% of the dose after the solution and 50.9% of the dose after the tablet. Hence $f \simeq 1$. The final linear regressions of the log of urinary excretion rates against time had a half-life of 5 h corresponding to an α_N value of 0.1386 h^{-1}. The ratio of the intercepts was 0.7. Substitution of these values into Eq. (4.55) gives k_r as 0.462 h^{-1}. When release (dissolution) from the dosage is the rate-limiting step in drug absorption, this method gives an estimate of the absorption rate constant since under these conditions $k_r \simeq k_a$.

The usefulness of the intercept method is greatest when intravenous data are not available (so that the Loo-Riegelman or deconvolution method cannot be applied) and when the oral data clearly indicate that the drug distributes in a multicompartment manner (so that the Wagner-Nelson method may not be applied). The weaknesses of the method include the assumption of first-order absorption and the need for α_N to be essentially the same for both studies. Also, this method may yield unusual and misleading results if the drug precipitates in the gut after administration of the solution dosage form.

EXTENT OF ABSORPTION

Although the standard definition of bioavailability includes both rate and extent of drug absorption, bioavailability and the alternative terms, *availability* and *systemic availability,* are often used to signify solely the extent of absorption or the amount of drug reaching the systemic circulation because this is often the principal concern of comparative bioavailability studies. Since the average steady-state concentration of drug in plasma on repetitive dosing is directly proportional to the amount absorbed, administering a drug in a formulation from which the extent of absorption is lower than from another formulation is the same as administering a lower dose.

The amount of drug reaching the systemic circulation after oral administration is often less than the administered dose. There are many reasons for this. Poor formulations may release only a part of the dose before reaching the colon. This is found most often with formulations of poorly water soluble drugs or with special formulations that are designed deliberately to delay release of the drug. However, oral administration of even the best formulation of a drug may result in less than completely availability. Some drugs are so polar that permeation of the gastrointestinal epithelium is limited. Other drugs are subject to chemical or enzymatic degradation before reaching the systemic circulation; this may occur in the gut lumen, in the gut wall, or in the liver during the first pass.

The systemic availability of a drug after oral administration of a formulation rarely exceeds that found with a solution. In almost all cases the performance of a dosage form or formulation can be evaluated by comparison with that of a solution. However, equivalent availability does not imply complete availability. For example, Wagner et al. [20] have shown that the availability of propoxyphene is the same after oral administration of a commercially available capsule and an aqueous solution, but the systemic availability of propoxyphene is less than 25% of the administered dose largely because of first-pass metabolism [21]. Although relative availability studies are useful for characterizing the formulation, one must determine absolute availability to characterize the drug.

Estimation of absolute availability after oral administration almost always requires comparison with data obtained after intravenous administration. In the case of water-soluble drugs, data after intramuscular administration may be acceptable as an absolute standard. Various oral standards have been used to determine relative availability. These include aqueous and nonaqueous solutions, carefully formulated suspensions and certain commercial formulations that are generally accepted as standards.

Almost all bioavailability studies are concerned with the systemic availability or relative availability of a drug after oral administration. However, the extent of absorption may also be of concern when administering a drug by any extravascular route, for example when giving a drug suspension intramuscularly or when giving a solution of drug that is likely to precipitate in the muscle depot on injection. Although it is reasonable to assume that the entire dose of an intramuscularly administered drug will be absorbed eventually, absorption may be so slow that, effectively, availability may be considered incomplete.

This may occur if the release of a fraction of the dose in the muscle depot is so slow as to give drug concentrations in plasma below that which one can measure. Availability is also a consideration after intravenous administration of a chemical derivative of a drug (a prodrug) that is intended to produce the drug itself in the body. If the prodrug is both converted to the drug and eliminated by other routes, the availability of the drug is less than complete. This is the case for chlorampehnical after intravenous administration of chloramphenical succinate [22].

Systemic or relative availability of a drug may be determined based on drug concentrations in plasma, urinary excretion of un-metabolized drug, or pharmacologic effects. The last mentioned is considered briefly in Chap. 6. In some instances availability esti-mates may be based on metabolite or total radioactivity in plasma or urine.

Drug Concentrations in Plasma

The most commonly used method for estimating availability is the comparison of the total area under the drug concentration in plasma versus time curve, AUC, after oral administration of the test formula-tion and after administration of the standard.

In referring to the availability of a drug after oral administration we will use the term *systemic availability* F when the standard is an intravenous solution and the term *relative availability* F_r when the standard is an oral formulation. An example of the results of a rela-tive availability study is shown in Fig. 4.5. Formulation (a) is con-sidered to be the reference standard.

By definition,

$$F = \frac{(\int_0^\infty C \; dt)_{oral}}{(\int_0^\infty C \; dt)_{i.v.}} = \frac{AUC_{oral}}{AUC_{i.v.}} \qquad (4.56)$$

when equal doses are given intravenously and orally;

$$F = \frac{D_{i.v.} \cdot AUC_{oral}}{D_{oral} \cdot AUC_{i.v.}} \qquad (4.57)$$

when different doses D are given intravenously and orally; and

$$F_r = \frac{AUC_{test}}{AUC_{standard}} \qquad (4.58)$$

assuming that equal doses are given in the test formulation and the standard.

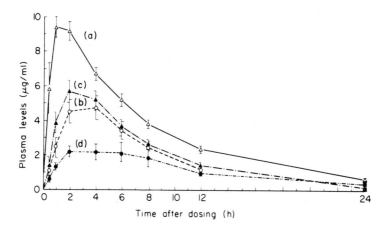

Fig. 4.5 Average chloramphenicol concentrations in plasma for groups of 10 healthy volunteers who received single 0.5 g oral doses of the drug in various commercial preparations (a, b, c, or d). Product (a) is considered the standard. (From Ref. 23.)

It is easily shown for any multicompartment model with linear processes that the ratio of areas after intravenous and oral administration is equal to F. Since

$$AUC_{oral} = \frac{FD_{oral}}{(V_{\beta}\lambda_n)_{oral}} \tag{4.59}$$

and

$$AUC_{i.v.} = \frac{D_{i.v.}}{(V_{\beta}\lambda_n)_{i.v.}} \tag{4.60}$$

it follows that

$$\frac{AUC_{oral}}{AUC_{i.v.}} = \frac{FD_{oral}(V_{\beta}\lambda_n)_{i.v.}}{D_{i.v.}(V_{\beta}\lambda_n)_{oral}} \tag{4.61}$$

Assuming that the same dose was given intravenous and orally, and the clearance of the drug, $V_{\beta}\lambda_n$, was the same in each study, Eq. (4.61) can be reduced to Eq. (4.56).

The proximity of the estimated average value of F or F_r as derived from either Eq. (4.56) or (4.58) to the true value of F or F_r depends on the assumption that average drug clearance is the same in each of the comparative studies. This is unlikely to be the case if different panels of subjects are used for each trial since inter-subject variability in drug clearance can often be pronounced. This variability can be reduced (but not eliminated) by carefully matching the subjects with respect to sex, body weight, age, health status, and other factors. A still better solution is to use the same subjects in both trials. Furthermore, by using the same subjects and by alternating the order of drug administration (i.e., a crossover study), we can avoid subject effects and period effects.

Today, almost all bioavailability studies are carried out in a crossover fashion with a single panel of subjects. Hence the average values of F or F_r determined from these studies are usually good estimates of the true value. However, these studies are still sometimes plagued by intrasubject variability; that is, an individual's ability to clear a drug may differ demonstrably from one administration of drug to the next. It is likely that the larger the intrasubject variability in drug elimination, the larger the standard deviation associated with the estimated value of F or F_r. Large standard deviations make it difficult to differentiate products, an important purpose of bioavailability studies. Differentiation at an appropriate level of confidence under conditions where there is considerable intrasubject variability may require a very large panel of subjects.

There is considerable interest in reducing the effect of intrasubject variability in bioavailability studies. This would be accomplished if we could somehow account for differences in clearance in the same individual from one treatment to another [see Eq. (4.61)]. Unfortunately, this is not possible because one cannot determine clearance without making some assumption concerning bioavailability. Alternatively, one can assume that the apparent volume of distribution in a given individual is invariant from trial to trial and then correct for differences in half-life [24].

Rearranging Eq. (4.61), assuming that $(V_\beta)_{i.v.} = (V_\beta)_{oral}$, and recognizing that $t_{1/2} = 0.693/\lambda_n$ yields

$$F = \frac{D_{i.v.}(t_{1/2})_{i.v.} \cdot AUC_{oral}}{D_{oral}(t_{1/2})_{oral} \cdot AUC_{i.v.}} \qquad (4.62)$$

This so-called half-life correction method assumes that a change in $t_{1/2}$ from one study to the next in the same subject reflects solely a change in clearance and is not mediated by a change in apparent volume of distribution. It is probably reasonable to attempt the half-life correction in most bioavailability studies but to accept it only when it results in a substantial decrease in the standard deviation of the mean value of F or F_R. The half-life correction method must never be used when a change in $t_{1/2}$ reflects more persistent or prolonged absorption of drug from one dosage form than another [25].

An alternative correction for intrasubject variability called the Kwan-Till method is based on variability in renal clearance and requires both plasma concentration and urinary excretion data [26]. This method assumes that changes in total clearance are solely the result of changes in renal clearance and that nonrenal clearance remains constant from study to study. It appears to be most useful for but not limited to drugs that are substantially excreted unchanged in the urine. The total plasma or systemic clearance is given by

$$Cl_s = \frac{D_{i.v.}}{AUC_{i.v.}}$$

(4.63)

but may also be expressed as

$$Cl_s = Cl_r + Cl_{nr}$$

(4.64)

that is, as the sum of renal clearance Cl_r and nonrenal clearance Cl_{nr}. The renal clearance of a drug is given by

$$Cl_r = \frac{f_u D}{AUC}$$

(4.65)

where f_u is the fraction of the administered dose that is ultimately excreted unchanged in the urine;

$$f_u = \frac{X_u^\infty}{D}$$

(4.66)

Equation (4.61) may be rearranged and expressed as

$$F = \frac{(Cl_s)_{oral} D_{i.v.} \cdot AUC_{oral}}{(Cl_s)_{i.v.} D_{oral} \cdot AUC_{i.v.}} = \frac{(Cl_{nr} + Cl_r)_{oral} D_{i.v.} \cdot AUC_{oral}}{(Cl_{nr} + Cl_r)_{i.v.} D_{oral} \cdot AUC_{i.v.}}$$

(4.67)

Assuming that nonrenal clearance is the same for both the oral and intravenous study, and recognizing that Cl_{nr} is equal to the difference between Eqs. (4.63) and (4.65), we can state that

$$F = \frac{(D_{i.v.}/AUC_{i.v.} - f_{u,i.v.} D_{i.v.}/AUC_{i.v.} + f_{u,oral} D_{oral}/AUC_{oral}) AUC_{oral} D_{i.v.}}{(D_{i.v.}/AUC_{i.v.} - f_{u,i.v.} D_{i.v.}/AUC_{i.v.} + f_{u,i.v.} D_{i.v.}/AUC_{i.v.}) AUC_{i.v.} D_{oral}}$$

(4.68)

which can be simplified to

$$F = \left(\frac{D_{i.v.}}{AUC_{i.v.}} - \frac{f_{u,i.v.} D_{i.v.}}{AUC_{i.v.}} + \frac{f_{u,oral} D_{oral}}{AUC_{oral}} \right) \frac{AUC_{oral}}{D_{oral}}$$

$$= \frac{AUC_{oral} D_{i.v.} (1 - f_{u,i.v.})}{AUC_{i.v.} D_{oral}} + f_{u,oral}$$

(4.69)

Even if the assumption regarding the constancy of nonrenal clearance
from one study to the next were incorrect, it would be of little consequence if the drug were substantially excreted unchanged, since
Cl_{nr} would represent a small fraction of Cl_S. This method has recently been used for estimating the availability of fluoride from tablets [27]. Calculating F by means of Eq. (4.57) and (4.69) yielded
values of 107.8 ± 27.2 and 100.8 ± 9.2 %, respectively. Applying the
correction factor reduced the apparent variability of the estimate.
In this case, nonrenal clearance was about 60% of total clearance.
The Kwan-Till method outlined above applies exactly only when an
intravenous reference is available. In the absence of such data, an
approximation has been proposed and evaluated [26, 28].

The correction method described above assigns the variability
in total plasma clearance to renal clearance and assumes no variability
in nonrenal clearance. Since there is no way to measure nonrenal
clearance independently, one may alternatively assume that the nonrenal clearance varies in direct proportion to changes in renal
clearance, so that

$$F = \frac{(Cl_r)_{oral} D_{i.v.} \cdot AUC_{oral}}{(Cl_r)_{i.v.} D_{oral} \cdot AUC_{i.v.}} \qquad (4.70)$$

Calculating the availability of fluoride for the example cited above [27]
using Eq. (4.70) yields $F = 101.5 \pm 24.0$%. The correction reduces the
average bioavailability to a more realistic absolute estimate, but is
has no effect on the standard deviation. Although this method is
not useful for fluoride, it may apply to other drugs and may be used
in the absence of an intravenous reference.

A systemic (integrated) approach to the estimation of bioavailability
using both model-independent (Kwan-Till) and pharmacokinetic
(half-life correction) techniques has been presented [29]. The methods
of Kwan-Till [26] and Wagner-Nelson [6] or Loo-Riegelman [7] are
integrated such that one is able to check many of the assumptions
inherent in these techniques and make adjustments for apparent deviations. This integrated approach as well as the Kwan-Till method
requires that plasma and urine be obtained during the bioavailability
study; the half-life correction method requires one or the other, not
both.

In the typical single-dose bioavailability study, blood sampling is
usually terminated before the entire drug concentration in plasma
versus time curve is characterized (see Fig. 4.6). In such cases the
estimation of $\int_0^\infty C\, dt$ or AUC requires an extrapolation. The available
data are first used to calculate $\int_0^t C\, dt$, where t is the time the last
sample was obtained, using the trapezoidal rule (see Appendix D) or
some other method [30]. The data are then plotted on semilogarithmic
coordinates to estimate K or λ_n (see Fig. 4.6). It is assumed that the
drug concentration-time curve after time t is described by

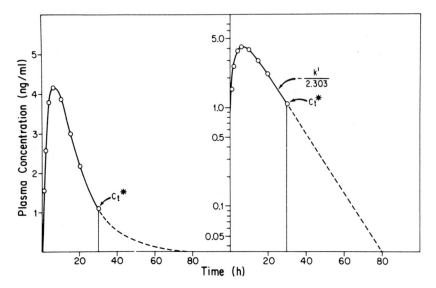

Fig. 4.6 Rectilinear and semilogarithmic plots of drug concentration
in plasma versus time after a single oral dose. The last blood sample
was taken before drug concentration had declined to a negligible
level, requiring that part of the total area under the curve be estimated
[see Eq. (4.75).]

$$C = C_0 e^{-Kt} \qquad (4.71)$$

or

$$C = C_0 e^{-\lambda_n t} \qquad (4.72)$$

Integrating these expressions from t to infinity yields

$$\int_t^\infty C\,dt = \frac{C_t}{K} \qquad (4.73)$$

or

$$\int_0^t C\,dt = \frac{C_t}{\lambda_n} \qquad (4.74)$$

where C_t is the concentration at the last sampling time. The total
area under the drug concentration in plasma versus time curve for a
multicompartment model is given by

$$\text{AUC} = \int_0^\infty C \, dt = \int_0^t C \, dt + \frac{C_t}{\lambda_n} \qquad (4.75)$$

This technique is useful but does not reduce the need for obtaining blood samples for as long as possible after dosing. The smaller the contribution of the extrapolation area term (C_t/K or C_t/λ_n) to the total area, the more accurate the estimation of total area.

The treatment described above suggests that the minimum time required for sampling in a bioavailability study is that which assures a reliable estimate of the elimination rate constant (i.e., three to four elimination half-lives after dosing). In some instances, however, considerably shorter sampling periods appear adequate. Lovering et al. [31] determined for different formulations of many drugs that the ratio of areas under the drug concentration-time curve changed little between the apparent end of the absorption period and the time when blood sampling was terminated. They concluded that for a wide range of conditions the area ratios for any two formulations at a time equal to about twice that required for the apparent termination of absorption are within a few percentage points of the area ratios at infinite time. The theoretical basis for these observations is complex, but the work of Kwan and colleagues [32–34] provides some insight. In general, we can state for all cases that sampling should not be terminated until some time after absorption is complete. For a one-compartment model with first-order absorption and elimination, the closer the values of the absorption rate constants for two formulations, the shorter is the sampling time required for the ratio of areas to approximate the ratio at infinite time. For the same model the greater the difference between k_a and K, the shorter is the time required to determine an area ratio that approximates the ratio at infinite time. For example, for two formulations each with $k_a/K \geq 5$, the area ratio after a time equal to one elimination half-life is usually within 80% of the ratio at infinite time. When the values of the absorption rate constants are closer, the approximation is better. When the sampling interval is equal to two elimination half-lives, the area ratio is within 90% of the ratio at infinite time if $k_a/K \geq 5$ for both formulations. It appears that the use of partial areas in comparative bioavailability studies will be most successful for drugs with long half-lives and for formulations from which these drugs are relatively rapidly absorbed. Although we can rationalize results such as those found with digoxin [35], where for certain formulations the area measured over the interval 0 to 5 h correlates extremely well with the area measured over the interval 0 to 96 h, the prospective use of partial areas cannot be encouraged. One is always faced with the uncertainty of deciding when absorption has effectively stopped. If sampling is terminated before absorption is complete, comparison of partial areas will be misleading. For this reason we favor sampling as long as possible after administration and the application of Eq. (4.75) where appropriate.

There are times when the estimation of the availability of a drug after a single dose is difficult. For example, single-dose bioavailability studies in patients who require the drug necessitate stopping drug therapy. Also, the usual dose of some drugs produce such low drug concentrations in plasma after a single dose that it may be impossible to determine concentrations for more than a few hours after administration. In such cases it may be desirable to estimate bioavailability after repetitive dosing. Drug concentrations in plasma at steady state are often considerably higher than those found after a single dose. We have shown in Chap. 3 that the area under the drug concentration in plasma versus time curve over a dosing interval at steady state after repetitive dosing of a fixed dose at a fixed interval is equal to the total area resulting from that dose in a single-dose study. Therefore,

$$F_r = \frac{(\int_0^\tau C_{ss} \, dt)_{test}}{(\int_0^\tau C_{ss} \, dt)_{standard}} \tag{4.76}$$

where C_{ss} denotes drug concentrations at steady state and τ is the dosing interval. Equation (4.76) assumes that the dosage regimen was the same for both studies. One advantage of this method is that fewer data points are required to characterize the area because the time course of change in drug concentrations in plasma at steady state is less precipitous than after a single dose and sampling times are bounded by the dosing interval. A second advantage is that patients or normal subjects may be crossed over from one formulation to another without a drug washout period. It is necessary, however, upon a change of formulation that the drug be given for four to seven elimination half-lives before estimating $\int_0^\tau C_{ss} \, dt$ to assure attainment of the new steady state. Table 4.6 summarizes the results of a steady-state bioavailability study with digoxin [36]. The study consisted of a randomized crossover design, in six healthy volunteers, with three 2-week treatment periods. Digoxin was given once daily at 8:00 a.m. Drug concentrations in plasma were determined during the final dosing interval (day 14). Figure 4.7 shows average drug concentration-time curves during a dosing interval at steady state for three quindine formulations [37].

Attempts to estimate availability by comparing single steady-state drug concentrations in plasma after different formulations rather than areas over the dosing interval may lead to incorrect results. For example, consider a one-compartment model with first-order absorption and elimination. The drug concentration at the end of any dosing interval at steady state is given by

Table 4.6 Estimation of Digoxin Bioavailability Using Steady-State
Plasma or Urine Data (see Ref. 36)

Dosage Form	$\int_0^\tau C_{ss}\,dt$ (ng-h/ml)	F	X_u^{ss} (mg)	F
Intravenous solution	37.6	1.00	105.0	1.00
Oral solution	25.6	0.68	94.7	0.90
Oral tablet	21.8	0.58	89.7	0.85

Notes: In each case, 0.25 mg of digoxin was given every 24 h for
2 weeks. Each value represents the mean of six subjects.

$$C_{min}^{ss} = \frac{k_a FX_0}{V(k_a - K)} \frac{1}{1 - e^{-K\tau}} e^{-K\tau} \qquad (4.77)$$

assuming that each dose is given postabsorption. The ratio of
trough or minimum concentrations at steady state for two formulations
in the same individual is given by

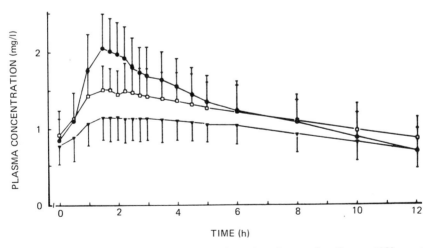

Fig. 4.7 Mean quinidine concentrations in plasma for three different
products during a dosing interval at steady state. The drug was given
every 12 h for 6 days before sampling. Comparison of the areas under
the curves during the dosing interval, adjusted for administered dose,
permits an assessment of relative bioavailability. (From Ref. 37,
reprinted with permission.)

$$\frac{(C_{min}^{ss})_{test}}{(C_{min}^{ss})_{standard}} = \frac{[k_a F/(k_a - K)]_{test}}{[k_a F/(k_a - K)]_{standard}} \tag{4.78}$$

assuming that K, V, τ, and X_0 are the same in both cases. Clearly, the ratio of trough concentrations is equal to F_r (i.e., $F_{test}/F_{standard}$) only if the absorption rate constants for each formulation are the same or if absorption from both formulations is such that $k_a \gg K$ in each case. Further examination of Eq. (4.78) reveals that if drug is absorbed from two formulations to the same extent but at different rates, the ratio of trough levels cannot be unity. For example, if the standard were absorbed faster than the test formulation but to the same extent, the ratio will exceed unity and one could incorrectly conclude that the test formulation is better absorbed.

The principal disadvantage of the steady-state method for estimating availability is that the clinical aspects are much more difficult to control and execute. It may take many days to achieve steady state. In any prolonged study, the potential lapses in subject compliance increase with time. As an alternative, Kwan and colleagues [32–34] have proposed a comprehensive method to permit bioavailability estimates under quasi- or non-steady state conditions. The basic strategy is to effect sufficient drug accumulation to facilitate assessment of bioavailability without unduly prolonging the clinical phase of the study. Only one aspect of this method will be considered here. The reader is directed to the original publications for mathematical derivations.

Consider that two treatments of the same drug are to be compared by administering sequentially ℓ doses of a standard formulation followed immediately by m doses of a test formulation according to the same dosage regimen. Under certain conditions it can be shown that [32]

$$F_r = \frac{F_{test}}{F_{standard}} = \left[\frac{(\int_0^\tau C \, dt)_{m+\ell}}{(\int_0^\tau C \, dt)_\ell} - e^{-mK\tau}\right] \frac{1 - e^{-\ell K\tau}}{1 - e^{-mK\tau}} \tag{4.79}$$

where the integral term in the numerator represents the area under the drug concentration in plasma versus time curve over the dosing interval after the last dose of the test formulation and the one in the denominator represents the area over the dosing interval after the last dose of the standard. If m = ℓ, Eq. (4.79) reduces to

$$F_r = \frac{(\int_0^\tau C \, dt)_{m+\ell}}{(\int_0^\tau C \, dt)_\ell} - e^{-mK\tau} \tag{4.80}$$

For a multicompartment system K is replaced by λ_n. The derivation of Eq. (4.79) is based on a linear model with first-order absorption, and requires that $k_a \gg K$ or λ_n for both formulations, where K or λ_n represents the slope of the terminal linear phase of a semilogarithmic plot of plasma concentration versus time. Alternatively, it requires that k_a is the same for both formulations. If neither of these conditions is satisfied, Eqs. (4.79) and (4.80) are approximations. The validity of the approximation depends on (1) the difference between the two absorption rate constants (the smaller the difference, the better the approximation); (2) the difference between the absorption rate constant for each formulation and the elimination rate constant of the drug (the larger these differences, the better the approximation); and (3) the proximity of $\ell \tau$ and $(m + \ell)\tau$ to the time required to achieve steady state (the closer one is to steady state, the better the approximation). Kwan presents several strategies to improve the approximations as well as alternative strategies to compare different formulations under a variety of quasi- and non-steady state conditions [32–34]. Based on his experience with this method, Kwan [33] concludes: "In general, the relative bioavailability between two formulations in a crossover study is a function of the ratio of respective mean plasma concentration at quasi- and nonsteady-state. Appropriate correction factors may be introduced to compensate for the effects of dose, dosing sequence, half-life, sampling interval, and residuals. Each of these elements can be readily identified in the equations developed for each design variation."

Although it is widely accepted that the absolute availability F of a drug after oral administration can be determined only by reference to results obtained after intravenous administration, there is an interesting exception. A method has been proposed for estimating the absolute availability of drugs with renal clearances that are reproducibly perturable, without reference to an intravenous dose [38].

Consider the oral administration of a drug under two conditions, X and Y, which results in different renal clearances. These conditions may be the coadministration of agents that acidify or alkalinize the urine or that inhibit tubular secretion. Total clearance is the sum of renal and nonrenal clearances. We shall assume that nonrenal clearance and the fraction of dose absorbed are the same under both conditions. Therefore,

$$(Cl_s)_X = (Cl_r)_X + (Cl_{nr})_X \tag{4.81}$$

and

$$(Cl_s)_Y = (Cl_r)_Y + (Cl_{nr})_Y \tag{4.82}$$

where $(Cl_{nr})_X = (Cl_{nr})_Y$. Subtracting Eq. (4.82) from (4.81) yields

$$\Delta Cl_s = \Delta Cl_r \tag{4.83}$$

where $\Delta Cl_s = (Cl_s)_X - (Cl_s)_Y$ and $\Delta Cl_r = (Cl_r)_X - (Cl_r)_Y$. For each condition, total clearance is given by

$$(Cl_s)_X = \frac{FD}{AUC_X}$$

(4.84)

and

$$(Cl_s)_Y = \frac{FD}{AUC_Y}$$

(4.85)

where $F = F_X = F_Y$ and the dose $D = D_X = D_Y$. It follows that

$$\Delta Cl_r = \frac{FD}{AUC_X} - \frac{FD}{AUC_Y}$$

(4.86)

and

$$F = \frac{\Delta Cl_r}{D} \frac{AUC_X \cdot AUC_Y}{AUC_Y - AUC_X}$$

(4.87)

Since all the terms on the right-hand side of Eq. (4.87) can be determined from the two experiments, it is evident that under certain conditions F can be determined without resorting to an intravenous study.

This method was tested using intravenous furosemide data from a furosemide-probenecid interaction study [39]. If the method were valid, an F value of unity should be obtained. A mean value of $F = 1.05 \pm 0.11$ was determined. The method has also been used to estimate the availability of tocainide [40] and lithium [41].

Urinary Excretion Data

It is sometimes advantageous or necessary to determine systemic or relative availability from urinary excretion data. The basis for this determination is that the ratio of the total amount of unchanged drug excreted in the urine after oral administration to that following intravenous administration of the same dose is a measure of the absorption (systemic availability) of the drug. This relationship is valid for all linear models. Since

$$X_u^\infty = \frac{FDCl_r}{Cl_s}$$

(4.88)

it follows that

$$F = \frac{(X_u^\infty)_{oral}(Cl_s)_{oral}(Cl_r)_{i.v.} D_{i.v.}}{(X_u^\infty)_{i.v.}(Cl_s)_{i.v.}(Cl_r)_{oral} D_{oral}}$$

(4.89)

If we assume that there is a crossover design with a single panel of subjects and that there is no intrasubject variability in Cl_r and Cl_s from one study to the next, Eq. (4.89) reduces to

$$F = \frac{(X_u^\infty)_{oral} D_{i.v.}}{(X_u^\infty)_{i.v.} D_{oral}} \qquad (4.90)$$

or

$$F = \frac{(X_u^\infty)_{oral}}{(X_u^\infty)_{i.v.}} \qquad (4.91)$$

when equal doses are administered intravenously and orally. In a similar manner we can show under similar conditions that

$$F_r = \frac{(X_u^\infty)_{test}}{(X_u^\infty)_{standard}} \qquad (4.92)$$

An example of the data required to estimate relative bioavailability from urinary excretion studies is shown in Fig. 4.8.

The Kwan-Till method may be used in conjunction with urinary excretion data to reduce the standard deviation of the mean value of F or F_r. One of two corrections based on experimental estimates of renal clearance may be applied. First, one may assume that although renal clearance is different from one study to the next, this change is compensated for by changes in nonrenal clearance so that total (systemic) clearance is the same. In this case Eq. (4.89) reduces to

$$F = \frac{(X_u^\infty)_{oral}}{(X_u^\infty)_{i.v.}} \frac{D_{i.v.}}{D_{oral}} \frac{(Cl_r)_{i.v.}}{(Cl_r)_{oral}} \qquad (4.93)$$

Alternatively, one may assume that nonrenal clearance Cl_{nr} remains the same. In this case Eq. (4.89) may be written as

$$F = \frac{(X_u^\infty)_{oral}}{(X_u^\infty)_{i.v.}} \frac{D_{i.v.}}{D_{oral}} \frac{(Cl_{nr} + Cl_r)_{oral}(Cl_r)_{i.v.}}{(Cl_{nr} + Cl_r)_{i.v.}(Cl_r)_{oral}} \qquad (4.94)$$

Recognizing that nonrenal clearance is the difference between Cl_s and Cl_r and that $(Cl_{nr})_{oral} = (Cl_{nr})_{i.v.}$, we obtain

$$F = \frac{(X_u^\infty)_{oral}}{(X_u^\infty)_{i.v.}} \frac{D_{i.v.}}{D_{oral}} \frac{(Cl_s)_{i.v.} - (Cl_r)_{i.v.} + (Cl_r)_{oral}}{(Cl_s)_{i.v.} - (Cl_r)_{i.v.} + (Cl_r)_{i.v.}} \frac{(Cl_r)_{i.v.}}{(Cl_r)_{oral}}$$

$$(4.95)$$

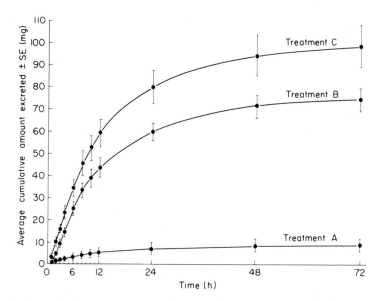

Fig. 4.8 Average cumulative amounts of tetracycline excreted in the urine of six subjects after a single 250 mg dose of the drug (see Ref. 42). The upper curve (C) was the result of administering an oral aqueous solution of the drug to fasting subjects. The middle curve (B) was observed after oral administration of the solution to the same subjects after breakfast. Curve A was obtained after rectal administration of the aqueous solution.

Rearrangement of Eq. (4.88) yields

$$(Cl_s)_{i.v.} = \frac{(Cl_r)_{i.v.}}{(f_u)_{i.v.}} \tag{4.96}$$

where $(f_u)_{i.v.} = (X_u^\infty)_{i.v.}/D_{i.v.}$. Substituting for Cl_s in Eq. (4.95) according to (4.96) and simplifying, we obtain

$$F = \frac{(X_u^\infty)_{oral}}{(X_u^\infty)_{i.v.}} \, \frac{D_{i.v.}}{D_{oral}} \, \frac{(Cl_r/f_u)_{i.v.} - (Cl_r)_{i.v.} + (Cl_r)_{oral}}{(Cl_r/f_u)_{i.v.}}$$

$$\times \frac{(Cl_r)_{i.v.}}{(Cl_r)_{oral}} \tag{4.97}$$

which further simplifies to

$$F = \frac{(X_u^\infty)_{oral}}{(X_u^\infty)_{i.v.}} \, \frac{D_{i.v.}}{D_{oral}} \, \frac{(Cl_r/f_u)_{i.v.} - (Cl_r)_{i.v.} + (Cl_r)_{oral}}{(Cl_r)_{oral}/(f_u)_{i.v.}} \tag{4.98}$$

The principal drawback in using urinary excretion data for estimating availability is the need for collecting urine until virtually all of the drug has been excreted. With some drugs this may require several days of collection. Some investigators have observed with certain drugs that the ratio of amounts excreted over a relatively short period of time after administration of two formulations is similar to the ratio obtained on prolonged urine collection. For example, Greenblatt et al. [43] found that the 1-day and 6-day excretion of digoxin after intravenous and oral administration of many preparations were highly correlated (r = 0.94) and the overall variability in the two measures was nearly identical, despite the fact that less than half of the cumulative 6-day urinary digoxin excretion was recovered on the first day of collection. A similar observation has been made by Bates and Sequeira [44] with respect to the urinary excretion of total 6-desmethylgriseofulvin after administration of more than 20 formulations of griseofulvin which varied about fourfold in availability (see Fig. 4.9). Theory predicts that the ratio of amounts excreted in the urine in a comparative bioavailability study are asymptotic with time. For drugs with long half-lives and for formulations from which these drugs are relatively rapidly absorbed, the ratio will closely approximate the asymptotic value long before the drug is completely excreted. The use of partial urine collections for estimating comparative bioavailability may be appropriate if the pharmacokinetics of the drug are well characterized, but the prospective use of this method requires too many assumptions to be reasonable.

Systemic or relative availability of a drug may also be estimated from urinary excretion data at steady state. In theory the amount excreted over a dosing interval at steady state is equal to the total amount excreted to infinity after a single dose of the drug. Therefore,

$$F_r = \frac{(X_u^{ss})_{test}}{(X_u^{ss})_{standard}} \qquad (4.99)$$

where X_u^{ss} denotes the amount of drug excreted in the urine from time zero to τ during any dosing interval at steady state. Equation (4.99) assumes that the dosage regimen was the same for both studies. A principal advantage of steady-state studies compared to single-dose studies is that the urine collection period is bounded by the dosing interval. Patients or normal subjects may be crossed over from one formulation to another without a drug washout period but, on a change of formulation, the drug must be given for four to seven elimination half-lives before determining X_u^{ss} to assure that the new steady state has been reached. Table 4.6 compares the bioavailability of digoxin from different formulations as estimated from the area under serum

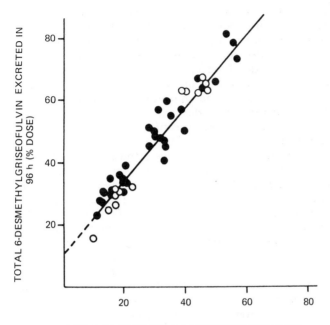

TOTAL 6-DESMETHYLGRISEOFULVIN EXCRETED
IN 24 h (% DOSE)

Fig. 4.9 Relationship between 24 h and 96 h cumulative urinary excretion of 6-desmethylgriseofulvin after a single 500 mg dose of griseofulvin in various products to healthy volunteers. In the case of
griseofulvin it appears that bioavailability estimates based on a 24 h
urine collection are equivalent to those based on a complete (96 h)
collection of urine. $y = 1.20x + 11.2$, $n = 47$, $r = 0.965$, $P < 0.001$.
(From Ref. 44, reprinted with permission.)

digoxin concentration-time curves over a dosing interval at steady
state and from steady-state digoxin excretion in urine.

**Bioavailability Estimates Based on Radioactivity, Nonspecific Assays,
or Metabolite Levels**

In the early studies of a new drug candidate, a specific assay may not
be available at a time when one wishes to evaluate the absorption of
the drug from test formulations. In this case it is not uncommon for
investigators to use nonspecific assays which detect drug as well as
one or more metabolites (i.e., "apparent" drug) or to administer
radiolabeled drug and to determine total radioactivity in plasma or
urine. Nonspecific assays have also been applied to drugs that are
used in very small doses and have relatively large apparent volumes

of distribution, so that drug concentrations in plasma are unusually
low and below the sensitivity of common assay methods. Some bioavailability studies have been based on the appearance of a major
metabolite of the drug in plasma or urine. This is often the case
when a drug is very rapidly metabolized and intact drug is difficult
or impossible to detect.

For linear pharmacokinetic systems, estimates of relative availability based on the area under the concentration of total radioactivity,
apparent drug, or metabolite in plasma versus time curve or based
on cumulative urinary excretion of total radioactivity, apparent drug
or metabolite may provide a useful measure of the relative performance
of the test formulation. The use of nonspecific assays is not appropriate for nonlinear systems. In such cases the total area under the
intact drug concentration in plasma-time curve is a function of the
rate of absorption and the amount absorbed, and estimates of availability based on total radioactivity or other nonspecific methods may be
misleading. Nonspecific assays should never be used for estimating
systemic or absolute availability. The approach fails to detect pre-
systemic metabolism in the gut or liver during absorption since drug
and metabolites are not differentiated. Consequently, systemic
availability will be overestimated.

Many other useful comments regarding the use of isotopes in bio-
abailability studies are found in a scientific commentary by Riegelman
et al. [45].

STATISTICAL CONSIDERATIONS IN COMPARATIVE BIOAVAILABILITY STUDIES

An aspect of bioavailability testing that is of concern to the scientist
and that has broad socioeconomic implications is the interpretation of
the results. Metzler notes that very often bioavailability is a problem
in equivalence [46]. Is the test formulation equivalent to the standard?
What constitutes inequivalence? The answers to these questions must
be based on a consideration of pharmacokinetics, clinical implications,
and statistics. An extensive discussion of the subject is beyond the
scope of this text, but a limited consideration is appropriate. The
reader is referred to commentaries by Metzler [46] and Westlake [47]
for a more detailed treatment.

The traditional statistical methodology which has been applied to
scientific experiments is designed to show that a difference exists
between two treatments. The null hypothesis of no difference is
formulated in the expectation that the results of the experiment will
be inconsistent with the null hypothesis and the alternative hypothesis
of some difference could be accepted. If this is not the case, we accept the null hypothesis, which is quite different from proving it.

Bioavailability studies present some nontraditional problems.
Sometimes we are interested in proving that the test formulation is

Table 4.7 Comparison of Confidence Interval and Hypothesis Testing (see Ref. 46)

Test Formulation	Results of Experiment: Comparative Bioavailability of Test Formulation to Standard Formulation with 95% Confidence Limits (Statistical)	Confidence Limit (95%) Criterion for Acceptance and Decision Reached by a Knowledgeable Pharmacologist, Physician, etc.	Decision Based on Hypothesis Testing, $\alpha = 0.05$ One-sided test
		Drug A: *Lower limit must be 80% or more*	
A-1	92% (82% or more)	Acceptable	Acceptable
A-2	92% (85% or more)	Acceptable because lower limit exceeds 80%	Unacceptable
A-3	100% (55% or more)	100% looks good, but data are insufficient, unacceptable	Acceptable

A-4	95% (78% or more)	Unacceptable because the lower limit is less than 80%; may become acceptable with more data	Acceptable
A-5	120% (105% or more)	Acceptable, even though more available than standard, because lower limit is greater than 80%	Acceptable
		Drug B: Lower limit must be greater than 85%, and upper limit must be less than 115%	*Two-sided test*
B-6	105% (97% and 113%)	Acceptable	Acceptable
B-7	110% (95% and 125%)	Unacceptable because upper limit is greater than 115%	Acceptable
B-8	96% (93% and 99%)	Acceptable	Unacceptable

different from the standard, but at other times we are interested in
"proving" that they are equivalent. Obviously, the most expedient
approach to accepting the null hypothesis is poorly designed experiments with few subjects and large variability. Even in the more
traditional situation where we are seeking differences between formulations we may find statistically significant differences that are in
fact trivial from a clinical point of view. What we really want to learn
from all bioavailability studies, irrespective of our expectation, is
the difference between the test formulation and the standard and
whether or not the difference is acceptable. The latter is largely a
clinical question but also of concern to compendias and others who
are interested in establishing standards. Thus it appears reasonable
to conclude that the evaluation of bioavailability data should be based
on a confidence interval method rather than hypothesis testing [46,
47]. The clinician or some other appropriate party can specify that
the bioavailability of the new formulation relative to the standard must
be within a certain range and that this must be known with a certain
level of confidence. For example, it might be specified that, with
95% confidence, the new formulation should be between 80 and 120% as
available as the standard. A comparison of decisions based on confidence intervals and hypothesis testing for several comparative bioavailability studies is presented in Table 4.7. If it is known that the
standard formulation is completely available, it is only necessary to
specify lower limits for the formulation (see drug A in Table 4.7).
In most cases both lower and upper limits would be specified (see
drug B in Table 4.7). The confidence interval method is gaining wide
acceptance as the appropriate statistical approach for evaluating
comparative bioavailability studies.

SUSTAINED RELEASE

The therapeutic index TI of a drug has classically been defined as
the ratio of the median toxic or lethal dose to the median effective
dose. For clinical purposes, a better definition is the ratio of the
maximum drug concentration in plasma at which the patient is free of
adverse effects of the drug to the minimum drug concentration in
plasma required to elicit a minimally adequate therapeutic response.
In principle, a drug should be given with sufficient frequency so
that the ratio of maximum to minimum drug concentrations in plasma
at steady state is less than the therapeutic index and at a high enough
dose to produce effective concentrations [48]. For a linear, one-
compartment system with repetitive intravenous dosing (constant dose,
constant dosing interval τ) the ratio of maximum to minimum drug
concentrations in plasma at steady state is given by

$$\frac{C_{max}^{ss}}{C_{min}^{ss}} = e^{K\tau} \qquad (4.100)$$

where K is the first-order elimination rate constant. It follows that

$$e^{K\tau} \le TI \tag{4.101}$$

and

$$\tau \le t_{1/2} \frac{\ln TI}{\ln 2} \tag{4.102}$$

where TI is the therapeutic index. When the therapeutic index of a drug is 2, the dosing interval should be equal to no more than one biologic half-life of the drug. For drugs with short half-lives ($t_{1/2} \le 6$ h) and low therapeutic indices ($TI \le 3$), the proper dosing schedule requires the drug to be given unreasonably frequently. This situation prevails with theophylline and procainamide, among other drugs. Sustained-release dosage forms may alleviate this problem, since the slower the absorption of a drug, the smaller the ratio of C_{max} to C_{min} over a dosing interval at steady state. In theory a drug that must be given every 3 h at a dose of 100 mg can be given every 6 h (D = 200 mg), every 12 h (D = 400 mg), or every 24 h (D = 800 mg) simply by reducing the absorption rate constant of the drug to maintain the C_{max} to C_{min} ratio. This may be accomplished by modifying the formulation to reduce the release rate of drug relative to that of a conventional formulation. Many sustained-release products are commercially available from which drug is absorbed in an apparent first-order fashion but at a considerably lower rate than observed after conventional tablets or capsules (see Fig. 4.10).

Although mathematical theory sets no limit as to how infrequently we can give a drug in a sustained-release formulation, a very stringent limit is imposed on oral formulations by the finite time over which a drug may be absorbed in the gastrointestinal tract after administration. The literature on drug absorption, gastric emptying, and intestinal motility suggests to us that within 9 to 12 h after administration of most prolonged-release dosage forms, the drug will be at a site in the intestine from which absorption is poor and ineffective. With this effective absorption time range in mind, it follows that the maximum absorption half-life should be 3 to 4 h. Formulations that release drug more slowly are likely to result in unacceptably low availability in a significant number of patients. In principle, a formulation that releases a well-absorbed drug in a first-order fashion with a half-life of 4 h will result in bioavailabilities ranging from about 80 to 90% of the dose if absorption time is limited to 9 to 12 h. A formulation with a 3 h half-life for drug release yields availabilities of about 90 to 95% of the dose over these absorption times. Shorter effective absorption times require still more conservative estimates of maximum half-lives.

Assuming maximum absorption half-lives of 3 or 4 h, to ensure adequate availability, we have calculated C_{max} to C_{min} ratios at

Table 4.8 Calculated Steady-State Data for Drugs with Different Elimination Half-Lives Given in One of Two Sustained-Release Formulations (see Ref. 50)

Elimination Half-Life (h)	Dose	τ	t_{max}^{ss}	C_{max}^{ss}	C_{min}^{ss}	$C_{max}^{ss}/C_{min}^{ss}$
		Formulation A: release half-time = 3 h				
1.98	400	8	2.6	17.3	9.5	1.8
	600	12	3.1	20.7	6.0	3.4
	1200	24	3.5	35.6	0.9	41.0
3.15	400	8	2.9	25.8	17.5	1.5
	600	12	3.6	29.4	12.8	2.3
	1200	24	4.3	46.4	3.0	15.3
4.01	400	8	3.0	31.9	23.5	1.4
	600	12	3.8	35.6	18.4	1.9
	1200	24	4.8	53.2	5.8	9.2
4.95	400	8	3.0	38.7	30.2	1.3
	600	12	4.0	42.4	24.8	1.7
	1200	24	5.2	60.3	9.8	6.2
5.97	400	8	3.1	46.1	37.5	1.2
	600	12	4.1	49.8	31.9	1.6
	1200	24	5.5	67.1	15.0	4.5

4 / Absorption Kinetics and Bioavailability

Formulation B: release half-time = 4 h

1.98	400	8	2.7	16.5	10.6	1.6
	600	12	3.3	19.1	7.6	2.5
	1200	24	3.9	30.4	1.9	15.8
3.15	400	8	3.0	25.0	18.7	1.3
	600	12	3.8	27.7	14.8	1.9
	1200	24	4.9	40.4	4.9	8.2
4.01	400	8	3.1	31.2	24.8	1.3
	600	12	4.1	33.9	20.6	1.6
	1200	24	5.4	47.6	8.2	5.8
4.95	400	8	3.2	38.0	31.5	1.2
	600	12	4.2	40.7	27.1	1.5
	1200	24	5.9	54.7	12.8	4.3
5.97	400	8	3.2	45.4	38.9	1.2
	600	12	4.4	48.1	34.2	1.4
	1200	24	6.2	62.2	18.4	3.4

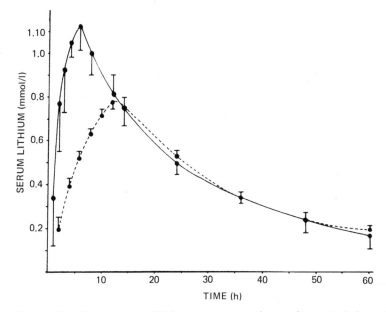

Fig. 4.10 Mean serum lithium concentrations after administration of a single 1.8 g dose to four manic patients (see Ref. 49). The drug was given either as a conventional preparation (——) or as a sustained-release preparation (---).

steady state for drugs with elimination half-lives ranging from 1 to 6 h given at a dosing rate of 50 mg/h at intervals of 8, 12, or 24 h. The maximum concentration in plasma at steady state was determined from

$$C_{max}^{ss} = \frac{D}{V} \frac{1}{1 - e^{-K\tau}} e^{-Kt_{max}^{ss}} \tag{4.103}$$

assuming complete absorption, where

$$t_{max}^{ss} = \frac{2.3 \log [k_a(1 - e^{-K\tau})/K(1 - e^{-k_a\tau})]}{k_a - K} \tag{4.104}$$

and the minimum concentration in plasma at steady state from

$$C_{min}^{ss} = \frac{k_a D}{V(k_a - K)} \left(\frac{1}{1 - e^{-K\tau}} e^{-K\tau} - \frac{1}{1 - e^{-k_a\tau}} e^{-k_a\tau} \right) \tag{4.105}$$

The results are summarized in Table 4.8. It is evident, in general, that drugs with short half-lives and low therapeutic indices must be given no less frequently than twice a day. Once-a-day dosing with sustained-release dosage forms is appropriate for drugs with higher therapeutic indices or with longer half-lives. However, the need for sustained release formulations of such drugs is not as great since adequate therapy can be achieved at reasonable dosing intervals.

Drugs with pronounced multicompartment characteristics after oral administration often show large C_{max} to C_{min} ratios. Some must be dosed at intervals considerably less than the biologic half-life to avoid adverse effects that are associated with high drug concentrations in plasma (central compartment). A relatively modest reduction in the absorption rate constant of such drugs by appropriate formulation may substantially reduce the maximum to minimum drug concentrations in plasma at steady state and may permit considerably less frequent administration of the drug. In essence, the reduced absorption rate may eliminate the "spike" of drug concentration in plasma associated with rapid absorption and slow distribution [50]. The principal advantage of less frequent drug administration is the potential improvement in patient compliance with the prescribed regimen.

Pharmacokinetic theory suggests that the ultimate method for reducing the C_{max} to C_{min} ratio is to have zero-order absorption. Once steady state is achieved under these conditions, drug concentration in plasma is constant as long as absorption persists. Several

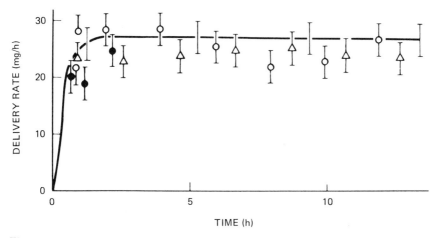

Fig. 4.11 In vitro (——) and in vivo ($\triangle$, $\bigcirc$, $\bullet$) release rates of potassium chloride from a dosage form that utilizes the principle of the elementary osmotic pump. The in vivo data were obtained in three different dogs. Bars show experimental error. (From Ref. 54, reprinted with permission.)

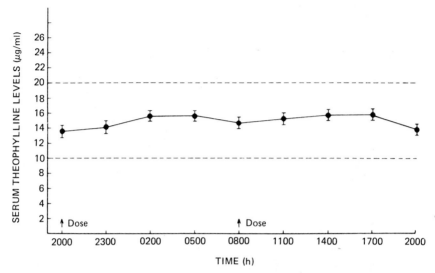

Fig. 4.12 Mean steady-state serum levels of theophylline in 20 asthmat-
ic children who were receiving an oral sustained-release preparation
of the drug every 12 h. The very small difference between peak and
trough concentrations suggests that absorption of the drug from this
dosage form can be described, at least on the average, by zero-
order kinetics. (From Ref. 55. © 1980 American Academy of
Pediatrics.)

investigators have discussed the application of pharmacokinetic principles to the design of sustained-release formulations that release
drug in a zero-order fashion [51–53]. An example of such a system
is the elementary osmotic pump [54]. The in vivo release rate of KCl
from this dosage form in the gastrointestinal tract of dogs is shown
in Fig. 4.11. Such dosage forms, however, are still limited by considerations of effective residence time of drug at absorption sites in
the gastrointestinal tract. Accordingly, a drug with a short half-
life must usually be given no less frequently than twice a day.

    In our view the most important criteria for the evaluation of
sustained-release products are bioavailability and C_{max} to C_{min} ratios
at steady state. It is certainly desirable to have a bioavailability of
at least 80% relative to the conventional dosage form. Where appropriate, the peak-to-trough ratio at steady state should be no greater
than the therapeutic index of the drug. In all cases, this ratio
should not exceed that observed after repetitive administration of
the conventional dosage form at shorter intervals. The data in Fig.
4.12 indicate exemplary performance of a sustained-release product
of theophylline. The C_{max} to C_{min} ratio at steady state resulting from

administration of this dosage form every 12 h is smaller than that found on administration of a conventional dosage form of theophylline every 6 h.

REFERENCES

1. R. E. Notari, J. L. DeYoung, and R. H. Reuning. Effect of parallel first-order drug loss from site of administration on calculated values for absorption rate constants. *J. Pharm. Sci.* *61*:135 (1972).
2. J. A. Clements, R. C. Heading, W. S. Nimmo, and L. F. Prescott. Kinetics of acetaminophen absorption and gastric emptying in man. *Clin. Pharmacol. Ther.* *24*:420 (1978).
3. D. Perrier and M. Gibaldi. Calculation of absorption rate constants for drugs with incomplete availability. *J. Pharm. Sci.* *62*:225 (1973).
4. R. A. Ronfeld and L. Z. Benet. Interpretation of plasma concentration-time curves after oral dosing. *J. Pharm. Sci.* *66*:178 (1977).
5. J. G. Wagner. "Absorption rate constants" calculated according to the one-compartment open model with first-order absorption: Implications in in vivo-in vitro correlations. *J. Pharm. Sci.* *59*:1049 (1970).
6. J. G. Wagner and E. Nelson. Kinetic analysis of blood levels and urinary excretion in the absorptive phase after single doses of drug. *J. Pharm. Sci.* *53*:1392 (1964).
7. J. C. K. Loo and S. Riegelman. New Method for calculating the intrinsic absorption rate of drugs. *J. Pharm. Sci.* *57*:918 (1968).
8. E. Nelson. Per cent absorbed versus time plots from metabolite level in blood. *J. Pharm. Sci.* *54*:1075 (1965).
9. J. G. Wagner. Method for estimating rate constants for absorption, metabolism, and elimination from urinary excretion data. *J. Pharm. Sci.* *56*:489 (1967).
10. J. G. Wagner. *Fundamentals of Clinical Pharmacokinetics.* Drug Intelligence Publications, Hamilton, Ill., 1975.
11. H. G. Boxenbaum and S. A. Kaplan. Potential source of error in absorption rate calculations. *J. Pharmacokinet. Biopharm.* *3*:257 (1975).
12. J. G. Wagner. Application of the Loo-Riegelman absorption method. *J. Pharmacokinet. Biopharm.* *3*:51 (1975).
13. J. M. Strong, J. S. Dutcher, W. K. Lee, and A. J. Atkinson, Jr. Absolute bioavailability in man of N-acetylprocainamide determined by a novel stable isotope method. *Clin. Pharmacol. Ther.* *18*:613 (1975).

14. P. J. Murphy and H. R. Sullivan. Stable isotopes in pharmacokinetic studies. *Annu. Rev. Pharmacol. Toxicol.* *20*:609
(1980).

15. A. Rescigno and G. Segre. *Drug and Tracer Kinetics.* Blaisdell, Waltham, Mass., 1966.

16. J. G. Wagner. Do you need a pharmacokinetic model, and, if
so, which one? *J. Pharmacokinet. Biopharm.* *3*:457 (1975).

17. D. P. Vaughan and M. Dennis. Mathematical basis of point-
area deconvolution method for determining in vivo input functions. *J. Pharm. Sci.* *67*:663 (1978).

18. L. Z. Benet and C.-W. N. Chiang. The use of deconvolution
methods in pharmacokinetics. In *Abstracts of Papers Presented
at the 13th National Meeting of the APhA Academy of Pharmaceutical Sciences,* vol. 2, Chicago, 1972, p. 169.

19. D. P. Vaughan. A model independent method for estimating
the in vivo release rate constant of a drug from its oral formulations. *J. Pharm. Pharmacol.* *28*:505 (1976).

20. J. G. Wagner, P. G. Welling, S. B. Roth, E. Sakmar, K. P.
Lee, and J. E. Walker. Plasma concentrations of propoxyphene
in man following oral administration of the drug in solution and
capsule forms. *Int. J. Clin. Pharmacol.* *5*:371 (1972).

21. D. Perrier and M. Gibaldi. Influence of first-pass effect on the
systemic availability of propoxyphene. *J. Clin. Pharmacol.*
12:449 (1972).

22. R. L. Slaughter, J. A. Pieper, F. B. Cerra, B. Brodsky, and
J. R. Koup. Chloramphenical sodium succinate kinetics in
critically ill patients. *Clin. Pharmacol. Ther.* *28*:69 (1980).

23. A. J. Glazko, A. W. Kinkel, W. C. Alegnani, and G. L. Holmes.
An evaluation of the absorption characteristics of different
chloramphenicol preparations in normal human subjects. *Clin.
Pharmacol. Ther.* *9*:472 (1968).

24. J. G. Wagner. Method of estimating relative absorption of a
drug in a series of clinical studies in which blood levels are
measured after single and/or multiple doses. *J. Pharm. Sci.*
56:652 (1967).

25. J. R. Koup and M. Gibaldi. Some comments on the evaluation
of bioavailability data. *Drug. Intell. Clin. Pharm.* *14*:327
(1980).

26. K. C. Kwan and A. E. Till. Novel method for bioavailability
assessment. *J. Pharm. Sci.* *62*:1494 (1973).

27. J. Ekstrand, M. Ehrenbo, and L. O. Boreus. Fluoride bioavailability after intravenous and oral administration: Importance
of renal clearance and urine flow. *Clin. Pharmacol. Ther.*
23:329 (1978).

28. S. Hwang and K. C. Kwan. Further considerations on model-
independent bioavailability estimation. *J. Pharm. Sci.* *69*:77
(1980).

29. A. E. Till, L. Z. Benet, and K. C. Kwan. An integrated approach to the pharmacokinetic analysis of drug absorption. *J. Pharmacokinet. Biopharm.* *2*:525 (1974).

30. K. C. Yeh and K. C. Kwan. A comparison of numerical integrating algorithms by trapezoidal, Lagrange, and spline approximation. *J. Pharmacokinet. Biopharm.* *6*:79 (1978).

31. E. G. Lovering, I. J. McGilveray, I. McMillan, and W. Tostowaryk. Comparative bioavailabilities from truncated blood level curves. *J. Pharm. Sci.* *64*:1521 (1975).

32. K. C. Kwan, J. V. Bondi, and K. C. Yeh. Bioavailability assessment under quasi- and nonsteady-state conditions: I. Theoretical considerations. *J. Pharm. Sci.* *64*:1639 (1975).

33. K. C. Yeh and K. C. Kwan. Bioavailability assessment under quasi- and nonsteady-state conditions: II. Study design. *J. Pharm. Sci.* *65*:512 (1976).

34. J. V. Bondi, H. B. Hucker, K. C. Yeh, and K. C. Kwan. Bioavailability assessment under quasi- and nonsteady-state conditions: III. Application. *J. Pharm. Sci.* *65*:1657 (1976).

35. J. G. Wagner, M. Christensen, E. Sakmar, D. Blair, J. D. Yates, P. W. Willis, A. J. Sedman, and R. G. Stoll. Equivalence lack in digoxin plasma levels. *JAMA* *224*:199 (1973).

36. D. H. Huffman, C. V. Manion, and D. L. Azarnoff. Absorption of digoxin from different oral preparations in normal subjects during steady-state. *Clin. Pharmacol. Ther.* *16*:310 (1974).

37. T. Huynh-Ngoc, M. Chabot, and G. Sirois. Bioavailability of three commercial sustained-release tablets of quinidine in maintenance therapy. *J. Pharm. Sci.* *67*:1456 (1978).

38. D. Lalka and H. Feldman. Absolute drug bioavailability: Approximation without comparison to parenteral dose for compounds exhibiting perturbable renal clearance. *J. Pharm. Sci.* *63*:1813 (1974).

39. D. Lalka, P. duSouich, A. J. McLean, and M. Gibaldi. Absolute drug bioavailability: II. Evaluation of renal clearance perturbation method using literature data assuring a fraction absorbed of unity. *J. Pharm. Sci.* *67*:591 (1978).

40. D. Lalka, M. B. Meyer, B. R. Duce, and A. T. Elvin. Kinetics of the oral antiarrhythmic lidocaine congener, tocainide. *Clin. Pharmacol. Ther.* *19*:757 (1976).

41. R. I. Poust, A. G. Mallinger, J. Mallinger, J. M. Himmelhoch, J. F. Neil, and I. Hanin. Absolute availability of lithium. *J. Pharm. Sci.* *6*:609 (1977).

42. J. G. Wagner, L. G. Leslie, and R. S. Grove. Relative absorption of both tetracycline and penicillin G administered rectally and orally in aqueous solution. *Int. J. Clin. Pharmacol.* *2*:44 (1969).

43. D. J. Greenblatt, D. W. Duhme, J. Koch-Weser, and T. W.
    Smith. Comparison of one- and six-day urinary digoxin excre-
    tion in single dose bioavailability studies. *Clin. Pharmacol.
    Ther.* *16*:813 (1974).
44. T. R. Bates and J. A. L. Sequeira. Use of 24 hr. urinary
    excretion data to assess bioavailability of griseofulvin in
    humans. *J. Pharm. Sci.* *64*:709 (1975).
45. S. Riegelman, M. Rowland, and L. Z. Benet. Use of isotopes
    in bioavailability testing. *J. Pharmacokinet. Biopharm.* *1*:83
    (1973).
46. C. M. Metzler. Bioavailability—A problem in equivalence.
    Biometrics *30*:309 (1974).
47. W. J. Westlake. The design and analysis of comparative blood-
    level trials. In *Current Concepts in the Pharmaceutical Sciences:
    Dosage Form Design and Bioavailability,* J. Swarbrick (Ed.),
    Lea & Febiger, Philadelphia, 1973.
48. F. Theeuwes and W. Bayne. Dosage form index: An objective
    criterion for evaluation of controlled-release drug delivery
    systems. *J. Pharm. Sci.* *66*:1388 (1977).
49. D. P. Thornhill. Pharmacokinetics of ordinary and sustained-
    release lithium carbonate in manic patients after acute dosage.
    Eur. J. Clin. Pharmacol. *15*:267 (1978).
50. M. Gibaldi and P. J. McNamara. Steady-state concentrations
    of drugs with short half-lives when administered in oral sus-
    tained-release formulations. *Int. J. Pharm.* *2*:167 (1979).
51. M. Rowland and A. H. Beckett. Mathematical treatment of
    oral sustained release drug formulations. *J. Pharm. Pharma-
    col.* *16*:156T (1964).
52. J. R. Robinson and S. P. Erikson. Theoretical formulations
    of sustained-release dosage forms. *J. Pharm. Sci.* *55*:1254
    (1966).
53. M. R. Dobrinska and P. G. Welling. Blood levels from a
    sustained-release dosage form. *J. Pharm. Sci.* *64*:1728
    (1975).
54. F. Theeuwes. Elementary osmotic pump. *J. Pharm. Sci.*
    64:1987 (1975).
55. H. W. Kelly and S. Murphy. Efficacy of a 12-hour sustained-
    release preparation in maintaining therapeutic serum theophyl-
    line levels in asthmatic children. *Pediatrics* *66*:97 (1980).

5

Apparent Volume of Distribution

The proportionality constant relating drug concentration in blood or plasma to the amount of drug in the body has been termed the apparent volume of distribution. There has been considerable confusion concerning the estimation and meaning of the apparent volume of distribution of a drug. A principal cause of this confusion is the fact that there is no obvious relationship between the apparent and real volume of distribution of a drug.

The real distribution volume of a drug is related to body water and cannot exceed total body water (i.e., about 58% of body weight in the normal adult human). Body water may be divided into at least three distinct compartments: the vascular fluid or blood, the extracellular fluid, and the intracellular fluid. In humans, extracellular fluid is about one-third of total body water and includes the plasma, which is about 4% of body weight. Blood volume, which includes the intracellular fluid of the erythrocytes and other formed elements, is about twice the plasma volume.

Some high molecular weight substances, such as Evans blue or indocyanine green, are essentially confined to the circulating plasma after intravenous administration and can be used to estimate plasma volume (or blood volume if the hematocrit is determined). Certain ions, such as chloride or bromide, rapidly distribute throughout the extracellular fluid but do not easily cross cell membranes, so they may be used to estimate extracellular water. The volume of total body water may be estimated by means of heavy water or certain lipid-soluble substances, such as antipyrine, which distribute rapidly throughout the total body water.

The apparent volume of distribution of each of these tracers approximates its true volume of distribution because binding to plasma proteins and tissues is negligible. For most substances this is not the case. Most drugs are significantly bound in either the vascular or extravascular space, or both. Drugs that are predominantly bound to plasma proteins have apparent volumes of distribution that are

smaller than their real volumes of distribution, whereas drugs that
are predominantly bound to extravascular tissues have apparent volumes of distribution that are larger than their real distribution space.
For different drugs, volumes of distribution may range from about
0.04 to more than 20 liters/kg.

RELATIONSHIP BETWEEN VOLUME OF DISTRIBUTION, DRUG BINDING AND ELIMINATION, AND ANATOMIC VOLUME

A quantitative expression relating apparent volume of distribution,
real distribution space, and binding may be developed using the model
shown in Fig. 5.1. The model consists of two physiologic spaces, the
vascular or blood space and the extravascular or tissue space. Linear
binding occurs in both spaces and the concentration of free drug is
the same throughout the total body water. After administration of
drug into the vascular space by intravenous bolus injection, distribution is assumed to be instantaneous. Elimination occurs in a first-

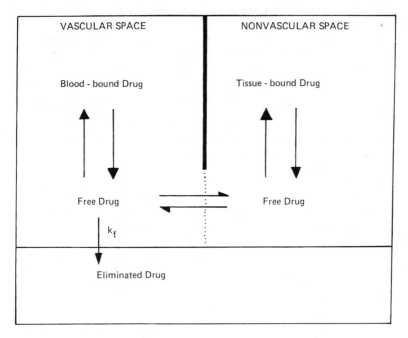

Fig. 5.1 One-compartment pharmacokinetic model with two linear binding sites. Initially, a bolus dose of drug is introduced in the vascular
space; binding and distribution is assumed to be instantaneous. The
rate of drug elimination is given by the product of k_f and free drug
concentration.

order fashion at a rate proportional to the free drug concentration.
The model is, in one sense, a one-compartment system in that drug
distribution between the two physiologic spaces is assumed to be instantaneous. However, in another sense, the model is a two-compartment system since vascular binding sites (such as plasma proteins)
and tissue binding sites are restricted to separate spaces.

In the case of linear binding in the vascular space (blood),

$$C_{Bb} = bC_f \tag{5.1}$$

and

$$A_{Bb} = bV_B C_f = bA_{Bf} \tag{5.2}$$

where C_{Bb} is the concentration of drug bound in the blood at time t;
b is a proportionality constant relating free (unbound) drug concentration C_f to bound drug concentration in the blood; A_{Bb} and A_{Bf}
are the amounts of drug bound and free, respectively, in the blood
at time t; and V_B is blood volume.

Since the free drug concentration at any time is the same throughout the system, it follows that the amount of free drug in the blood
is given by

$$A_{Bf} = \frac{V_B}{V_f} A_f \tag{5.3}$$

where V_f is the volume of distribution of free (unbound) drug and is
equal to the sum of V_B and V_T (where V_T is the volume of the tissue
or extravascular space), and A_f is the amount of free drug in the
body at time t. It follows that

$$A_{Bb} = b \frac{V_B}{V_f} A_f \tag{5.4}$$

In the case of linear binding in the extravascular space,

$$C_{Tb} = BC_f \tag{5.5}$$

and

$$A_{Tb} = BV_T C_f = BA_{Tf} \tag{5.6}$$

where C_{Tb} is the concentration of drug bound in the extravascular
space at time t; B is a proportionality constant relating free drug
concentration to bound drug concentration in the extravascular space;
A_{Tb} and A_{Tf} are the amounts of drug bound and free, respectively,
in the extravascular space at time t; and V_T is the volume of the
extravascular space. Since the free drug concentration at any time
is the same in both spaces, it follows that

$$A_{Tf} = \frac{V_T}{V_f} A_f \tag{5.7}$$

and

$$A_{Tb} = B \frac{V_T}{V_f} A_f \tag{5.8}$$

At any time after administration, the entire dose D can be accounted for by the sum of the amounts bound in the vascular and extravascular space, the amount of free drug in the body, and the amount eliminated:

$$D = A_f + A_{Bb} + A_{Tb} + k_f \int_0^t A_f \, dt \tag{5.9}$$

where k_f is the first-order elimination rate constant and the term $k_f \int_0^t A_f \, dt$ represents the amount eliminated up to time t. Differentiation of Eq. (5.9) with respect to time yields

$$\frac{dA_f}{dt} + \frac{dA_{Bb}}{dt} + \frac{dA_{Tb}}{dt} + k_f A_f = 0 \tag{5.10}$$

By differentiating Eqs. (5.4) and (5.8), we obtain

$$\frac{dA_{Bb}}{dt} = b \frac{V_B}{V_f} \frac{dA_f}{dt} \tag{5.11}$$

and

$$\frac{dA_{Tb}}{dt} = B \frac{V_T}{V_f} \frac{dA_f}{dt} \tag{5.12}$$

Therefore, Eq. (5.10) may be transformed to

$$\frac{dA_f}{dt} \left(1 + b \frac{V_B}{V_f} + B \frac{V_T}{V_f} \right) + k_f A_f = 0 \tag{5.13}$$

Rearrangement yields

$$\frac{-dA_f}{dt} \left(1 + b \frac{V_B}{V_f} + B \frac{V_T}{V_f} \right) = k_f A_f \tag{5.14}$$

Since $A_f = V_f C_f$, it follows that

$$\frac{-dC_f}{dt} = \frac{k_f}{1 + b(V_B/V_f) + B(V_B/V_f)} C_f = \beta C_f \tag{5.15}$$

where β is the apparent elimination rate constant and is given by

$$\beta = \frac{k_f}{1 + b(V_B/V_f) + B(V_T/V_f)}$$ (5.16)

If we define a new term, f, as the fraction of the total amount of drug in the body which is free, then

$$f = \frac{A_f}{A_f + A_{Bb} + A_{Tb}} = \frac{1}{1 + (A_{Bb}/A_f) + (A_{Tb}/A_f)}$$ (5.17)

Rearranging Eq. (5.4) gives a term for A_{Bb}/A_f and rearranging Eq. (5.8) gives a term for A_{Tb}/A_f. Substituting these terms in Eq. (5.17) yields

$$f = \frac{1}{1 + b(V_B/V_f) + B(V_T/V_f)}$$ (5.18)

Substituting this expression in Eq. (5.16) gives

$$\beta = fk_f$$ (5.19)

It is evident that the apparent elimination rate constant β is the product of the instrinsic elimination rate constant for free drug k_f and the fraction of the total amount of drug in the body that is free, f. Ordinarily, we cannot measure f in humans and it is very difficult to measure in animals. On the other hand, we can determine the fraction free in the vascular space (i.e., the fraction unbound in blood) by relatively simple binding experiments. This parameter, f_B, is defined as

$$f_B = \frac{C_f}{C_f + C_{Bb}} = \frac{V_B C_f}{V_B C_f + V_B C_{Bb}} = \frac{A_{Bf}}{A_{Bf} + A_{Bb}}$$ (5.20)

Comparison of Eqs. (5.17) and (5.20) suggests that the relationship between f and f_B is complex and nonlinear. It follows that β will not be a linear function of f_B.

Integration of Eq. (5.15) yields

$$C_f = C_f^\circ e^{-\beta t}$$ (5.21)

where C_f° is the concentration of free drug at time zero (i.e., immediately after injection).

The total drug concentration in the blood C_B is given by

$$C_B = C_f + C_{Bb} = C_f + bC_f = (1 + b)C_f$$ (5.22)

It follows that

$$C_B = C_B^\circ e^{-\beta t}$$ (5.23)

The initial condition at time zero for the model is given by the equation

$$A_f^o + A_{Tb}^o + A_{Bb}^o = D \qquad (5.24)$$

The ratio of A_B^o to dose D is

$$\frac{A_B^o}{D} = \frac{V_B C_B^o}{D} = \frac{A_{Bf}^o + A_{Bb}^o}{A_f^o + A_{Tb}^o + A_{Bb}^o} \qquad (5.25)$$

Therefore,

$$C_B^o = \frac{A_{Bf}^o + A_{Bb}^o}{A_f^o + A_{Tb}^o + A_{Bb}^o} \frac{D}{V_B} \qquad (5.26)$$

Equations (5.17) and (5.20) apply equally at the initial condition and at any time t. Therefore, the ratio of f to f_B is given by

$$\frac{f}{f_B} = \frac{A_{Bf}^o + A_{Bb}^o}{A_f^o + A_{Bb}^o + A_{Tb}^o} \frac{A_f^o}{A_{Bf}^o} \qquad (5.27)$$

Since A_f^o/A_{Bf}^o is equal to V_f/V_B, according to Eq. (5.3), it follows that on rearrangement of Eq. (5.27), we obtain

$$\frac{A_{Bf}^o + A_{Bb}^o}{A_f^o + A_{Bb}^o + A_{Tb}^o} = \frac{V_B}{V_f} \frac{f}{f_B} \qquad (5.28)$$

Substituting Eq. (5.28) into Eq. (5.26) yields

$$C_B^o = \frac{f}{f_B} \frac{D}{V_B} \frac{V_B}{V_f} = \frac{f}{f_B} \frac{D}{V_f} \qquad (5.29)$$

The systemic (blood) clearance of a drug, Cl_S, is calculated from the ratio of the dose to the total area under the blood concentration-time curve:

$$Cl_S = \frac{D}{\int_0^\infty C_B \, dt} \qquad (5.30)$$

Integration of Eq. (5.23) from t = 0 to t = ∞, followed by substitution for C_B^o from Eq. (5.29) and for β from Eq. (5.19), gives

$$\int_0^\infty C_B \, dt = \frac{C_B^o}{\beta} = \frac{D}{f_B V_f k_f} \qquad (5.31)$$

Substituting this term in Eq. (5.30) yields

$$Cl_S = f_B (V_f k_f) \qquad (5.32)$$

where $V_f k_f$ is the intrinsic clearance. Thus we see the classic relationship between systemic clearance and the fraction of drug free in the blood, which was first described by Levy and Yacobi [1].

By definition, systemic clearance is the product of the apparent volume of distribution and the apparent elimination rate constant:

$$Cl_s = V\beta \tag{5.33}$$

Therefore,

$$V = \frac{Cl_s}{\beta} \tag{5.34}$$

Substituting for Cl_s from Eq. (5.32) and for β from Eq. (5.19) gives

$$V = \frac{f_B}{f} V_f \tag{5.35}$$

Equation (5.35) indicates that in the absence of drug binding (i.e., $f = f_B = 1$), $V = V_f$. This is the case for antipyrine; the apparent volume of distribution of antipyrine closely approximates total body water.

From Eqs. (5.17) and (5.20) it can be shown that

$$\frac{f_B}{f} = \frac{A_{Bf}}{A_{Bf} + A_{Bb}} \frac{A_f + A_{Bb} + A_{Tb}}{A_f} \tag{5.36}$$

Since in all cases an amount term is the product of a concentration term and a volume term,

$$\frac{f_B}{f} = \frac{V_B C_f}{V_B C_f + V_B C_{Bb}} \frac{V_f C_f + V_B C_{Bb} + V_T C_{Tb}}{V_f C_f} \tag{5.37}$$

which simplifies to

$$\frac{f_B}{f} = \frac{V_f C_f + V_B C_{Bb} + V_T C_{Tb}}{C_f + C_{Bb}} \frac{1}{V_f} \tag{5.38}$$

Therefore,

$$\frac{f_B}{f} V_f = \frac{V_f C_f + V_B C_{Bb} + V_T C_{Tb}}{C_f + C_{Bb}} \tag{5.39}$$

Substituting Eq. (5.39) in Eq. (5.35) and rearranging terms yields

$$V(C_f + C_{Bb}) = V_f C_f + V_B C_{Bb} + V_T C_{Tb} \tag{5.40}$$

Dividing each term in Eq. (5.40) by C_f gives

$$\frac{V(C_f + C_{Bb})}{C_f} = V_f + \frac{V_B C_{Bb}}{C_f} + \frac{V_T C_{Tb}}{C_f} \tag{5.41}$$

It is helpful to define a new term f_T (i.e., the fraction free in the extravascular space), which is, by analogy to f_B [see Eq. (5.20)], given by

$$f_T = \frac{C_f}{C_f + C_{Tb}} \tag{5.42}$$

By rearranging terms in Eqs. (5.20) and (5.42), we can show that

$$\frac{C_{Bb}}{C_f} = \frac{1 - f_B}{f_B} \tag{5.43}$$

and

$$\frac{C_{Tb}}{C_f} = \frac{1 - f_T}{f_T} \tag{5.44}$$

Substituting Eqs. (5.20), (5.43), and (5.44) into Eq. (5.41) yields

$$\frac{V}{f_B} = V_f + \frac{1 - f_B}{f_B} V_B + \frac{1 - f_T}{f_T} V_T \tag{5.45}$$

Recognizing that V_f is simply the sum of V_B and V_T, and multiplying each term in Eq. (5.45) by f_B gives the following expression:

$$V = f_B(V_B + V_T) + (1 - f_B)V_B + f_B \frac{1 - f_T}{f_T} V_T \tag{5.46}$$

Expanding each term yields

$$V = f_B V_B + f_B V_T + V_B - f_B V_B + \frac{f_B - f_B f_T}{f_T} V_T \tag{5.47}$$

which simplifies to

$$V = V_B + \frac{f_B}{f_T} V_T \tag{5.48}$$

Experimentally, drug binding is determined, by one of several methods, in plasma or serum rather than in blood. Hence one determines f_p, the fraction of drug unbound (free) in the plasma, rather than f_B. However, f_p values can be easily converted to f_B values by multiplying f_p by the ratio of drug concentrations in plasma and in whole blood [i.e., $f_B = f_p(C_p/C_B)$].

In the event that no information is available concerning the partitioning of drug between plasma and red blood cells, an alternative expression for calculating apparent volume of distribution is as follows:

$$V' = V_p + V_T' \frac{f_p}{f_T'}$$ (5.49)

In Eq. (5.49), V' is the apparent volume of distribution relating the total amount of drug in the body to the total drug concentration in plasma, V_p is plasma volume, and V_T' is the volume of the extravascular space plus the erythrocyte volume. Drug binding to erythrocytes contributes to f_T'.

The derivation outlined above resulting in Eq. (5.48) or (5.49) was first presented by Gibaldi and McNamara [2] and leads to a relationship identical to that proposed by Wilkinson and Shand [3] based on the work of Gillette [4]. This relationship is conceptually very useful. It is evident that ordinarily, the smallest apparent volume of distribution of a drug is blood volume. This value is approached when there is extensive binding in the vascular space (i.e., $f_B \to 0$) and little binding in the extravascular space (i.e., $f_T \to 1$). A highly polar drug, restricted to the vascular space because of molecular weight considerations, may have an apparent volume of distribution equal to plasma volume. Lipid-soluble drugs such as dicumarol that are highly bound to plasma proteins but less bound to tissues (i.e., $f_B/f_T < 1$) have apparent volumes of distribution that are between the values of blood volume and the volume of total body water. Many basic drugs, including amphetamine, are preferentially bound to extravascular tissues (i.e., $f_B/f_T > 1$) and have apparent volumes of distribution that exceed the volume of total body water. Drugs that are negligibly bound (i.e., $f_B = f_T = 1$) have apparent volumes of distribution that approximate the volume of total body water in the cases of lipid-soluble compounds (e.g., antipyrine) or the volume of the extracellular space in the case of poorly lipid soluble compounds.

Equation (5.48) predicts a linear relationship between apparent volume of distribution V and fraction free in the blood f_B when the fraction free in the extravascular space is constant. Thus if certain perturbations such as disease state, concomitant drug therapy, or genetic factors affect plasma protein binding of a drug but have no effect on tissue binding, a plot of V versus f_B will be linear with a positive slope and an intercept equal to V_B (see Fig. 5.2). If the perturbation produces a parallel but smaller effect on tissue binding, an apparently linear plot may result, but the value of the intercept will be greater than V_B. If the effects on plasma protein and tissue binding are quantitatively similar, V is independent of f_B. Both of these cases are also shown in Fig. 5.2. Perturbations that principally

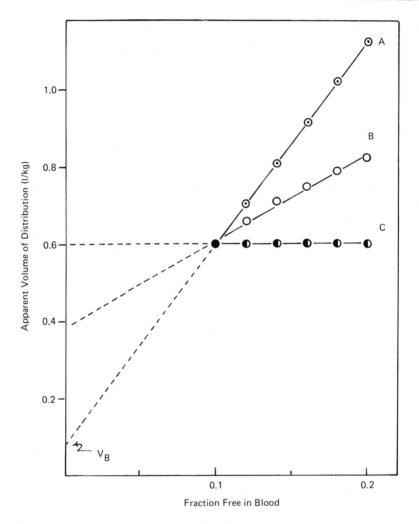

Fig. 5.2 Apparent volume of distribution as a function of free fraction of drug in blood, f_B. Blood volume is equal to 75 ml/kg. Total body water is equal to 600 ml/kg. Case A: f_B varies from 0.1 to 0.2, f_T is constant at 0.1. Case B: f_B varies from 0.1 to 0.2, f_T varies from 0.1 to 0.14 such that $f_T = 0.4\, f_B + 0.06$. Case C: Both f_B and f_T vary from 0.1 to 0.2 such that f_B/f_T is constant. (Data from Ref. 2.)

affect plasma protein binding will produce an increase in V, whereas those that principally affect tissue binding will result in a decrease in V. An example of the latter situation is found with digoxin in patients with renal disease [5].

TISSUE BINDING

Although the fraction free in the extravascular space, f_T, cannot be determined directly in humans, it may be possible, under certain circumstances, to estimate it indirectly by using a rearranged form of Eq. (5.48):

$$f_T = \frac{f_B V_T}{V - V_B} \tag{5.50}$$

By determining V and f_B experimentally and by using appropriate estimates of V_B and V_T, we can readily calculate f_T. Therefore, we can assess whether a perturbation that affects plasma protein binding also affects tissue binding. Using this approach it has been found that uremia and nephrosis, both of which significantly decrease the plasma protein binding of phenytoin in humans, have no effect on the apparent tissue binding of the drug. On the other hand, apparently genetically related differences in plasma protein binding of warfarin in individual rats are paralleled by differences in tissue binding [6].

Clarification of the role of tissue (extravascular) binding in drug disposition and drug effects requires further investigation, but it is clear that the systemic clearance of a drug is independent of tissue binding [see Eq. (5.32)]. On the other hand, tissue binding appears to be a principal determinant of the apparent elimination rate constant β or half-life of a drug.

By rearrangement of Eq. (5.33), we can show that

$$\beta = \frac{Cl_s}{V} \tag{5.51}$$

Substituting for Cl_s according to Eq. (5.32), and for V according to Eq. (5.48), yields

$$\beta = \frac{f_B V_f k_f}{V_B + (f_B/f_T)V_T} \tag{5.52}$$

If we assume a situation where drug binding to erythrocytes is negligible, and define apparent volume of distribution in terms of drug concentration in plasma rather than blood, we may rewrite Eq. (5.52) as

$$\beta = \frac{f_p V_f k_f}{V_p + (f_p/f_T)V_T'} \tag{5.53}$$

Since plasma volume is only about 40 ml/kg, it follows that for drugs with an apparent volume of distribution greater than 400 ml/kg, $V - V_p \backsimeq V \backsimeq V_T'(f_p/f_T)$ and

$$\beta \overset{\sim}{-} \frac{f_p V_f k_f}{(f_p / f_T) V_T'} = \frac{f_T V_f k_f}{V_T'} \tag{5.54}$$

As we have noted, the product of V_f and k_f is usually designated as intrinsic clearance or Cl_I and reflects the intrinsic ability of the eliminating organ(s) (e.g., the liver or kidneys or both) to clear the drug from the blood. Therefore,

$$\beta \overset{\sim}{-} \frac{f_T Cl_I}{V_T} \tag{5.55}$$

and

$$t_{1/2} \overset{\sim}{-} \frac{0.693 V_T}{f_T Cl_I} \tag{5.56}$$

Equation (5.56) shows that, for many drugs, half-life is a function of the body's intrinsic ability to eliminate the drug and of the degree of binding of the drug in the extravascular space, and that half-life is independent of plasma protein binding. Although Eq. (5.56) applies rigorously only to drugs with apparent volumes of distribution exceeding 400 ml/kg, it has been shown for drugs with apparent volumes ranging from 100 to 400 ml/kg that, under the conditions stated half-life is largely dependent on tissue binding and less dependent on plasma protein binding [7]. The half-lives of drugs with apparent volumes of distribution of less than 100 ml/kg are highly dependent on plasma protein binding.

It should be recognized that f_T is a hybrid constant and reflects the weighted average of drug binding to different organs and tissues in the extravascular space. As noted by Gillette [4], Eq. (5.48) is more appropriately expressed as

$$V = V_B + \frac{f_B \sum_{i=1}^{n} (C_T)_i (V_T)_i}{C_f} \tag{5.57}$$

where C_f is the concentration of free (unbound) drug at steady state, $(C_T)_i$ is the total (bound and unbound) drug concentration in a given tissue or organ at steady state, and $(V_T)_i$ is the anatomic volume of the given organ or tissue. Since C_f / f_B is equal to total drug concentration in blood C_B, it follows that

$$V = V_B + \sum_{i=1}^{n} R_i (V_T)_i \tag{5.58}$$

where R_i is the partition coefficient or distribution ratio of drug between tissue and blood [i.e., $R_i = (C_T)_i / C_B$].

The fraction bound in the extravascular space, f_T, largely reflects the binding of drug to organs and tissues that contain large
fractions of the total amount of drug in the body. An assessment of
f_T by pharmacokinetic means [see Eq. (5.50)] to detect the effect
of a perturbation on tissue binding may fail to reveal even substantial
changes in drug binding to tissues or organs that contribute little to
the overall apparent volume of the extravascular space.

ESTIMATION OF APPARENT VOLUMES OF DISTRIBUTION

In principal, one can calculate the apparent volume of distribution
of drug in laboratory animals or in humans, on necropsy, by determining the distribution ratio between blood and each of the principal
organs and tissues that account for the total amount of drug in the
body, estimating the anatomic volume of each and using Eq. (5.58).
This has been carried out for lidocaine in the monkey [8] but is a
formidable task. Thus many other, considerably simpler, methods
have been devised to estimate the apparent volume of distribution of a
drug in the intact organism. All methods require that the drug be
given intravenously so that the amount reaching the systemic circulation will be equivalent to the administered dose and be known.

For the model described in Fig. 5.1, it can be shown that drug
concentrations in the vascular space (blood or plasma) decline
exponentially with time (see Fig. 1.1). Extrapolation of such data to
zero time on the drug concentration axis provides an estimate of the
initial drug concentration C_0 immediately after intravenous bolus injection but before any drug has been eliminated. It follows that

$$V = \frac{dose}{C_0} \tag{5.59}$$

The volume term calculated by this equation is often called $V_{extrapolated}$.
This equation must never be applied to data obtained after oral or
intramuscular administration, even if complete absorption or availability can be assumed.

In practice, however, few drugs show simple monoexponential decline immediately after injection; that is, our assumption regarding
instantaneous distribution throughout the body space seems rarely to
be true. In most cases, it appears that a finite time is required for a
drug to distribute throughout the body space, and most plots of log
drug concentration versus time after intravenous bolus injection must
be described by multiexponential equations (suggestive of a multicompartment system) rather than monoexponential equations (indicative of
one-compartment systems). Under these conditions extrapolation of
the linear portion of the log concentration versus time plot to the concentration axis yields a value which is less than the concentration of
drug in the blood immediately after injection. Furthermore, calculation of V according to Eq. (5.59) by assuming that the extrapolated

value is equal to C_0 will result in an overestimate of the apparent volume of distribution. Therefore, we may use Eq. (5.59) only when the deviation of the log concentration versus time plot from a mono-exponential expression is negligible.

A more general, and therefore more useful, approach for estimating V is to use the well-developed relationship between the total area under the drug concentration versus time curve, AUC, and the intravenous dose:

$$AUC = \frac{dose}{VK} \qquad (5.60)$$

or

$$AUC = \frac{dose}{V\beta} = \frac{dose}{V\lambda_n} \qquad (5.61)$$

where K is the first-order elimination rate constant (one-compartment model) and β or λ_n is the terminal slope (times 2.303) of the curve described by plotting log concentrations versus time for a drug in a linear multicompartment system. Upon rearrangement we obtain

$$V = \frac{dose}{K \cdot AUC} \qquad (5.62)$$

and

$$V = \frac{dose}{\beta \cdot AUC} = \frac{dose}{\lambda_n \cdot AUC} \qquad (5.63)$$

The volume term described by Eq. (5.62) is sometimes called V_{area}, whereas that described by Eq. (5.63) has been termed V_{area} or V_β. The terminology V_β arises from the fact that this volume term relates drug concentration in plasma or blood to the total amount of drug in the body during the terminal exponential phase (log-linear or β phase) of a log drug concentration in blood or plasma-time curve for any multicompartment model where elimination occurs from the central compartment [9]. Equation (5.62) or (5.63) may be applied to data obtained after oral administration of a drug *only* when complete absorption *and* complete systemic availability (i.e., no first-pass or gut metabolism) can be assumed.

An estimate of apparent volume of distribution that is equivalent to V_{area} or V_β may also be obtained from blood- or plasma-level data obtained after constant rate intravenous infusion for a sufficiently long period to attain steady state. The drug concentration in plasma or blood under these conditions, C_{ss}, is given by

$$C_{ss} = \frac{k_0}{Cl_s} \qquad (5.64)$$

where k_0 is the zero-order infusion rate constant and Cl_S is systemic clearance. For a one-compartment model, $Cl_S = VK$, and for a multi-compartment model, $Cl_S = V\beta$. Hence

$$V = \frac{k_0}{KC_{ss}}$$

(5.65)

or

$$V = \frac{k_0}{\beta C_{ss}}$$

(5.66)

If a one-compartment model can be assumed, an estimate of apparent volume of distribution may be obtained from data collected before steady state during constant rate intravenous infusion. Under these conditions

$$C = \frac{k_0}{VK} (1 - e^{-Kt})$$

(5.67)

where t is infusion time. V may be calculated from the slope of a plot of C versus $1 - e^{-Kt}$, which is equal to k_0/VK. The infusion rate k_0 is known and the rate constant K may be estimated from data collected after stopping the infusion. The volume term calculated by means of Eq. (5.65) or (5.66) has sometimes been termed $V_{infusion}$ (V_{inf}) or $V_{infusion\ equilibrium}$ ($V_{inf\ eq}$) but is, in fact, equivalent to V_{area} or V_β.

If the body may be viewed as a single compartment with respect to the distribution and elimination kinetics of a drug, the volume terms introduced above (i.e., $V_{extrapolated}$, V_{area}, $V_{inf\ eq}$) and the physiologically based apparent volume of distribution defined by Eq. (5.48) or (5.58) are equivalent. This physiologically based volume is equivalent to the apparent volume of distribution at steady state, V_{SS}.

In those situations where the body may not be viewed as a single compartment and where there is a finite time required for distribution to take place so that a multicompartment model is required to describe the kinetics of the drug, the volume terms are not equivalent. Under these circumstances, one finds that $V_{extrapolated} > V_{area}$ or $V_\beta = V_{inf\ eq} > V_{SS}$. Moreover, yet another volume term, V_c or V_1, the volume of the central compartment, is often used to describe multi-compartment models. By definition, $V_{SS} > V_c$. The only useful volume terms for multicompartment systems are V_β, V_c, and V_{SS}.

The β-phase apparent volume of distribution, V_β, may be calculated for any linear multicompartment model by determining the total area under the drug concentration in plasma or blood versus time curve, AUC, after a single intravenous administration and the slope of the long-linear or β phase and by applying Eq. (5.61). It can also be shown that $V_\beta = k_{10}V_c/\beta$, where k_{10} is the apparent elimination rate constant of drug from the central compartment. The product of V_β and β or V_c and k_{10} is systemic clearance.

The principal shortcoming of this apparent volume of distribution term as an index of drug distribution is that V_β may reflect the degree of equilibration of a drug under dynamic conditions rather than its apparent distribution volume. This is more easily appreciated when one recognizes that V_β is a function of the elimination kinetics of a drug [10]. An increase in the intrinsic elimination rate constant will cause an increase in V_β, whereas a decrease in elimination will cause a decrease in V_β. Hence a change in the V_β of a drug may not reflect a change in the actual distribution space or in the degree of binding but may signify merely a change in the degree of equilibration between central and peripheral compartments secondary to a change in elimination kinetics. For a multicompartment system with drug elimination occurring from the central compartment, characterized by the rate constant k_{10}, the limits of V_β are ∞ as $k_{10} \to \infty$, and V_{ss} as $k_{10} \to 0$.

Drug concentration C in a linear multicompartment model as a function of time after intravenous injection can always be described by an equation of the form

$$C = \sum_{i=1}^{n} C_i e^{-\lambda_i t} \qquad (5.68)$$

where C_i is the coefficient of the ith exponential term of the polyexponential equation and λ_i is the exponent multiplying time t in the exponential terms. Note that λ_1 is the largest λ_i (usually symbolized by α in a two-compartment model), λ_2 is the second largest, and so on. The term λ_n (or β) is used to denote the smallest value of λ_i. Under these conditions the apparent volume of the central compartment is given by

$$V_c = \frac{\text{intravenous dose}}{\Sigma C_i} \qquad (5.69)$$

For a two-compartment open model, V_c = intravenous dose/$(A + B)$. This volume term may be useful for estimating peak concentrations in plasma or blood for drugs that distribute relatively slowly in the body and are absorbed relatively rapidly after oral or intramuscular administration. Drugs with relatively small V_c/V_{ss} ratios may show unusually large peak-to-trough concentration ratios over a dosing interval even when administered relatively frequently.

The most useful volume term to describe the apparent distribution space in a multicompartment system is V_{ss}. As its name implies, V_{ss} relates the amount of drug in the body to the drug concentration in the plasma or blood at steady state, during repetitive dosing, or during constant rate infusion. V_{ss} is independent of drug elimination, and its relationship to anatomical space and drug binding has been described by Eqs. (5.48) to (5.50).

Equations to define and estimate V_{ss} have been developed in Chap. 2. A useful expression for calculating V_{ss} after rapid intravenous administration of a drug whose disposition is described by Eq. (5.68) is [11]

$$V_{ss} = \frac{D \sum\limits_{i=1}^{n} C_i/\lambda_i^{\ 2}}{\left(\sum\limits_{i=1}^{n} C_i/\lambda_i\right)^2} = \frac{D \sum\limits_{i=1}^{n} C_i/\lambda_i^{\ 2}}{(AUC)^2} \qquad (5.70)$$

Equation (5.70) is a general relationship that applies to any linear multicompartment model in which elimination occurs from the central compartment. For a two-compartment open model we may write Eq. (5.70) as

$$V_{ss} = \frac{D[(A/\alpha^2) + (B/\beta^2)]}{[(A/\alpha) + (B/\beta)]^2} \qquad (5.71)$$

Thus calculation of V_{ss} simply requires curve-fitting of drug concentration-time data after intravenous bolus injection, to estimate C_i and λ_i values, and application of Eq. (5.70).

Although (5.70) is a rather general expression, it does require the implicit elaboration of a compartment model. A still more general, model-independent approach for estimating V_{ss} has been proposed [12,13]. It can be shown that the term $\sum_{i=1}^{n} C_i/\lambda_i^2$ [see the numerator of Eq. (5.70)] is, in fact, equal to the area under the first moment of the drug concentration in blood or plasma curve, AUMC, that is, the area under the curve of the product of time t and drug concentration C from time zero to infinity. In other words,

$$V_{ss} = \frac{D[(\int_0^\infty tC \ dt]}{[\int_0^\infty C \ dt]^2} = \frac{D[AUMC]}{[AUC]^2} \qquad (5.72)$$

The principal assumptions required for developing Eq. (5.72) are that the system is linear and that drug elimination takes place from the measured site (i.e., the plasma, blood, or central compartment).

This method does not not require the assumption of a compartment model, nor does it require a curve-fitting procedure. To calculate V_{ss}, one must merely determine the total areas under the drug concentration versus time curve and under the first moment versus time curve (see Fig. 5.3) using the trapezoidal rule (see Appendix D) or some other convenient method.

Since many drugs are administered by a constant rate intravenous infusion over a short period of time rather than by a rapid intravenous injection, the following variant of Eq. (5.72) [14] is often useful:

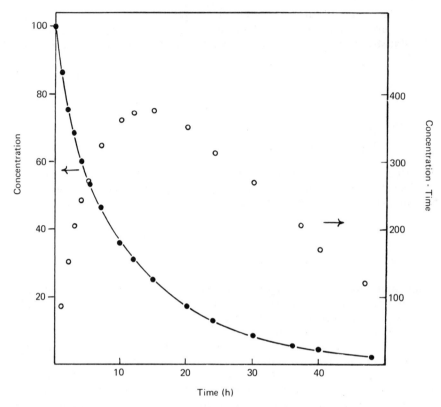

Fig. 5.3 Plots of concentration versus time (●) and of the product of concentration and time versus time (○) after intravenous bolus injection of a drug. The total area under the concentration versus time curve is AUC; the total area under the concentration-time versus time curve is AUMC.

$$V_{ss} = \frac{k_0 T \cdot AUMC}{(AUC)^2} - \frac{T(k_0 T)}{2 \cdot AUC} \tag{5.73}$$

where k_0 is the infusion rate, T the infusion time, and $k_0 T$ the administered dose.

For many drugs V_β [see Eq. (5.63)] provides a close approximation of V_{ss}. However, in at least two situations, V_β significantly overestimates V_{ss}. One case is that of drugs that are rapidly cleared from the central compartment with short half-lives. For example, it has been calculated for benzypenicillin in humans that V_β = 26 liters, whereas V_{ss} = 15 liters [10]. A second case occurs where most of the dose of a drug is eliminated relatively rapidly but a small fraction of the dose persists and gives rise to unusually long half lives. In such cases the area under the extrapolated line from the β phase to the drug concentration axis represent a relatively small fraction of the total area under the drug concentration versus time curve (see Fig. 2.9, curve Y). Based on data in the literature [15], it may be calculated that for gentamicin in humans, $V_\beta = 202$ liters, whereas $V_{ss} = 33$ liters. The latter value is a much more realistic and more useful estimate of the apparent distribution space of gentamicin.

In 1976, Niazi [16] suggested that the change in apparent distribution volume manifested by a drug in a multicompartment system as a function of time after intravenous administration might be a useful parameter for characterizing distribution kinetics (see Fig. 5.4). Immediately after injection the drug occupies a space we have termed V_c, the volume of the central compartment. V_c may also be thought of as a proportionality constant relating drug concentration in plasma or blood to the amount of drug in the body at $t = 0$ (i.e., the intravenous dose). The apparent volume or proportionality constant relating concentration and amount increases with time until it reaches a limiting value which we have termed V_β. We have noted that V_β is actually a proportionality constant relating drug concentration in plasma or blood to amount of drug in the body during the β phase and that $V_\beta > V_c$. The time-dependent volume of distribution V_t may be

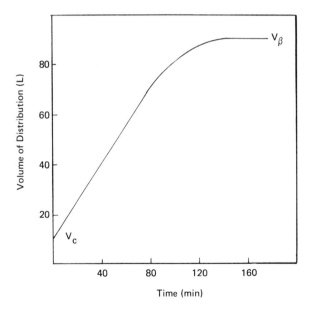

Fig. 5.4 Apparent volume of distribution of trichloromonofluoromethane as a function of time following intravenous administration in the dog. (Data from Ref. 16.)

defined as the ratio of the amount of drug in body at any time to the drug concentration in plasma or blood at that time and will vary in value from V_c to V_β. Since in a multicompartment model where the drug is eliminated only from the central compartment, the amount of drug remaining in the body as a function of time can be expressed in terms of fractional areas [17]. It can be shown that [16]

$$V_t = \frac{D \cdot AUC_{t \to \infty}}{C_t \cdot AUC_{0 \to \infty}} \qquad (5.74)$$

where D is the intravenous dose, C_t is the drug concentration at time t, and the AUC terms refer to either partial or total areas under the concentration-time plot. Comparative plots of V_t versus time for different individuals or different species receiving the same drug might be helpful in characterizing rates of distribution.

The idea of time-dependent changes in apparent volume of distribution is also useful for systems showing nonlinear plasma protein binding or tissue binding. Such changes may be quantified for one-compartment models but are difficult to describe quantitatively for multicompartment models. In principle, it can be shown that V decreases with time when nonlinear plasma protein binding occurs, whereas V increases with time when only nonlinear extravascular tissue binding occurs [18].

REFERENCES

1. G. Levy and A. Yacobi. Effect of plasma protein binding on elimination of warfarin. *J. Pharm. Sci.* *63*:805 (1974).
2. M. Gibaldi and P. J. McNamara. Apparent volumes of distribution and drug binding to plasma proteins and tissues. *Eur. J. Clin. Pharmacol.* *13*:373 (1978).
3. G. R. Wilkinson and D. G. Shand. A physiologic approach to hepatic drug clearance. *Clin. Pharmacol. Ther.* *18*:377 (1975).
4. J. R. Gillette. Factors affecting drug metabolism. *Ann. N.Y. Acad. Sci.* *179*:43 (1971).
5. R. H. Reuning, R. A. Sams, and R. E. Notari. Role of pharmacokinetics in drug dosage adjustment: I. Pharmacologic effect kinetics and apparent volume of distribution of digoxin. *J. Clin. Pharmacol.* *13*:127 (1973).
6. M. Gibaldi and P. J. McNamara. Tissue binding of drugs. *J. Pharm. Sci.* *66*:1211 (1977).
7. M. Gibaldi, G. Levy, and P. J. McNamara. Effect of plasma protein and tissue binding on the biologic half-life of drugs. *Clin. Pharmacol. Ther.* *24*:1 (1978).
8. N. Benowitz, R. P. Forsyth, K. L. Melmon, and M. Rowland. Lidocaine disposition kinetics in monkey and man: I. Prediction by a perfusion model. *Clin. Pharmacol. Ther.* *16*:87 (1974).

9. M. Gibaldi, R. Nagashima, and G. Levy. Relationship between drug concentration in plasma or serum and amount of drug in the body. *J. Pharm. Sci.* *58*:193 (1969).
10. W. J. Jusko and M. Gibaldi. Effects of change in elimination on various parameters of the two-compartment open model. *J. Pharm. Sci.* *61*:1270 (1972).
11. J. G. Wagner. Linear pharmacokinetic equations allowing direct calculation of many needed pharmacokinetic parameters from the coefficients and exponents of polyexponential equations which have been fitted to data. *J. Pharmacokinet. Biopharm.* *4*:443 (1976).
12. J. H. Oppenheimer, H. L. Schwartz, and M. I. Surks. Determination of common parameters of iodothyronine metabolism and distribution in man by noncompartmental analysis. *J. Clin. Endocrinol. Metab.* *41*:319 (1975).
13. L. Z. Benet and R. L. Galeazzi. Noncompartmental determination of the steady-state volume of distribution. *J. Pharm. Sci.* *68*:1071 (1979).
14. C. S. Lee, D. C. Brater, J. G. Gambertoglio, and L. Z. Benet. Disposition kinetics of ethambutol in man. *J. Pharmacokinet. Biopharm.* *8*:335 (1980).
15. W. A. Colburn, J. J. Schentag, W. J. Jusko, and M. Gibaldi. A model for the prospective identification of the prenephrotoxic state during gentamicin therapy. *J. Pharmacokinet. Biopharm.* *6*:179 (1978).
16. S. Niazi. Volume of distribution as a function of time. *J. Pharm. Sci.* *65*:452 (1976).
17. W. L. Chiou. A simple equation to estimate the fraction of drug remaining in the body after an intravenous injection. *J. Pharm. Pharmacol.* *34*:342 (1972).
18. P. J. McNamara, G. Levy, and M. Gibaldi. Effect of plasma protein and tissue binding on the time course of drug concentration in plasma. *J. Pharmacokinet. Biopharm.* *7*:195 (1979).

6

Kinetics of Pharmacologic Response

The type of relationship that exists between the plasma concentration of a drug and a given response is generally determined by two factors: whether concentration is directly or indirectly related to response, and whether the drug interacts with the receptor in a reversible or irreversible manner. The simplest type is where there is a direct relationship between plasma concentration and response, and where the interaction of the drug and the receptor is reversible. Many drugs (e.g., antiarrythmics, digitalis glycosides, theophylline, and neuromuscular blocking agents) appear to act directly and reversibly. A second type of concentration-response relationship is where the elicited response is not directly related to the plasma drug concentration. This is generally referred to as an indirect pharmacologic response, and is best exemplified by the coumarin anticoagulants. A third type is where the drug binds to the receptor irreversibly. Anticancer agents and bactericidal antibiotics are examples of drugs that exert their effects in this manner.

KINETICS OF DIRECTLY REVERSIBLE PHARMACOLOGIC RESPONSE

One-Compartment Model

The concept of a direct and rapidly reversible response implies that a given intensity of response is associated with a particular drug concentration at the site of action. By definition in the model under consideration, the drug concentration at the receptor site C_r is proportional to the drug concentration in the plasma C, and the interaction between the drug and receptor is reversible:

$$C \rightleftharpoons C_r + \text{receptor} \rightleftharpoons \frac{\text{drug-receptor}}{\text{complex}} \rightarrow \text{response}$$

The following relationship, known as the Hill equation, has been proposed to relate plasma concentration and response R under these circumstances:

$$R = \frac{R_m C^s}{(1/Q) + C^s} \tag{6.1}$$

where R_m is the maximum intensity of the pharmacologic response (i.e., $R \to R_m$ as $C \to \infty$), Q is a constant related to the affinity of the drug for the receptor, and s is a constant that relates the change in response to the change in concentration. One should also note that the term 1/Q is equal to the drug concentration in the plasma (raised to the sth power) at which response is 50% of maximal response, (i.e., $C_{50\%}^s$). The basis for Eq. (6.1) has been discussed in detail [1]. This equation will quantitatively and fully characterize the typical sigmoid curve resulting from a log C versus R-type plot. Rearranging terms and inverting both sides of (6.1) yields

$$\frac{R_m}{R} = \frac{1 + C^s Q}{C^s Q} \tag{6.2}$$

Subtracting unity from both sides of this equation (i.e., R/R from the left side and $C^s Q / C^s Q$ from the right side), collecting terms, and again inverting both sides of the equation gives

$$\frac{R}{R_m - R} = C^s Q \tag{6.3}$$

A linear form of this equation is

$$\log \frac{R}{R_m - R} = s \log C + \log Q \tag{6.4}$$

A plot of $R/(R_m - R)$ versus C on log-log graph paper will yield a straight line with a slope of s.

A more common approach relating response and concentration is based on the well-known empirical plot of response versus logarithm of dose, plasma concentration, or amount of drug in the body which yields the classical sigmoid curve shown in Fig. 6.1. Very often this curve manifests excellent linearity from at least 20 to 80% of the maximum attainable intensity of response, a region of particular interest and applicability under clinical conditions. This linear relationship may be expressed by

$$R = m \log C + r \tag{6.5}$$

where R and C are as described previously, m is the slope of the R versus log C plot, and r is a constant. Such linearity between response

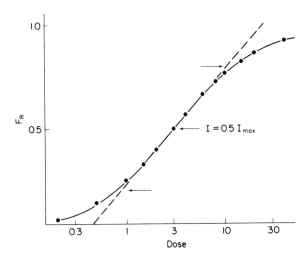

Fig. 6.1 Typical log dose-response curve calculated according to the relationship $F_R = D/(K + D)$, where K is a constant and F_R is the fraction of the maximum response of the system attained after a dose D. The plot is apparently linear in the region bounded by $F_R = 0.2$ and $F_R = 0.8$ (see arrows). A dose of 3 units is the median effective dose ED_{50} since it produces an intensity I of response that is 50% of the maximum intensity I_{max}. (Data from Ref. 2.)

and log C has been demonstrated for a number of drugs, examples of which are propranolol (Fig. 6.2) and theophylline (Fig. 6.3). Relating response to the logarithm of plasma concentration rather than the logarithm of dose should reduce the variability in the data by removing variability related to interpatient differences in drug absorption and elimination.

Rearrangement of (6.5) yields

$$\log C = \frac{R - r}{m} \tag{6.6}$$

In a one-compartment system, the plasma concentration of drug at any time following the administration of an intravenous bolus dose of a drug that is eliminated by first-order processes can be described by

$$\log C = \log C_0 - \frac{Kt}{2.303} \tag{6.7}$$

where C_0 is the plasma concentration at time zero, t is time, and K is the apparent first-order elimination rate constant of the drug. Based on the proposed model, the maximum response elicited by this dose, R_0, would be associated with a plasma concentration of C_0 [5]. Therefore, an equation analogous to (6.6) can be written:

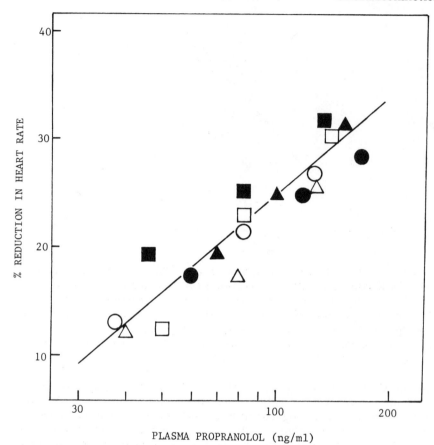

Fig. 6.2 Relationship between response (percent reduction in exer-
cise-induced tachycardia) and propranolol concentration in plasma
(log scale) after intravenous administration to healthy volunteers.
(Data from Ref. 3.)

$$\log C_0 = \frac{R_0 - r}{m} \qquad\qquad (6.8)$$

Substituting the values of log C and log C_0 from (6.6) and (6.8),
respectively, into (6.7) yields

$$\frac{R - r}{m} = \frac{R_0 - r}{m} - \frac{Kt}{2.303} \qquad\qquad (6.9)$$

This equation can be simplified to give

$$R = R_0 - \frac{mK}{2.303} t \qquad\qquad (6.10)$$

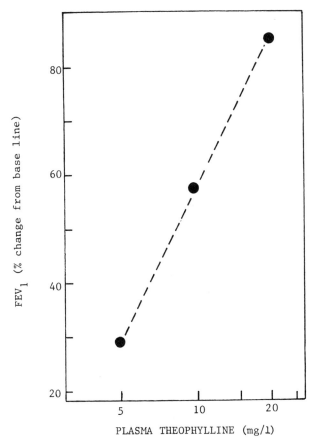

PLASMA THEOPHYLLINE (mg/l)

Fig. 6.3 Relationship between average response (normalized improve-ment in 1 s forced expiratory volume) and theophylline concentra-tion in plasma (log scale) after intravenous administration of the drug to patients. (Data from Ref. 4.)

This equation shows that, under the conditions stated, the intensity of response decreases at a constant rate that is a function of the ap-parent first-order elimination rate constant K and the slope of the response versus log C curve, m. It should be noted that the rate of decline in response is zero order even though the rate of decline in plasma concentration is first order. This linear or zero-order de-cline in response with time has been demonstrated for a number of drugs and an example is shown in Fig. 6.4.

It is also readily shown by substituting log C from Eq. (1.94) $[C = k_a F X_0 (e^{-Kt} - e^{-k_a t})/V(k_a - K)]$ into Eq. (6.5) that (6.10) also describes the decay of effect in the postabsorptive phase (i.e.,

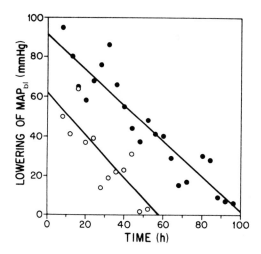

Fig. 6.4 Time course of hypotensive response (reduction in mean
arterial pressure) in a patient following 10 (O) and 25 (●) mg single
oral doses of minoxidil. Some time after administration, the intensity
of the drug's effect declines at a constant and similar rate after each
dose. (Data from Ref. 6.)

$e^{-k_a t} \rightarrow 0$) after oral or intramuscular drug administration. An example
is the zero-order loss of the stimulant effect of amphetamine after intramuscular administration (Fig. 6.5). Although the decline in pharmacologic response for many drugs that act directly and reversibly is
zero order, there are examples where the decline in response appears
to be first order. This type of decline has been observed with the
digitalis glycosides (Fig. 6.6).

This departure from theory may be related to the approximate
nature of Eq. (6.5). Although (6.10) predicts a linear decline of
pharmacologic response with time after intravenous administration,
combination of (6.1) with the appropriate pharmacokinetic expression
for drug elimination in a one-compartment model suggests that the
decline of pharmacologic response is curvilinear (see Fig. 6.7). Regions of this curve may be linearized on semilogarithmic coordinates.
Of particular importance is the fact that the response versus time
curves are *nearly* linear in the response range 20 to 80%. Hence, for
all practical purposes one would anticipate for a large number of drugs
that the loss of effect would indeed be essentially linear over a very
wide reponse range, as predicted by (6.10).

Regardless of the relationship between response and concentration, one can frequently demonstrate a relationship between the duration of a given response and the dose and half-life or elimination rate
constant of a drug [9]. Equation (6.7) can be readily converted to an

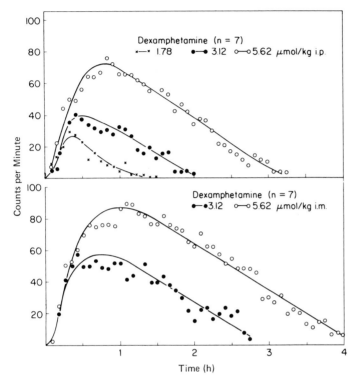

Fig. 6.5 Time course of central nervous sytem response (locomotor activity measured in counts per minute) after intraperitoneal and intramuscular administration of dexamphetamine sulfate to rats. Irrespective of dose and route of administration, the effect of the drug declines at a constant rate during the postabsorptive phase. (From Ref. 7.)

equation in terms of amount by multiplying the concentration terms by the apparent volume of distribution. This yields

$$\log X = \log X_0 - \frac{Kt}{2.303} \tag{6.11}$$

where X is the amount of drug in the body at time t and X_0 is the initial amount of drug in the body (i.e., the intravenous dose). If it is assumed that the intensity of a pharmacologic response is associated with a given amount of drug in the body, and that there is a minimum amount of drug in the body X_{min} necessary to elicit a response, the time necessary for the initial amount of drug in the body X_0 to decline to this minimum effective amount is the duration of response t_d. Substitution of X_{min} for X and t_d for t in (6.11) yields

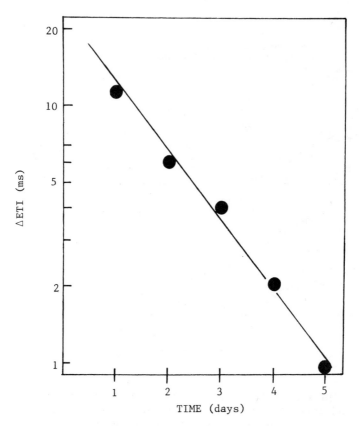

Fig. 6.6 Time course of cardiac response (change in ejection time index, plotted on log scale) after intravenous administration of digoxin. Exponential decline of response has also been observed with other cardiac glycosides, including ouabain, deslanoside C, and digitoxin. (Data from Ref. 8.)

$$\log X_{min} = \log X_0 - \frac{Kt_d}{2.303} \qquad (6.12)$$

which when solved for t_d is

$$t_d = \frac{2.303}{K} \log X_0 - \frac{2.303}{K} \log X_{min} \qquad (6.13)$$

Therefore, a plot of the duration of response versus the logarithm of the intravenous dose should be linear. The intercept on the log X_0 axis will be the minimum amount of drug in the body necessary to elicit a response, and the slope $-2.303/K$ will provide an estimate of the elimination rate constant. An example is shown in Fig. 6.8.

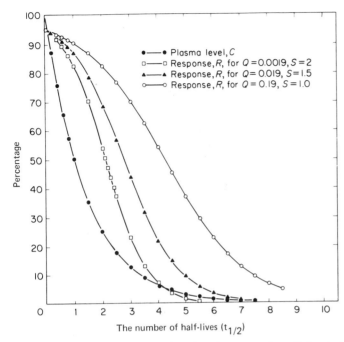

Fig. 6.7 Drug concentration in plasma and anticipated response curves under different conditions [see Eq. (6.1)] after intravenous administration. [From Ref. 1, © 1972 Academic Press, Inc. (London), Ltd., reprinted with permission.]

Equation (6.13) may be applied to determine the rate constant for drug elimination in instances where direct measurement of drug concentration as a function of time is not possible but where pharmacologic response can be measured adequately.

Under certain circumstances drugs may be dosed based on pharmacologic response. An example would be the use of neuromuscular blocking agents during anesthesia. If a drug confers on the body the pharmacokinetic properties of a one-compartment model, the administration of a second dose of a drug immediately after the apparent disappearance of the pharmacologic response from the initial dose is likely to produce a more intense and more prolonged response than the first dose. This is due to the fact that the second dose is superimposed on the minimum effective amount of drug remaining in the body from the first dose [11]. This phenomenon is readily expressed in mathematical terms by considering that the intensity of the response is related linearly to the logarithm of the amount of drug in the body (see Fig. 6.9). Hence

$$R = m(\log X - \log X_{min}) = m \log \frac{X}{X_{min}} \qquad (6.14)$$

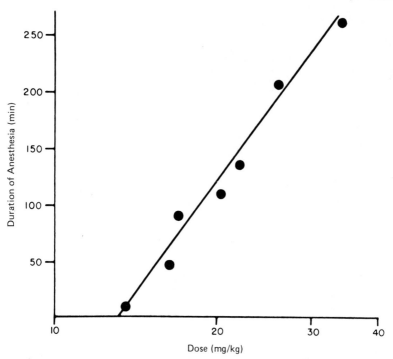

Fig. 6.8 Relationship between intravenous dose of pentobarbital
(x axis) and duration of anesthesia (y axis, in minutes) in monkeys.
X_{min}, the minimum dose required to elicit a measurable response, is
equal to 13 mg/kg. (From Ref. 10.)

This equation may be used to estimate the maximum intensity R_{01} of
the pharmacologic response elicited by an initial intravenous dose X_0:

$$R_{01} = m \log \frac{X_0}{X_{min}} \tag{6.15}$$

When a second (and equal) dose is administered immediately after
disappearance of the response of the first dose (i.e., when the
amount of drug in the body has declined to X_{min}), the maximum intensity of the response R_{02} would be

$$R_{02} = m \log \frac{X_0 + X_{min}}{X_{min}} \tag{6.16}$$

Obviously, $R_{02} > R_{01}$. The maximum response from a third and subsequent doses, if all were administered in the same manner as the
second dose, would be equal to the maximum response from the second
dose, and hence would be described by (6.16).

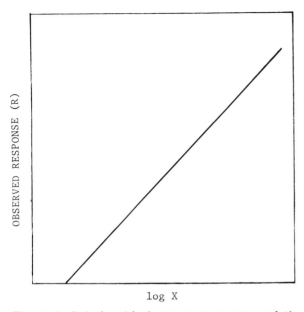

log X

Fig. 6.9 Relationship between response and the logarithm of the amount of drug in the body X, according to Eq. (6.14). The slope (m) of the line is the same as the slope of a log concentration-response plot [see Eq. (6.5)] and the X intercept corresponds to the minimum amount of drug in the body, X_{min}, needed to elicit a measurable response.

Similar reasoning may be applied to determine the effect of a second dose on the duration of a pharmacologic response. By rearranging (6.13), the duration of effect of the first dose can be written as

$$(t_d)_1 = \frac{2.303}{K} \log \frac{X_0}{X_{min}} \qquad (6.17)$$

It follows that the duration of effect of the second dose is

$$(t_d)_2 = \frac{2.303}{K} \log \frac{X_0 + X_{min}}{X_{min}} \qquad (6.18)$$

Again, it is apparent that $(t_d)_2 > (t_d)_1$. Equations (6.16) and (6.18) predict that there will be no further increase in the intensity and duration of response of third and subsequent doses. The predictable "potentiating" effect may be avoided by using $X_0 - X_{min}$ as the second and subsequent doses.

The total pharmacologic activity of a single dose of a drug has sometimes been represented as the area under the intensity of response

versus time curve (i.e., $\int_0^\infty R\ dt$). This index of total activity has
shortcomings for many drugs in that it does not define the maximum
intensity or duration of response. It is useful, however, in quanti-
tating such responses as diuresis, electrolyte excretion, and weight
loss. Since there is frequently a nonlinear relation between the
amount of drug in the body and the intensity of response [see, e.g.,
(6.1) and (6.5)] the *relative pharmacologic activity* of a drug (i.e.,
the total area under the effect versus time curve divided by the dose,
which upon intravenous administration is given by $\int_0^\infty R\ dt/X_0$) usually
decreases with increasing dose. Consequently, the total effect of a
fixed amount of drug per day may be affected by the dosage regimen
(i.e., the number of doses per day). Computer simulations using the
integrated form of (6.1) have shown that when the daily dose is divided, the total 24 h response is increased [1]. The greatest increase occurs with the first subdivision of the dose (i.e., two doses
a day compared with a single dose). It is of interest to note that the
administration of 1 g of chlorothiazide twice a day produces a significantly greater 24 h diuretic response than that observed after administration of a single dose of 2 g [12].

Multicompartment Models

Effect in the Central or Peripheral Compartment. The time course of
drug action in multicompartment systems depends on the location of the
site of action. Mathematically, the site may be located in the central
compartment or in the peripheral compartment or it may require representation as a separate compartment. The location of the site of
action may be determined by examining the relationship between the
intensity of response and the concentration of drug in the plasma or
the calculated amount of drug in a peripheral compartment. A relatively simple approach to this problem has been used with tubocurarine,
where effect data after several doses (over a fourfold range) were
available [13]. A detailed method to correlate response with either
plasma concentration or the "concentration" at some other site or
hypothetical compartment after a single dose has also been suggested
[14]. In essence, this method requires the following steps:

1. Measure the response and plasma concentration as a function
   of time until drug levels are no longer detectable.
2. By means of mathematical analysis, determine the appropriate
   pharmacokinetic model that rationalizes the concentration-
   time data.
3. Attempt to relate the response values to the instantaneous
   concentrations in the plasma compartment or peripheral compartments by means of some functional effect-concentration
   equation such as (6.1) or (6.5).

4. Once the appropriate pharmacokinetic model and functional
    equation are determined, *simultaneously* fit the observed drug
    concentration in the plasma, response, and time data, using a
    suitable nonlinear least-squares estimation program and a
    digital computer (Appendix H).

The significance of response correlations with drug "levels" in
hypothetical *peripheral* compartments of multicompartment models is
subject to challenge. Westlake [15] has demonstrated the large degree
of error that may be involved in calculating the amount of drug in the
peripheral compartment of a two-compartment model from drug concentration in the plasma versus time data after intravenous administration,
which can be rigorously fit to a biexponential equation. Still greater
error is involved if a more complex pharmacokinetic model is required
to rationalize the plasma concentration-time data. Additional error is
introduced when one considers that the quantitative assessment of response is often imprecise. Also, no single "response-concentration"
relationship has been universally accepted; rectilinear, log-linear,
or log-log plots have been used in arriving at these correlations.
Finally, the calculated time course of drug in a hypothetical peripheral
compartment reflects a type of weighted average of at least several
tissues. It is quite possible that the time course of drug at the site
of action and at some noneffector tissue having a relatively high
capacity for the drug may be significantly different, yet from a kinetic
point of view both the site of action and the noneffector tissue may
appear to be part of the same peripheral compartment.

If the site of action is associated with the central compartment,
a plot of response versus the logarithm of plasma concentration
should yield the same sigmoid-type curve as that shown in Fig. 6.1. A
similar relationship should also be observed when the response is
associated with a peripheral compartment and response is plotted
against the logarithm of the calculated amount of drug in a peripheral
compartment. Examples of these two possible situations are illustrated
in Figs. 6.10 and 6.11, respectively. When the site of action is associated with a peripheral compartment, and response is plotted as a
function of the logarithm of plasma concentration, response will increase with decreasing plasma concentration during the distributive
phase, reach a peak, then decrease during the postdistributive phase.
This type of response-concentration profile is depicted in Fig. 6.12.
The maximum response observed following a given dose will occur when
maximum drug levels are attained in the peripheral compartment.

In multicompartment systems the rate of decline of response is
likely to occur at a constant rate independent of dose during the postdistributive phase, irrespective of the apparent site of effect. However, drug concentrations in the postdistributive phase may be too

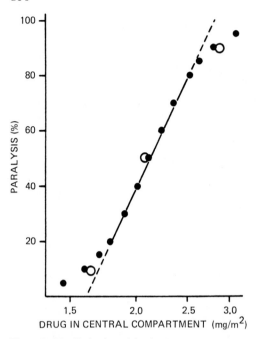

Fig. 6.10 Relationship between neuromuscular response (percent paralysis) and amount of drug in the central compartment of a multi-compartment system (log scale) after intravenous administration of tubocurarine. The closed circles were calculated based on a pharmaco-kinetic model and the open circles represent experimental data from normal volunteers. (From Ref. 16, reprinted with permission.)

low to be of clinical consequence. When the site of action is associated with the central compartment the maximum response will be observed shortly after administration of the intravenous dose (i.e., during the distributive phase). Since drug concentration during the distributive phase does not decline in a monoexponential fashion, one would not expect response to decline in a linear manner. Theory suggests that the decline of response to a drug showing multicompartment charac-teristics and apparently acting in the central compartment will be a curvilinear function of time after intravenous administration. Inter-estingly, the decline of effect of certain drugs such as tubocurarine which show pronounced multicompartment characteristics is apparently linear after a given dose, but the apparent zero-order rate of decay of effect decreases with increasing dose (see Fig. 6.13). This linearity merely reflects the fact that over the limited concentration range as-sociated with the range of intensities of pharmacologic effect, the curvilinear log C versus time plot can often be approximated by a straight line. The dose dependence results from the changing slope

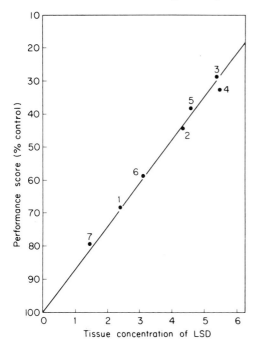

Fig. 6.11 Relationship between behavioral response (average performance scores on arithmetic tests) and amount of drug in the peripheral compartment of a two-compartment open model (or "tissue concentration") after intravenous administration of d-lysergic acid
diethylamide (LSD) to volunteer subjects. The number associated
with each data point denotes the blood sample number after drug administration (e.g., number 1 represents the "tissue concentration"
calculated from the drug concentration found in the first blood sample
taken after injection). (From Ref. 14.)

of the log C versus time curve in this concentration range as a function
of dose (see Fig. 6.14).

    In contrast to the relationships developed for the one-compartment
model in the first section of this chapter, the duration of effect of a
drug conferring multicompartment characteristics to the body is not a
linear function of the logarithm of the intravenous dose. Examples
are shown in Figs. 6.15 and 6.16. Apparently, linear relationships
between duration of effect and logarithm of dose can be obtained in a
restricted dose range, but the slope of the line is dependent on the
intensity of the effect used as the end point [18]. Moreover, for a
so-called two-compartment drug the slope of this apparently linear relationship after intravenous administration may approximate $1/\lambda_1$,
$1/\lambda_n$, or some other intermediate value. An additional observation is

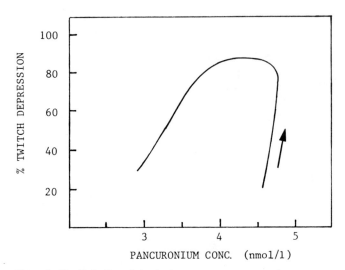

Fig. 6.12 Relationship between neuromuscular response (percent twitch depression) and pancuronium concentration in the plasma after intravenous administration of the drug. The arrow denotes the time course of the response. The results suggest that the locus of drug effect is at a site peripheral to the central compartment. (From Ref. 17, ⊚ 1978 Macmillan Journals Ltd., reprinted with permission.)

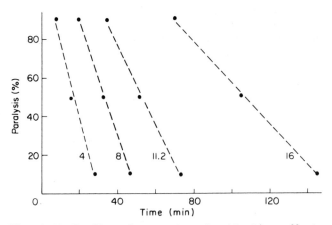

Fig. 6.13 Decline of neuromuscular blocking effects after intravenous administration of different doses of d-tubocurarine to human volunteers. Although the loss of effect is zero order, the rate is dose dependent. (From Ref. 16, reprinted with permission.)

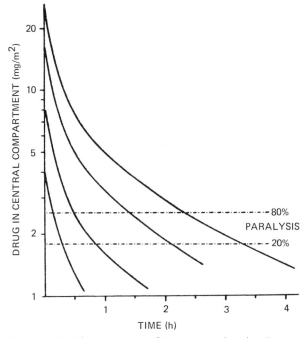

Fig. 6.14 Time course of tubocurarine in the central compartment of a multicompartment system after intravenous administration of different doses to healthy volunteers. The horizontal lines denote drug levels required to elicit 20% and 80% paralysis of the thumb adductor muscle. Although the deline of drug levels between 80% response and 20% response is approximately log linear in each case, the slope is dose dependent. (From Ref. 16, reprinted with permission.)

that the duration of a response associated with the central compartment of a multicompartment system will increase with successive doses when the drug is dosed according to response alone (Fig. 6.17). This is in contrast to a one-compartment system, where the duration of response increases from the first to the second dose but does not increase on subsequent doses. The maximum response increases from the first to the second dose in both systems but does not increase thereafter.

It is of theoretical interest to consider drug effects in a peripheral compartment of a multicompartment system which is poorly accessible to the central compartment. Drug moves in and out of such deep compartments rather slowly. If the site of drug action is in the deep compartment, the pharmacologic effect will be delayed and prolonged, and the relationship between drug levels in the plasma and effect may not be readily apparent. With this type of drug, repeated intravenous

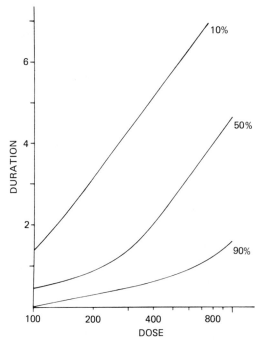

Fig. 6.15 Relationship between duration of response and intravenous dose (log scale), assuming that the site of effect is in the central compartment of a two-compartment model. The duration is measured in terms of the time required after administration of a given dose for the peak effect to decline to 90%, 50%, or 10% of the maximum attainable effect of the drug. It is evident that the shape of the curve depends on the end point. (From Ref. 18.)

administration of equal doses at constant time intervals will yield the concentration versus time patterns shown in Fig. 6.18 for the central and deep peripheral compartments. This simulation, with the assumed minimum detectable drug concentration in the central compartment and minimum pharmacologically effective drug concentration in the deep compartment, suggests certain clinically interesting characteristics. The pharmacologic effect appears only after the third dose, and the intensity of this effect increases beyond the tenth dose since drug levels in the deep compartment do, in fact, accumulate. When drug administration is stopped, the effect persists well beyond the last dose. There are pronounced pharmacologic effects at a time when there is no detectable drug concentration in the plasma. Thus the effects of drugs that act directly and reversibly in a deep compartment may sometimes be mistaken for indirect and/or irreversible drug effects.

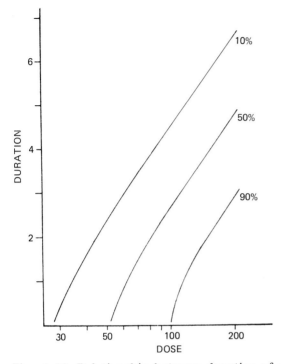

Fig. 6.16 Relationship between duration of response and intravenous dose (log scale), assuming that the site of effect is in the peripheral compartment of a two-compartment model. The end points used to determine duration of response are the same as in Fig. 6.15. For this particular simulation the curves are approximately linear and parallel. (From Ref. 18.)

Other Sites of Effect. A particular shortcoming of the pharmacodynamic modeling discussed in the preceding sections of this chapter is the required assumption that the plasma, central compartment, or some other pharmacokinetically identifiable compartment is associated with the pharmacologic effect. However, pharmacokinetic models concern themselves with the disposition of mass of drug in the body; a site receiving little mass is not described. There is no a priori reason to assume that the active site corresponds, kinetically, with a site receiving a large mass of drug. Accordingly, there is little reason to hope that the kinetics of drug in plasma, or another pharmacokinetically determined site, will parallel those at the active site. It has recently been proposed that the effect compartment be modeled as a separate compartment linked to the plasma compartment by a first-order process, and be one that receives a negligible mass of drug [19,20]. Therefore, one does not enter an additional exponential term into the phar-

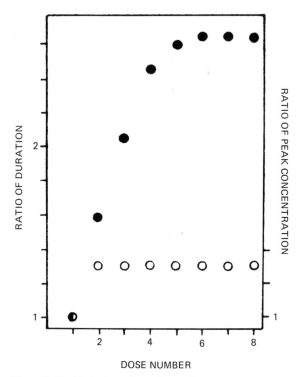

Fig. 6.17 Relative duration of response (●) and peak concentration (O) for a situation where equal intravenous doses are given repetitively as soon as a certain effect end point is reached, assuming that the site of effect is in the central compartment of a two-compartment model. (From Ref. 18.)

macokinetic solution for the mass of drug in the body to account for the effect compartment. The model is illustrated in Fig. 6.19. In this model a first-order rate constant k_{1e} connects the central to the effect compartment. Drug leaves the effect compartment by means of a first-order rate constant k_{e0}. By assuming k_{1e} to be very small relative to the magnitude of any other rate constant in the model (Fig. 6.19), the transfer of mass to the effect compartment is negligible, and consequently does not influence the plasma concentration versus time curve. Since a negligible amount of drug is transferred to the effect compartment, its return to the central compartment is inconsequential, and therefore may be taken to the outside rather than back into the system. The rate constant for drug removal from the effect compartment, k_{e0}, characterizes the temporal aspects of equilibrium between plasma concentration and response.

The following differential equation can be written for the amount of drug in the effect compartment, X_e:

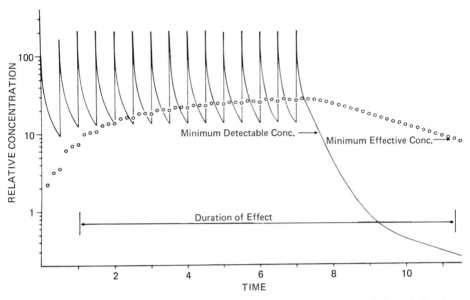

Fig. 6.18 Relative concentrations of a drug in the central (solid line) and deep peripheral (O) compartments of a multicompartment system during repetitive intravenous administration of equal doses at equal time intervals. (From Ref. 18.)

$$\frac{dX_e}{dt} = k_{1e}X_c - k_{e0}X_e \tag{6.19}$$

where k_{1e} and k_{e0} are as defined above and X_c is the amount of drug in the central compartment. The Laplace transform of (6.19) (see Appendix B) is

$$s(a_{s,e}) = k_{1e}a_{s,c} - k_{e0}a_{s,e} \tag{6.20}$$

Solving for $a_{s,e}$ and substituting the value of $a_{s,c}$ as given in (2.3) [i.e., $a_{s,c} = X_0 \prod_{i=2}^{n} (s + E_i)/\prod_{i=1}^{n} (s + \lambda_i)$] yields

$$a_{s,e} = \frac{k_{1e}X_0 \prod\limits_{i=2}^{n} (s + E_i)}{(s + k_{e0}) \prod\limits_{i=1}^{n} (s + \lambda_i)} \tag{6.21}$$

The anti-Laplace (see Appendix B) of (6.21) gives the following equation for the amount of drug in the effect compartment as a function of time:

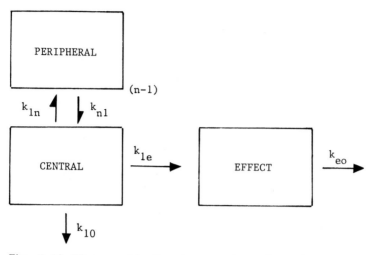

Fig. 6.19 Pharmacokinetic-pharmacodynamic model to describe that situation where the site of effect does not correspond to a pharmacokinetic compartment. (Data from Refs. 19 and 20.)

$$X_e = k_{1e}X_0 \frac{\prod\limits_{i=2}^{n} (E_i - k_{e0})}{\prod\limits_{i=1}^{n} (\lambda_i - k_{e0})} e^{-k_{e0}t}$$

$$+ k_{1e}X_0 \sum_{\ell=1}^{n} \frac{\prod\limits_{i=2}^{n} (E_i - \lambda_\ell)}{(k_{e0} - \lambda_\ell) \prod\limits_{\substack{i=1 \\ i\neq\ell}}^{n} (\lambda_i - \lambda_\ell)} e^{-\lambda_\ell t} \qquad (6.22)$$

where X_0 is the intravenous dose, E_i the sum of the exit rate constants from the ith compartment, n the number of compartments in the n-compartment mammillary model, and λ_i and λ_ℓ are disposition rate constants. Assuming that the amount of drug in the effect compartment is proportional to the concentration in this compartment, C_e:

$$X_e = V_e C_e \qquad (6.23)$$

where V_e is the apparent volume of the effect compartment, we can write (6.22) in terms of concentration as follows:

$$C_e = \frac{k_{1e} X_0}{V_e} \frac{\prod\limits_{i=2}^{n} (E_i - k_{e0})}{\prod\limits_{i=1}^{n} (\lambda_i - k_{e0})} e^{-k_{e0}t}$$

$$+ \frac{k_{1e} X_0}{V_e} \sum_{\ell=1}^{n} \frac{\prod\limits_{i=2}^{n} (E_i - \lambda_\ell)}{(k_{e0} - \lambda_\ell) \prod\limits_{\substack{i=1 \\ i \neq \ell}}^{n} (\lambda_i - \lambda_\ell)} e^{-\lambda_\ell t} \qquad (6.24)$$

By assuming that the rates of appearance of drug in and removal of drug from the effect compartment are governed by the same process, it follows that the clearance from the central to the effect compartment and the clearance out of the effect compartment are equal, and therefore

$$V_c k_{1e} = V_e k_{e0} \qquad (6.25)$$

Rearrangement of (6.25) to solve for k_{1e}/V_e (i.e., $k_{1e}/V_e = k_{e0}/V_c$) and substitution of k_{e0}/V_c for k_{1e}/V_e in (6.24) gives

$$C_e = \frac{k_{e0} X_0}{V_c} \frac{\prod\limits_{i=2}^{n} (E_i - k_{e0})}{\prod\limits_{i=1}^{n} (\lambda_i - k_{e0})} e^{-k_{e0}t}$$

$$+ \frac{k_{e0} X_0}{V_c} \sum_{\ell=1}^{n} \frac{\prod\limits_{i=2}^{n} (E_i - \lambda_\ell)}{(k_{e0} - \lambda_\ell) \prod\limits_{\substack{i=1 \\ i \neq \ell}}^{n} (\lambda_i - \lambda_\ell)} e^{-\lambda_\ell t} \qquad (6.26)$$

Multiexponential plasma concentration-time data after intravenous administration can be described by

$$C = \frac{X_0}{V_c} \sum_{\ell=1}^{n} \frac{\prod\limits_{i=2}^{n} (E_i - \lambda_\ell)}{\prod\limits_{\substack{i=1 \\ i \neq \ell}}^{n} (\lambda_i - \lambda_\ell)} e^{-\lambda_\ell t} \qquad (6.27)$$

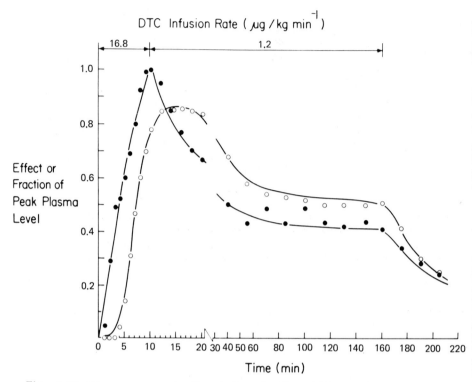

Fig. 6.20 Plasma concentration (●) and effect (O) relationships
during and after intravenous infusions of d-tubocurarine to a patient.
The solid lines represent the best fits of the proposed model to the
data. Note break in graph at 20 to 30 min, due to change of scale on
time axis. (From Ref. 19.)

Once plasma concentration-time data have been fitted, all the parameters in (6.27) and (6.26) (except for k_{e0}) can be generated. Substitution of C_e for C in (6.1) yields the following equation, which relates the observed pharmacologic response to concentrations in the
effect compartment:

$$R = \frac{R_m C_e^S}{(1/Q) + C_e^S} \tag{6.28}$$

where C_e is given by (6.26). Therefore, either response-time data
can be fitted after the concentration-time data have been fitted, generating values of R_m, s, Q, and k_{e0} [Eqs. (6.26) and (6.28)], or
response-time and concentration-time data can be fitted simultaneously
[Eqs. (6.26) to (6.28)], generating all pharmacokinetic and pharma-

codynamic parameters. This approach to the quantitative description of response-plasma concentration-time data has been used in the quantitative analysis of d-tubocurarine and disopyramide pharmacodynamics [19–21]. An example is presented in Fig. 6.20.

KINETICS OF INDIRECT PHARMACOLOGIC RESPONSE

The intensity of a pharmacologic response may not be due to a direct effect of the drug on the receptor; rather, it may be the net result of several processes only one of which is influenced by the drug. Under such circumstances a direct relationship between the plasma concentration of the drug and the measured pharmacologic response can generally not be obtained. If this is the case, the process that is influenced by the drug must be identified and an attempt made to relate plasma drug concentrations to changes in this process. A good example is the anticoagulant (hypoprothrombinemic) effect of the coumarin drugs, which inhibit the synthesis of certain vitamin K-dependent clotting factors (i.e., factors II, VII, IX, and X), but have no effect on the physiologic degradation of these factors. Thus the real effect of these drugs is inhibition of synthesis rate, and any correlation with plasma concentration must be based on this effect rather than on the degree of inhibition of clotting time [22]. Administration of warfarin or bishydroxycoumarin rapidly blocks the synthesis of prothrombin complex activity P [23], but significant anticoagulant effect will not be observed until normal circulating levels of P are reduced sufficiently. Hence it is not surprising that although peak levels of warfarin in the plasma are observed within several hours after oral administration, the maximum hypoprothrombinemic response does not appear until several days after administration (see Fig. 6.21).

The degree of anticoagulation is generally measured in terms of a prothrombin time PT. PT is a measure of the net effect of the rate of synthesis and the rate of degredation of the appropriate clotting factors. Prothrombin time is generally expressed as the percent of the normal prothrombin complex activity, and will be denoted by the symbol P. P can be determined employing the following relationship:

$$P = 100 \left(1 - \frac{PT_0 - PT_n}{PT_n} \right) \tag{6.29}$$

where PT_0 is the observed prothrombin time and PT_n is the normal prothrombin time. For example, if a prothrombin time of 19 s was measured, the prothrombin complex activity P would be 42% of normal, assuming a normal prothrombin time of 12 s.

The net rate of change of P at any time (i.e., dP/dt or R_{net}) may be described by

$$R_{net} = R_{syn} - R_{deg} \tag{6.30}$$

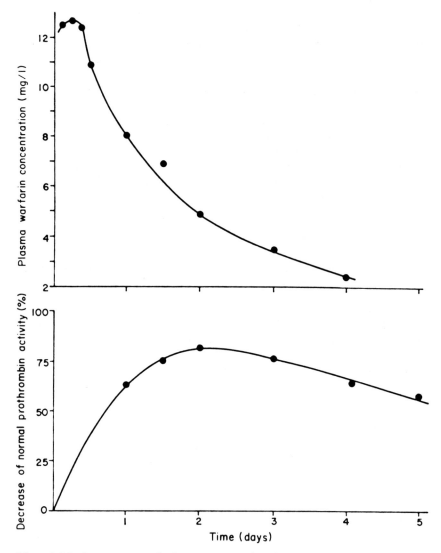

Fig. 6.21 Average warfarin concentration in plasma and depression of prothrombin complex activity after oral administration of warfarin to healthy subjects. (From Ref. 22.)

where R_{syn} and R_{deg} are the rates of P synthesis and degradation, respectively. The R values are measured in terms of percentage of normal activity per day since P is measured relative to the average P level of normal subjects.

As noted, the direct effect of coumarin anticoagulants is not reflected by changes in P but rather by changes in R_{syn} relative to its normal value. R_{syn} may be calculated from (6.30) if R_{deg} can be determined, since R_{net} is readily obtained from P (i.e., $R_{net} = dP/dt$). If it is assumed that the degradation of P is describable by first-order kinetics, then

$$R_{deg} = k_d P \tag{6.31}$$

where k_d is the apparent first-order degradation rate constant. This constant can be obtained experimentally from the slope of a log P versus time plot after administration of a synthesis blocking dose of a coumarin anticoagulant. Under these conditions R_{syn} in (6.30) equals zero. Therefore,

$$\frac{dP}{dt} = R_{net} = -R_{deg} \tag{6.32}$$

and hence

$$\frac{dP}{dt} = -k_d P \tag{6.33}$$

Integration of (6.33) yields

$$P = P_0 e^{-k_d t} \tag{6.34}$$

which in logarithmic terms is

$$\log P = \log P_0 - \frac{k_d t}{2.303} \tag{6.35}$$

where P_0 is the level of P prior to medication. Therefore, a plot of log P versus time should be a straight line, the slope of which will yield k_d (Fig. 6.22). In one study where a synthesis blocking dose of 1.5 mg/kg of warfarin was administered orally, an average value of k_d of 1.21 per day was determined [22]. This corresponds to an average half-life of 13.7 h.

Solving (6.30) for R_{syn} and substituting $k_d P$ for R_{deg} according to (6.31) and dP/dt for R_{net} according to (6.32) yields

$$R_{syn} = \frac{dP}{dt} + k_d P \tag{6.36}$$

Therefore, by knowing k_d and P as a function of time, R_{syn} can be determined.

The magnitude of response R at any given time can be expressed as the difference between the synthesis rate before medication R_{syn}° and R_{syn} at time t:

$$R = R_{syn}^\circ - R_{syn} \tag{6.37}$$

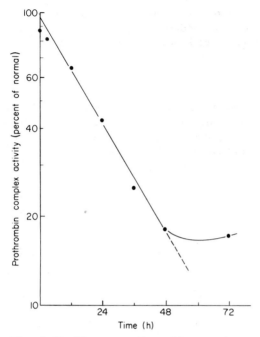

Fig. 6.22 Plasma prothrombin complex activity in a normal subject
after oral administration of 1.5 mg/kg dose of warfarin. (From
Ref. 22.)

As discussed above, the magnitude of many types of pharmacological
response is related to the logarithm of the plasma concentration of
the drug. Equation (6.14) can be converted to a concentration equation by dividing by volume of distribution to yield

$$R = m(\log C - \log C_{min}) \qquad (6.38)$$

where C_{min} is the minimum effective plasma concentration. Substituting
$R^\circ_{syn} - R_{syn}$ for R according to (6.37) in (6.38) and solving for R_{syn}
gives

$$R_{syn} = R^\circ_{syn} + m \log C_{min} - m \log C \qquad (6.39)$$

Therefore, a plot of R_{syn} versus log C should yield a straight line
with a slope of $-m$ (Fig. 6.23). According to (6.39), when R_{syn}
equals R°_{syn}, C equals C_{min}.

Prothrombin Complex Activity Versus Time. Although the direct
effect of the coumarin anticoagulants is on R_{syn}, the time course of
P is of interest since this is the actual response being measured. This
information can be obtained by incorporating the concepts expressed

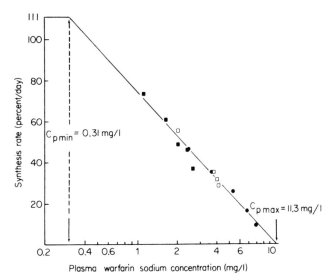

Fig. 6.23 Average synthesis rate of prothrombin complex activity as a function of plasma warfarin concentration in normal volunteers. Warfarin sodium dosing schedules: ●, a single oral dose of 1.5 mg/kg; ■, daily oral doses of 10 mg for 5 days; □, daily oral doses of 15 mg for 4 days. $C_{p\ min}$, the apparent minimum effective plasma warfarin sodium concentration; $C_{p\ max}$, the concentration of warfarin sodium in the plasma which apparently suppresses totally the synthesis of prothrombin complex activity. (From Ref. 22.)

in the preceding paragraphs into a single mathematical expression that permits the determination of P as a function of time and the initial plasma concentration (or dose) of the drug. Substitution of $dP/dt + k_dP$ for R_{syn} according to (6.36) in (6.39) and rearrangement yields

$$\frac{dP}{dt} = R^o_{syn} + m \log C_{min} - m \log C - k_dP \qquad (6.40)$$

Prior to the initiation of anticoagulant therapy, the circulating levels of P are constant at P^o, and at that time R^o_{syn} is given by

$$R^o_{syn} = k_dP^o \qquad (6.41)$$

[see (6.36)]. Substituting this value of R^o_{syn} in (6.40) results in

$$\frac{dP}{dt} = k_dP^o + m \log C_{min} - m \log C - k_dP \qquad (6.42)$$

It has been shown that after intravenous administration,

$$\log C = \log C_0 - \frac{Kt}{2.303} \qquad (6.7)$$

Accordingly,

$$\frac{dP}{dt} = k_d P^\circ - m \log \frac{C_0}{C_{min}} + \frac{mK}{2.303} t - k_d P \qquad (6.43)$$

Since the first two terms of (6.46) are constant for a given dose, they may be combined, and upon rearrangement,

$$\frac{dP}{dt} + K_d P = A_0 + \frac{mK}{2.303} t \qquad (6.44)$$

where $A_0 = k_d P^\circ - m \log (C_0/C_{min})$. Multiplying through by dt yields

$$dP + k_d P \, dt = A_0 \, dt + \frac{mK}{2.303} t \, dt \qquad (6.45)$$

The solution to this differential expression requires the use of an integrating factor.[+] In this case the appropriate integrating factor is $e^{\int k_d t}$, which is equivalent to $e^{k_d t}$. Multiplying through by this term yields

$$e^{k_d t} dP + k_d P e^{k_d t} dt = A_0 e^{k_d t} dt + \frac{mKt e^{k_d t}}{2.303} dt \qquad (6.46)$$

Since

$$d(Pe^{k_d t}) = e^{k_d t} dP + k_d P e^{k_d t} dt \qquad (6.47)$$

we may substitute $d(Pe^{k_d t})$ for the left-hand side of (6.46). Hence upon substitution and rearrangement, (6.46) may be rewritten as

$$d(Pe^{k_d t}) = \left(A_0 + \frac{mKt}{2.303} \right) e^{k_d t} dt \qquad (6.48)$$

The indefinite integral of this expression is

$$Pe^{k_d t} = \int \left(A_0 + \frac{mKt}{2.303} \right) e^{k_d t} dt + i \qquad (6.49)$$

where i is an integration constant. Upon rearrangement,

$$P = e^{-k_d t} \left[\int \left(A_0 + \frac{mKt}{2.303} \right) e^{k_d t} dt + i \right] \qquad (6.50)$$

[+]See L. M. Kells, *Elementary Differential Equations*, 6th ed. McGraw-Hill, New York, 1965, chap. 3, sec. 24, pp. 63–68.

The integral term of (6.50) may be expressed as

$$A_0 \int e^{k_d t} \, dt + \frac{mK}{2.303} \int te^{k_d t} \, dt$$

The first term of this expression is readily solved since

$$A_0 \int e^{k_d t} \, dt = \frac{A_0}{k_d} e^{k_d t} + i' \tag{6.51}$$

but the solution of the second term requires some effort. Considering the general relationship

$$xy = \int d(xy) = \int (x \, dy + y \, dx) = \int x \, dy + \int y \, dx \tag{6.52}$$

it follows that

$$\int x \, dy = xy - \int y \, dx \tag{6.53}$$

Now returning to the second term of the integral,

$$\frac{mK}{2.303} \int te^{k_d t} \, dt$$

and letting $t = x$ and $e^{k_d t} \, dt = dy$, it follows that $y = e^{k_d t}/k_d$.

Substituting these relationships in the second term of the integal yields

$$\int te^{k_d t} \, dt = \frac{te^{k_d t}}{k_d} - \int \frac{e^{k_d t}}{k_d} \, dt \tag{6.54}$$

which upon integration yields

$$\int te^{k_d t} \, dt = \frac{te^{k_d t}}{k_d} - \frac{e^{k_d t}}{k_d^2} + i'' \tag{6.55}$$

Upon further simplification,

$$\int te^{k_d t} \, dt = \frac{e^{k_d t}}{k_d^2} (k_d t - 1) + i'' \tag{6.56}$$

Accordingly,

$$\frac{mK}{2.303} \int te^{k_d t} \, dt = \frac{mKe^{k_d t}}{2.303 k_d^2} (k_d t - 1) + i'' \tag{6.57}$$

Summing (6.51) and (6.57) yields the integral term of (6.50):

$$\int \left(A_0 + \frac{mKt}{2.303} \right) e^{k_d t} \, dt = \frac{A_0}{k_d} e^{k_d t} + \frac{mKe^{k_d t}}{2.303k_d^2}(k_d t - 1) + i' + i''$$

(6.58)

Substituting the right-hand side of (6.58) for the integral terms in (6.50) and collecting the integration constants such that $i + i' + i'' = I$ yields

$$P = e^{-k_d t}\left[\frac{A_0}{K_d} e^{k_d t} + \frac{mKe^{k_d t}}{2.303k_d^2}(k_d t - 1) + I\right]$$

(6.59)

Upon simplification,

$$P = Ie^{-k_d t} + \frac{A_0}{k_d} - \frac{mK}{2.303k_d^2} + \frac{mK}{2.303k_d}t$$

(6.60)

Evaluation of I at $t = 0$, where $C = C_0$ and $P = P°$, yields

$$I = P° - \frac{A_0}{k_d} + \frac{mK}{2.303k_d^2}$$

(6.61)

Substituting for I and A_0 in (6.60) and simplifying the results gives

$$P = P° - a(1 - e^{-k_d t}) + bt$$

(6.62)

where

$$a = \frac{m \log (C_0/C_{min})}{k_d} + \frac{mK}{2.303k_d^2} \quad \text{and} \quad b = \frac{mK}{2.303k_d}$$

Equation (6.62) has a number of interesting features. Shortly after drug administration, when t is relatively small, the second term predominates over the third term and P decreases with time. At later times, the third term predominates and P increases with time. At some time later, $e^{-k_d t} \to 0$ and P increases linearly with time. Values of P calculated as a function of time after warfarin administration, by means of (6.62), agree exceedingly well with clinically observed values (see Fig. 6.24). A pharmacokinetic analysis by this method of the effect of a barbituate on the anticoagulant action of warfarin and bishydroxycoumarin has shown that the reduced efficacy of these drugs in

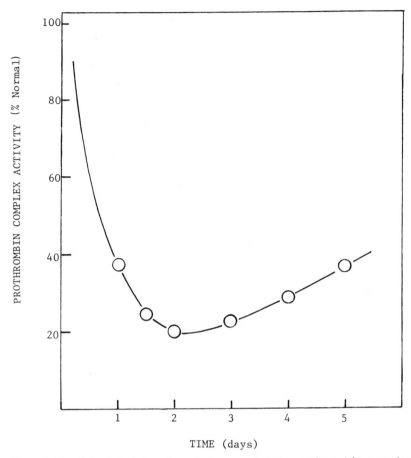

TIME (days)

Fig. 6.24 Calculated (——) and observed (O) prothrombin complex activity in healthy human subjects after a single oral dose of 1.5 mg/kg warfarin sodium. (From Ref. 22.)

humans during barbiturate administration is due to enhanced biotrans-formation of the coumarin drugs rather than to changes in distribu-tion or affinity to the pharmacologic receptors. Thus, whereas the biologic half-life of the coumarins was decreased significantly with the barbiturate, the relationship between effect and plasma-drug concen-tration remained unchanged [24,25]. On the other hand, phenyl-butazone, which also enhances the elimination of warfarin, has a pro-nounced effect on the relationship between synthesis rate of pro-thrombin complex activity and plasma-warfarin concentration [26]. These observations are consistent with the assumption that phenyl-butazone competitively displaces warfarin from nonspecific binding sites in the plasma and tissues and thereby increases the interaction

of the anticoagulant with its pharmacologic receptor and metabolizing
enzyme system.

KINETICS OF IRREVERSIBLE PHARMACOLOGIC RESPONSE

Although most drugs produce a response that is reversible, certain
antibiotics and anticancer agents cause cell death (an irreversible
effect) by the irreversible or covalent incorporation of drug into a
metabolic pathway of a cell. When discussing the kinetics of irreversible pharmacologic response, it is appropriate to consider two
classes of drugs, each of which affects the cell cycle and mitosis in
a different manner, one class which is nonphase specific in its cytoxic
effect and the other class which is phase specific.

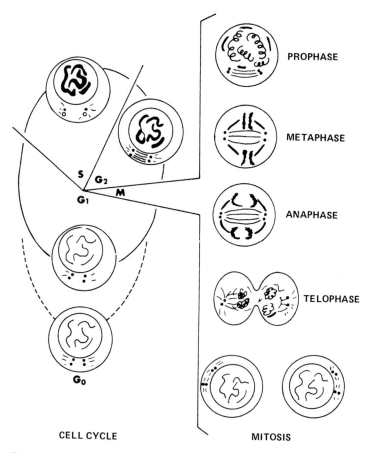

Fig. 6.25 Segments of the cell cycle and mitosis (see Ref. 27).

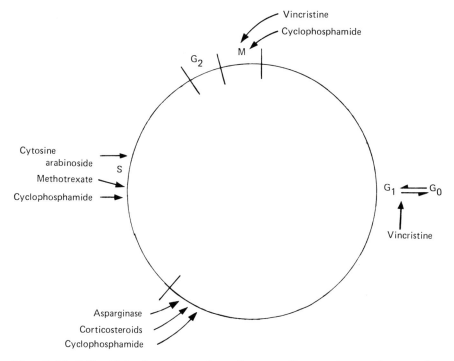

Fig. 6.26 Effect(s) of various chemotherapeutic agents on phases of the cell cycle. (From Ref. 28, reprinted with permission.)

The various segments of the cell cycle and mitosis are depicted in Fig. 6.25. Briefly, at the completion of mitosis M, the cells spend a variable period of time in a resting phase G_1. This is followed by the DNA synthesis period, the S phase. The cells cease DNA synthesis during the G_2 phase before reentry into mitosis. Each cytotoxic agent exerts its effect by disrupting one or more phases of the cell cycle. For example (see Fig. 6.26), methotrexate and cytosine arabinoside appear to inhibit DNA synthesis, while corticosteroids and L-asparginase inhibit the entry of cells into the S phase. Vincristine arrests mitosis and blocks the entry of resting cells into the mitotic cycle. Cyclophosphamide, on the other hand, appears to have several effects: inhibition of DNA synthesis, arrest of cells in mitosis, and inhibition of cells from entering DNA synthesis.

Nonphase Specific Drugs

The proposed model in Fig. 6.27 is an expansion of the model in Fig. 6.19, and is a slight modification of one presented previously [29]. This model permits an evaluation of the influence of cell cycle non-

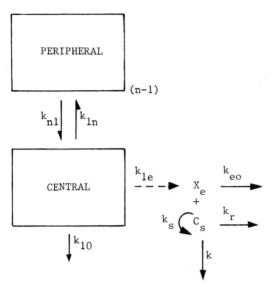

Fig. 6.27 Pharmacokinetic-cytotoxic model for nonphase specific drugs. (Data from Ref. 29.)

specific drugs on cell cytotoxicity. In this model X_e is the amount of drug in the effect compartment, C_s the concentration of proliferating target cells, k_s the rate constant for natural mitotic growth, k_r the rate constant for normal physiologic degradation, and k the rate constant for cell kill. All other parameters are as defined previously. As with the model in Fig. 6.19, the effect compartment is assumed to receive a negligible amount of the total drug in the body (i.e., k_{1e} is very small) and therefore does not influence the plasma concentration versus time curve. Nor does it enter into the pharmacokinetic solution for the amount of drug in the body.

Based on the model in Fig. 6.27, the following equation can be written for the rate of change of target cells:

$$\frac{dC_s}{dt} = k_s C_s - k_r C_s - kC_s X_e \tag{6.63}$$

Rearrangement yields

$$\frac{dC_s}{C_s} = (k_s - k_r)\, dt - kX_e\, dt \tag{6.64}$$

which when integrated becomes

$$\ln C_s = (k_s - k_r)\, t - k \int_0^t X_e\, dt + i \tag{6.65}$$

where i is a constant of integration. At $t = 0$, $i = \ln C_S^o$, where C_S^o is the concentration of target cells before the initiation of therapy. Substitution of $\ln C_S^o$ for i in (6.65) and rearrangement produces the following relationship:

$$\ln \frac{C_S}{C_S^o} = (k_s - k_r)t - k \int_0^t X_e \, dt \qquad (6.66)$$

Since most anticancer drugs have relatively short half-lives, it is suggested that the pharmacokinetic events (i.e., absorption, distribution, and elimination) are essentially over before much happens to the cells. Therefore,

$$\int_0^t X_e \, dt = \int_0^\infty X_e \, dt \qquad (6.67)$$

The amount of drug in the effect compartment as a function of time is given by

$$X_e = k_{1e} X_0 \frac{\prod\limits_{i=2}^{n} (E_i - k_{e0})}{\prod\limits_{i=1}^{n} (\lambda_i - k_{e0})} e^{-k_{e0}t}$$

$$+ k_{1e} X_0 \sum_{\ell=1}^{n} \frac{\prod\limits_{i=2}^{n} (E_i - \lambda_\ell)}{(k_{e0} - \lambda_\ell) \prod\limits_{\substack{i=1 \\ i \neq \ell}}^{n} (\lambda_i - \lambda_\ell)} e^{-\lambda_\ell t} \qquad (6.22)$$

Integration of (6.22) from zero to infinity yields

$$\int_0^\infty X_e \, dt = k_{1e} X_0 \left[\frac{\prod\limits_{i=2}^{n} (E_i - k_{e0})}{k_{e0} \prod\limits_{i=1}^{n} (\lambda_i - k_{e0})} \right.$$

$$\left. + \sum_{\ell=1}^{n} \frac{\prod\limits_{i=2}^{n} (E_i - \lambda_\ell)}{\lambda_\ell (k_{e0} - \lambda_\ell) \prod\limits_{\substack{i=1 \\ i \neq \ell}}^{n} (\lambda_i - \lambda_\ell)} \right] \qquad (6.68)$$

The same solution for $\int_0^\infty X_e \, dt$ [Eq. (6.72)] results regardless of the value of n. Therefore, arbitrarily setting n = 2 in (6.68) gives

$$\int_0^\infty X_e \, dt = k_{1e}X_0 \left[\frac{E_2 - k_{e0}}{k_{e0}(\lambda_1 - k_{e0})(\lambda_2 - k_{e0})} \right.$$

$$+ \frac{E_2 - \lambda_1}{\lambda_1(k_{e0} - \lambda_1)(\lambda_2 - \lambda_1)}$$

$$\left. + \frac{E_2 - \lambda_2}{\lambda_2(k_{e0} - \lambda_2)(\lambda_1 - \lambda_2)} \right] \qquad (6.69)$$

Bringing (6.69) to a common denominator, expanding the resulting numerator, canceling common terms, substituting k_{21} for E_2, and factoring out k_{21} produces

$$\int_0^\infty X_e \, dt = k_{1e}k_{21}X_0 \frac{\lambda_1^2\lambda_2 - \lambda_1\lambda_2^2 + \lambda_2^2 k_{e0} - \lambda_2 k_{e0}^2 - \lambda_1^2 k_{e0} + \lambda_i k_{e0}^2}{\lambda_1\lambda_2 k_{e0}(\lambda_1 - \lambda_2)(k_{e0} - \lambda_1)(k_{e0} - \lambda_2)}$$

$$(6.70)$$

Recognizing that the numerator of (6.70) is equal to $(\lambda_1 - \lambda_2)(k_{e0} - \lambda_1)(k_{e0} - \lambda_2)$ permits (6.70) to be simplified to

$$\int_0^\infty X_e \, dt = \frac{k_{1e}k_{21}X_0}{\lambda_1\lambda_2 k_{e0}} \qquad (6.71)$$

Since $\lambda_1\lambda_2 = k_{21}k_{10}$ [Eq. (2.100)], $k_{21}k_{10}$ can be substituted for $\lambda_1\lambda_2$ in (6.71) and k_{21} canceled to give

$$\int_0^\infty X_e \, dt = \frac{k_{1e}X_0}{k_{e0}k_{10}} \qquad (6.72)$$

Substitution of $k_{1e}X_0/k_{e0}k_{10}$ for $\int_0^t X_e \, dt$, according to (6.67) and (6.66) yields

$$\ln \frac{C_s}{C_s^0} = (k_s - k_r)t - \frac{kk_{1e}}{k_{e0}k_{10}} X_0 \qquad (6.73)$$

or

$$\log \frac{C_s}{C_s^0} = \frac{k_s - k_r}{2.303} t - \frac{kk_{1e}}{2.303 k_{e0}k_{10}} X_0 \qquad (6.74)$$

Equation (6.74) can be given as

$$\log \frac{C_s}{C_s^o} = \frac{k_s - k_r}{2.303} t - K_L X_0 \tag{6.75}$$

where

$$K_L = \frac{kk_{1e}}{2.303k_{e0}k_{10}} \tag{6.76}$$

Therefore, a plot of the logarithm of the fraction of surviving cells (C_s/C_s^o) versus dose should be linear. An example is presented in Fig. 6.28. The slope of the line K_L is a function of the affinity of the target cell for the drug, k, the elimination rate constant of the drug, k_{10}, and the constants responsible for the appearance and disappearance of drug in the effect compartment.

The reciprocal of K_L (i.e., $1/K_L$) has been defined as a lethality constant ED90, which is the dose increment of drug required to reduce the fraction of surviving cells (C_s/C_s^o) by one order of magnitude [29]. This lethality constant can be used to compare the cytotoxic effects of a drug on various cell systems or effects of various drugs on a single-cell system. For example, a comparison of the curves in Fig. 6.28 would suggest that cyclophosphamide has a smaller lethality constant for or is more potent against osteosarcoma cells than chimera spleen cells.

Cell-Cycle-Specific Drugs

There are some anticancer drugs which are cytotoxic only during a specific phase of the cell cycle. For this class of drugs the model in Fig. 6.29 is proposed. Again, this model is slightly modified from one presented previously [30]. C_s represents the concentration (or number) of cells sensitive to the drug, and C_r is the concentration (or number) of insensitive cells. Cells in each group are interconvertible with transformation rate constants k_{rs} and k_{sr}. All other terms are as defined previously. As can be seen from the model, the cell proliferation rate constant k_s is assumed to act only on C_s cells, and the rate constant for cell loss k_r acts only on C_r cells. This model is analogous to systems in which C_s and C_r represent proliferative and resting cells, respectively.

The rate of change in the number of target or proliferating cells and insensitive or resting cells can be written as the following differential equations:

$$\frac{dC_s}{dt} = k_s C_s - kX_e C_s - k_{sr} C_s + k_{rs} C_r \tag{6.77}$$

and

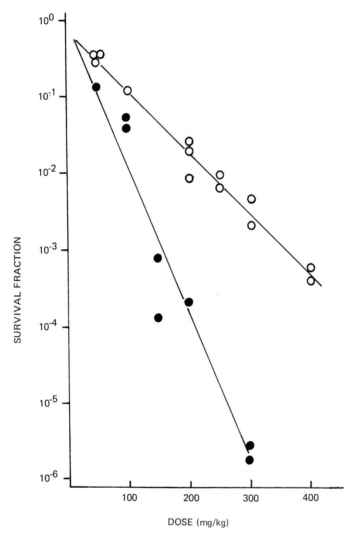

Fig. 6.28 Survival curves for chimera spleen cells (O) and osteo-sarcoma cells (●) after intraperitoneal administration of single doses of cyclophosphamide. (From Ref. 29, reprinted with permission.)

$$\frac{dC_r}{dt} = k_{sr}C_s - k_{rs}C_r - k_r C_r \tag{6.78}$$

The problem encountered in trying to solve (6.77) and (6.78) is the time-dependent nature of X_e. This problem can be overcome by numerical integration of the specific differential equations that describe

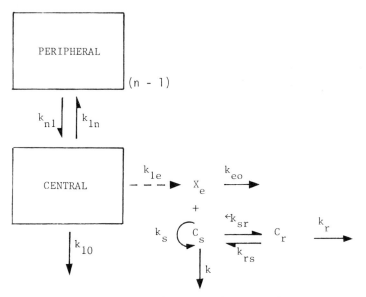

Fig. 6.29 Pharmacokinetic-cytotoxic model for cell-cycle-specific drugs. (Data from Ref. 30.)

the model [i.e., Eqs. (6.77) and (6.78), plus the differential equations for X_e and other compartments (see Fig. 6.29)]. Such an approach has been applied to arabinosylcytosine data (see Fig. 6.30).

If X_e in (6.77) is assumed to remain constant, a specific equation for (6.77) can be obtained quite readily. Assuming that X_e can be approximated by the average amount of drug in the effect compartment during a dosing interval at steady state, $\overline{X}_e$, where

$$\overline{X}_e = \frac{\int_0^\tau X_e \, dt}{\tau} \tag{6.79}$$

(see Chap. 3), then

$$X_e \sim \frac{\int_0^\tau X_e \, dt}{\tau} \tag{6.80}$$

where τ is the dosing interval and $\int_0^\tau X_e \, dt$ is the area under the X_e versus t curve during a dosing interval at steady state. Since $\int_0^\tau X_e \, dt$ equals $\int_0^\infty X_e \, dt$ (see Chap. 3), $k_{1e}X_0/k_{e0}k_{10}$ can be substituted for $\int_0^\tau X_e \, dt/\tau$ in (6.80) [see Eq. (6.72)] to give

$$X_e \sim \frac{k_{1e}X_0}{k_{e0}k_{10}\tau} \tag{6.81}$$

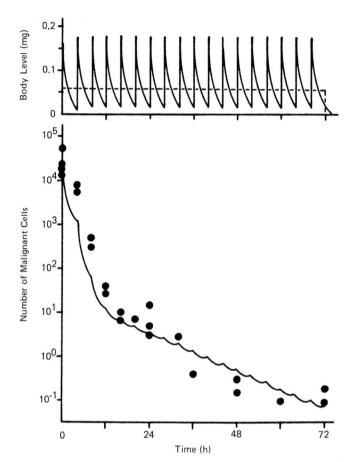

Fig. 6.30 Time course of drug levels and survival of lymphoma cells in mouse femur on multiple dosing of arabinosylcytosine (Ara-C). The upper graph shows the calculated body levels of Ara-C when doses of 0.167 mg are given every 4 h (assuming a biologic half-life of 1 h) as well as the average body level of Ara-C (dashed line). The solid line in the lower graph is calculated from the model using numerical integration. (From Ref. 30, © 1971 Plenum Publishing Corp.)

Substitution of this value of X_e for X_e in (6.77) yields

$$\frac{dC_s}{dt} = k_s C_s - \frac{kk_{1e} X_0 C_s}{k_{e0} k_{10} \tau} - k_{sr} C_s + k_{rs} C_r \qquad (6.82)$$

The solutions for C_s and C_r are provided in the appendix to this chapter.

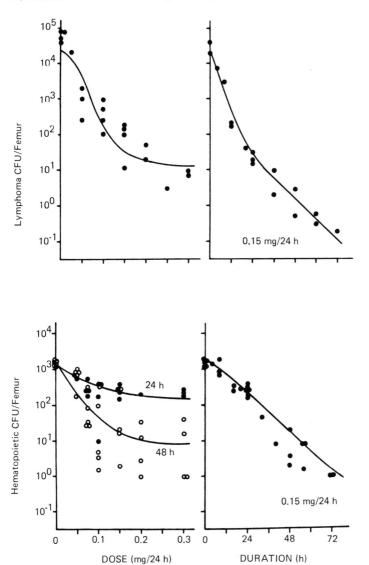

Fig. 6.31 Dose- and time-dependent cell survival curves for the effects of vinblastine on hematopoietic and lymphoma cells in the mouse femur. (From Ref. 30, © 1971 Plenum Publishing Corp.)

Of interest is the total number of cells in the system C_T as a function of time and of dose. This is given by

$$C_T = A_1 e^{-\alpha_1 t} + A_2 e^{-\alpha_2 t} \tag{6.83}$$

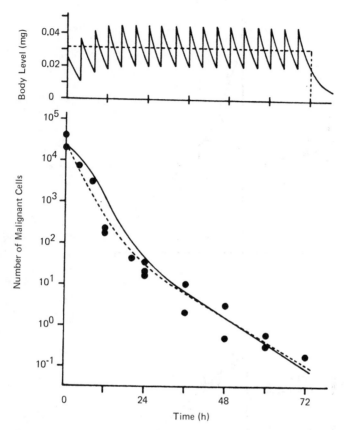

Fig. 6.32 Time course of drug levels and survival of lymphoma cells in mouse femur on multiple dosing of vinblastine. The upper graph shows the calculated body levels (solid line) of vinblastine when doses of 0.025 mg are given every 4 h (assuming a biologic half-life of 3.5 h) as well as the average body level of vinblastine at steady state (dashed line). The solid line in the lower graph is calculated from the model using numerical integration; the dashed line is based on average body levels. (From Ref. 30, © 1971 Plenum Publishing Corp.)

where t is time, α_1 and α_2 are disposition rate constants,

$$A_1 = \frac{C^\circ_s(k_{rs} + k_r + k_{sr} - \alpha_1) + C^\circ_r(KX_0 + k_{sr} - k_s + k_{rs} - \alpha_1)}{\alpha_2 - \alpha_1}$$

(6.84)

and

$$A_2 = \frac{C_s^\circ(k_{rs} + k_r + k_{sr} - \alpha_2) + C_r^\circ(KX_0 + k_{sr} - k_s + k_{rs} - \alpha_2)}{\alpha_1 - \alpha_2}$$

$$(6.85)$$

and C_s° and C_r° are the respective concentrations or numbers of sensitive and insensitive cells at time zero. Derivations of these equations may also be found in the appendix to this chapter.

The approximation that resulted in the solution for (6.83) allows the characterization of the average effect of a given dose of a drug, rather than the time course of effect of the dose, and is precise only at the instant that all of the drug has been lost from the body and tumor site [30]. An example of the application of Eq. (6.83) with regard to the effect of dose and time on hematopoietic and lymphoma cells in the mouse femur is illustrated in Fig. 6.31. Figure 6.32 demonstrates the good agreement between the approximate solution and a more rigorous kinetic treatment.

Although the data are limited, there are examples in the literature, as illustrated above, that demonstrate the application of the relationships developed in cancer chemotherapy. Unfortunately, there remains a paucity of information concerning the effect of duration of antibiotic therapy and dose on bacterial cell growth.

APPENDIX: SOLUTIONS FOR C_s, C_r, AND C_T FOR CELL SYSTEMS SENSITIVE TO DRUGS THAT ARE CELL CYCLE SPECIFIC

The differential equations for C_s and C_r [Eqs. (6.86) and (6.81), respectively] are

$$\frac{dC_s}{dt} = k_s C_s - KX_0 C_s - k_{sr} C_s + k_{rs} C_r \qquad (A6.1)$$

and

$$\frac{dC_r}{dt} = k_{sr} C_s - k_{rs} C_r - k_r C_r \qquad (A6.2)$$

where

$$K = \frac{kk_{1e}}{k_{e0} k_{10} \tau} \qquad (A6.3)$$

The respective Laplace transforms of these equations are (see Appendix A)

$$s\overline{C}_s - C_s^\circ = (k_s - KX_0 - k_{sr})\overline{C}_s + k_{rs}\overline{C}_r \qquad (A6.4)$$

and

$$s\overline{C}_r - C_r^\circ = k_{sr}\overline{C}_s - (k_{rs} + k_r)\overline{C}_r \tag{A6.5}$$

where C_s° and C_r° are the concentrations or numbers of sensitive and insensitive cells at time zero. Collecting common terms in these two equations yields the following:

$$(s + KX_0 + k_{sr} - k_s)\overline{C}_s = k_{rs}\overline{C}_r + C_s^\circ \tag{A6.6}$$

$$(s + k_{rs} + k_r)\overline{C}_r = k_{sr}\overline{C}_s + C_r^\circ \tag{A6.7}$$

Multiplying Eq. (A6.6) by $(s + k_{rs} + k_r)$ and (A6.7) by k_{rs}, adding the resulting expressions, and solving for $\overline{C}_s$ yields

$$\overline{C}_s = \frac{(s + k_{rs} + k_r)C_s^\circ + k_{rs}C_r^\circ}{\begin{array}{c}s^2 + s(KX_0 + k_{sr} + k_{rs} + k_r - k_s) \\ + (k_{rs} + k_r)(KX_0 + k_{sr} - k_s) - k_{rs}k_{sr}\end{array}} \tag{A6.8}$$

If we consider the identity

$$s^2 + s(KX_0 + k_{sr} + k_{rs} + k_r - k_s) + (k_{rs} + k_r)(KX_0 + k_{sr} - k_s)$$
$$- k_{rs}k_{sr} = (s + \alpha_1)(s + \alpha_2) \tag{A6.9}$$

Eq. (A6.8) can be rewritten as follows:

$$\overline{C}_s = \frac{(s + k_{rs} + k_r)C_s^\circ + k_{rs}C_r^\circ}{(s + \alpha_1)(s + \alpha_2)} \tag{A6.10}$$

where

$$\alpha_1 + \alpha_2 = KX_0 + k_{sr} + k_{rs} + k_r - k_s \tag{A6.11}$$

and

$$\alpha_1\alpha_2 = (k_{rs} + k_r)(KX_0 + k_{sr} - k_s) - k_{rs}k_{sr} \tag{A6.12}$$

Solving (A6.10) for C_s using a table of Laplace transforms (Appendix A) gives

$$C_s = \frac{(k_{rs} + k_r - \alpha_1)C_s^\circ + k_{rs}C_r^\circ}{\alpha_2 - \alpha_1}e^{-\alpha_1 t}$$
$$+ \frac{(k_{rs} + k_r - \alpha_2)C_s^\circ + k_{rs}C_r^\circ}{\alpha_1 - \alpha_2}e^{-\alpha_2 t} \tag{A6.13}$$

C_r can be solved for in a similar manner. Multiplying (A6.6) by k_{sr} and (A6.7) by $\underline{s} + KX_0 + k_{sr} - k_s$, adding the resulting expressions, solving for $\overline{C}_r$, and considering the identity given by (A6.9) yields

$$\overline{C}_r = \frac{(s + KX_0 + k_{sr} - k_s)C_r^\circ + k_{sr}C_s^\circ}{(s + \alpha_1)(s + \alpha_2)} \tag{A6.14}$$

The following equation for C_r as a function of time can be determined using a table of Laplace transforms (Appendix A):

$$C_r = \frac{(KX_0 + k_{sr} - k_s - \alpha_1)C_r^\circ + k_{sr}C_s^\circ}{\alpha_2 - \alpha_1} e^{-\alpha_1 t}$$

$$+ \frac{(KX_0 + k_{sr} - k_s - \alpha_2)C_r^\circ + k_{sr}C_s^\circ}{\alpha_1 - \alpha_2} e^{-\alpha_2 t} \tag{A6.15}$$

An expression for the total number of cells in the system, C_T, can be obtained by adding (A6.13) and (A6.15). Addition followed by simplification yields

$$C_T = C_s + C_r = A_1 e^{-\alpha_1 t} + A_2 e^{-\alpha_2 t} \tag{A6.16}$$

where

$$A_1 = \frac{C_s^\circ(k_{rs} + k_r + k_{sr} - \alpha_1) + C_r^\circ(KX_0 + k_{sr} - k_s + k_{rs} - \alpha_1)}{\alpha_2 - \alpha_1} \tag{A6.17}$$

and

$$A_2 = \frac{C_s^\circ(k_{rs} + k_r + k_{sr} - \alpha_2) + C_r^\circ(KX_0 + k_{sr} - k_s + K_{rs} - \alpha_2)}{\alpha_1 - \alpha_2} \tag{A6.18}$$

REFERENCES

1. J. G. Wagner. Kinetics of pharmacologic response: I. Proposed relationships between response and drug concentration in the intact animal and man. *J. Theor. Biol.* 20:173 (1968).

2. M. Gibaldi. Measurement and interpretation of certain biopharmaceutic and pharmacodynamic parameters. *Chemotherapy* 13:1 (1968).

3. D. G. McDevitt and D. G. Shand. Plasma concentrations and
    the time-course of beta blockade due to propranolol. *Clin.*
    Pharmacol. Ther. 18:708 (1975).
4. K. M. Piafsky and R. I. Olgivie. Dosage of theophylline in
    bronchial asthma. *N. Engl. J. Med. 292*:1218 (1975).
5. G. Levy. Relationship between elimination rate of drugs and
    rate of decline of their pharmacologic effects. *J. Pharm. Sci.*
    53:342 (1964).
6. D. Shen, K. O'Malley, M. Gibaldi, and J. L. McNay. Pharma-
    codynamics of minoxidil as a guide for individualizing dosage
    regimens in hypertension. *Clin. Pharmacol. Ther. 17*:593
    (1975).
7. J. M. Van Rossum and A. T. J. Van Koppen. Kinetics of
    psychomotor stimulant drug action. *Eur. J. Pharmacol. 2*:405
    (1968).
8. A. Weissler, J. R. Synder, C. D. Schoenfeld, and S. Cohen.
    Assay of digitalis glycosides in man. *Am. J. Cardiol. 17*:768
    (1966).
9. G. Levy and E. Nelson. Theoretical relationship between dose,
    elimination rate and duration of pharmacologic effect of drugs.
    J. Pharm. Sci. 54:812 (1965).
10. G. Levy. Kinetics of pharmacologic effects. *Clin. Pharmacol.*
    Ther. 7:362 (1966).
11. G. Levy. Apparent potentiating effect of a second dose of
    drug. *Nature 206*:517 (1965).
12. J. Murphy, W. Casey, and L. Lasagna. The effect of dosage
    regimen on the diuretic efficacy of chlorothiazide in human
    subjects. *J. Pharmacol. Exp. Ther. 134*:286 (1961).
13. M. Gibaldi, G. Levy, and W. Hayton. Kinetics of the elimination
    and neuromuscular blocking effect of d-tubocurarine in man.
    Anesthesiology 36:213 (1972).
14. J. G. Wagner. Relations between drug concentrations and re-
    sponse. *J. Mond. Pharm. 4*:14 (1971).
15. W. J. Westlake. Problems associated with analysis of pharma-
    cokinetic models. *J. Pharm. Sci. 60*:882 (1971).
16. M. Gibaldi and G. Levy. Dose-dependent decline of pharma-
    cologic effects of drugs with linear pharmacokinetic character-
    istics. *J. Pharm. Sci. 61*:567 (1972).
17. C. J. Hull, H. B. H. Van Beem, K. McLeod, A. Sibbald, and
    M. J. Watson. A pharmacokinetic model for pancuronium. *Br.*
    J. Anesthesiol. 50:1113 (1978).
18. M. Gibaldi, G. Levy, and H. Weintraub. Drug distribution and
    pharmacologic effects. *Clin. Pharmacol. Ther. 12*:734 (1971).
19. L. B. Sheiner, D. R. Stanski, S. Vozeh, R. D. Miller, and
    J. Ham. Simultaneous modeling of pharmacokinetics and phar-
    macodynamics: Application to d-tubocurarine. *Clin. Pharmacol.*
    Ther. 25:358 (1979).

20. B. Whitting, N. H. G. Holford, and L. B. Sheiner. Quantitative analysis of the disopyramide concentration-effect relationship. *Br. J. Clin. Pharmacol. 9*:67 (1980).
21. D. R. Stanski, J. Ham, R. D. Miller, and L. B. Sheiner. Pharmacokinetics and pharmacodynamics of d-tubocurarine during nitrous oxide-narcotic and halothane anesthesia in man. *Anesthesiology 51*:235 (1979).
22. R. Nagashima, R. A. O'Reilly, and G. Levy. Kinetics of pharmacologic effects in man: The anticoagulant action of warfarin. *Clin. Pharmacol. Ther. 10*:22 (1969).
23. R. A. O'Reilly, P. M. Aggeler, and L. S. Leong. Studies of the courmarin anticoagulant drugs: The pharmacodynamics of warfarin in man. *J. Clin. Invest. 42*:1542 (1963).
24. G. Levy, R. A. O'Reilly, and P. M. Aggeler. Pharmacokinetic analysis of the effect of barbiturate on the anticoagulant action of warfarin in man. *Clin. Pharmacol. Ther. 11*:372 (1970).
25. R. A. O'Reilly and G. Levy. Kinetics of the anticoagulant effect of bishydroxycoumarin in man. *Clin. Pharmacol. Ther. 11*:378 (1970).
26. R. A. O'Reilly and G. Levy. Pharmacokinetic analysis of potentiating effect of phenylbutazone on anticoagulating action of warfarin in man. *J. Pharm. Sci. 59*:1258 (1970).
27. V. T. DeVita. Cell kinetics and the chemotherapy of cancer. *Cancer Chemother. Rep. Pt. 3,2*:23 (1971).
28. B. C. Lampkin, N. B. McWilliams, and A. M. Mauer. Cell kinetics and chemotherapy of acute leukemia. *Semin. Hematol. 9*:211 (1972).
29. W. J. Jusko. Pharmacodynamics of chemotherapeutic effects: Dose-time-response relationships for phase-nonspecific agents. *J. Pharm. Sci. 60*:892 (1971).
30. W. J. Jusko. A pharmacodynamic model for cell-cycle-specific chemotherapeutic agents. *J. Pharmacokinet. Biopharm. 1*:175 (1973).

7

Nonlinear Pharmacokinetics

At therapeutic or nontoxic plasma concentrations, the pharmacokinetics of most drugs can be adequately described by first-order or linear processes. However, there are a small number of well-documented examples of drugs which have nonlinear absorption or distribution characteristics [e.g., ascorbic acid [1] and naproxen [2,3], respectively], and several examples drugs that are eliminated from the body in a nonlinear fashion.

MICHAELIS-MENTEN KINETICS

Drug biotransformation, renal tubular secretion, and biliary secretion usually require enzyme or carrier systems. These systems are relatively specific with respect to substrate and have finite capacities (i.e., they are said to be capacity limited). Frequently, the kinetics of these capacity-limited processes can be described by the Michaelis-Menten equation:

$$-\frac{dC}{dt} = \frac{V_m C}{K_m + C} \tag{7.1}$$

where $-dC/dt$ is the rate of decline of drug concentration at time t, V_m the theoretical maximum rate of the process, and K_m the Michaelis constant. It is readily seen by determining C when $-dC/dt = (1/2)V_m$ that K_m is in fact equal to the drug concentration at which the rate of the process is equal to one-half its theoretical maximum rate. Equation (7.1) can be derived based on the following scheme (see Appendix G for derivation):

$$E + C \underset{k_1}{\overset{k_{-1}}{\rightleftharpoons}} EC \overset{k_2}{\longrightarrow} E + M$$

In this scheme C is the concentration of drug, E the concentration of
enzyme, EC the concentration of the enzyme-drug complex, and M the
concentration of metabolite. The constants k_2 and k_{-1} are first-order
rate constants, and k_1 is a second-order rate constant. The Michaelis-
Menten equation is of value for describing in vitro and in situ as well
as certain in vivo rate processes. For in vivo systems the constants
V_m and K_m are affected by distributional and other factors and therefore must be viewed as functional, model-dependent constants.

SOME PHARMACOKINETIC CHARACTERISTICS OF MICHAELIS-MENTEN PROCESSES

There are two limiting cases of the Michaelis-Menten equation. If K_m
is much larger than C, (7.1) reduces to

$$- \frac{dC}{dt} = \frac{V_m}{K_m} C \qquad (7.2)$$

This equation has the same form as that describing first-order elimination of a drug: (1) after intravenous administration in a one-compartment model, (2) in the postabsorptive phase after some other route of
administration in a one-compartment model, or (3) in the postabsorptive, postdistributive phase in a multicompartment model. Assuming
apparent first-order elimination of a drug which confers one-compartment characteristics to the body and which is eliminated by a single
biotransformation process, the first-order rate constant K is actually
V_m/K_m. As shown in (7.2), if treatment with an enzyme inducer
causes an increase in the amount of enzyme (and therefore of V_m), the
apparent first-order rate constant of the process will also be increased.
Given the fact that drug elimination is so frequently observed to follow
apparent first-order kinetics, one must conclude that the drug concentration in the body (or, more correctly, at the site of an active
process) resulting from the usual therapeutic dosage regimens of
most drugs is well below the K_m of the processes involved in the disposition of these drugs.

There are some notable exceptions to this generalization and among
them are ethanol [4], salicylate [5,6], and phenytoin [7]. The elimination kinetics of phenytoin [8] and ethanol [9] appear to be adequately described by a single Michaelis-Menten expression, while
salicylate elimination [6] may be described by two capacity-limited
and three linear processes. Marked deviations from apparent first-
order drug elimination have also been noted frequently in cases of
drug intoxications. In the latter situation there is often some ambiguity as to whether the deviations are due to capacity-limited biotransformation of the high drug levels in the body [described by (7.1)] or
due to some toxicologic effect of the drug.

Another limiting case of the Michaelis-Menten equation is that which results when the drug concentration is considerably greater than K_m. Equation (7.1) then reduces to

$$- \frac{dC}{dt} = V_m \qquad (7.3)$$

Under these conditions, the rate is independent of drug concentration, so that the process occurs at a constant rate V_m. The kinetics of biotransformation of ethanol [4] have been observed to approach the condition described by (7.3) even at drug levels in the body that are appreciably lower than those considered to be toxic.

Based on the discussion above, if $-dC/dt$ is plotted as a function of plasma concentration, $-dC/dt$ would initially increase linearly with concentration, indicating first-order kinetics (Fig. 7.1). As the concentration increases further, $-dC/dt$ would increase at a rate less than proportional to concentration, and eventually asymptote at a

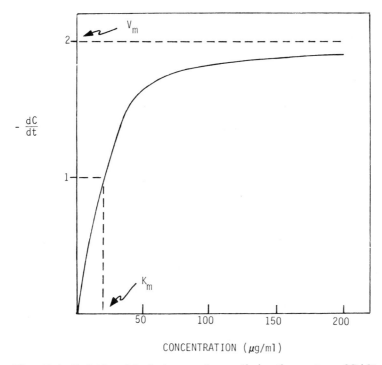

CONCENTRATION (μg/ml)

Fig. 7.1 Relationship between drug elimination rate $-dC/dt$ and drug concentration C for a Michaelis-Menten process. In this particular example the Michaelis constant K_m is equal to 10 μg/ml and the maximum rate V_m is equal to $2(\mu g/ml)h^{-1}$.

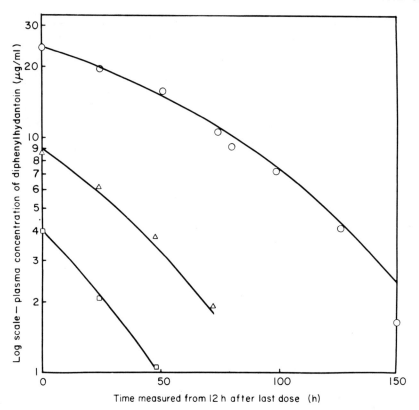

Fig. 7.2 Phenytoin (diphenylhydantoin) concentration in plasma 12 h after the last dose of a 3 day regimen of the drug at three different daily doses. The data are described by Eq. (7.9). O: 7.9 mg/kg; △: 4.7 mg/kg; □: 2.3 mg/kg. (From Ref. 10, © 1972 PJD Publications Ltd., reprinted with permission.)

rate equal to V_m which would be independent of concentration (i.e., a zero-order rate).

The time course of drug plasma concentration after intravenous injection of a drug that is eliminated only by a single capacity-limited process can be described for a one-compartment system by the integrated form of the Michaelis-Menten equation. Rearrangement of (7.1) yields

$$- \frac{dC}{C} (C + K_m) = V_m \, dt \tag{7.4}$$

or

$$-dC - \frac{K_m \, dC}{C} = V_m \, dt \tag{7.5}$$

Integration of this equation gives the expression

$$-C - K_m \ln C = V_m t + i \qquad (7.6)$$

where i is an integration constant. Evaluating i at t = 0, where $C = C_0$, yields

$$i = -C_0 - K_m \ln C_0 \qquad (7.7)$$

Substituting this expression for i in (7.6) and rearranging terms gives

$$t = \frac{C_0 - C}{V_m} + \frac{K_m}{V_m} \ln \frac{C_0}{C} \qquad (7.8)$$

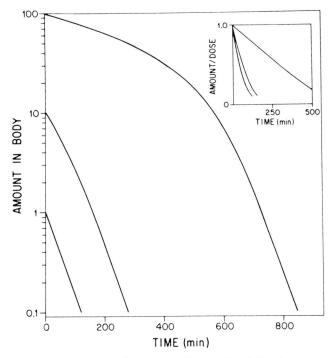

Fig. 7.3 Amount of drug in the body following intravenous administration of 1, 10, and 100 mg doses of a drug that is eliminated by a
single Michaelis-Menten process. A one-compartment system is assumed; $K_m = 10$ mg and $V_m = 0.2$ mg/min. The inset shows a plot of
amount of drug in the body divided by administered dose versus time
to show that the principle of superposition does not apply.

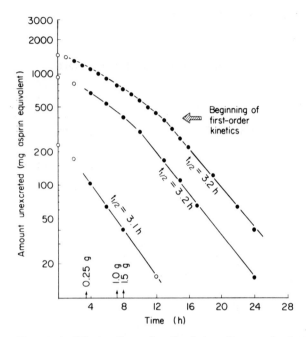

Fig. 7.4 Elimination of salicylate after oral administration of 0.25, 1.0, and 1.5 g doses of aspirin. Vertical arrows on the time axis indicate $t_{50\%}$, the time to eliminate 50% of the dose. (From Ref. 5, reprinted with permission.)

Unfortunately, it is not possible to solve this equation explicitly for C. Rather, one must determine the time t at which the initial concentration C_0 has decreased to C. A modified form of (7.8), that is,

$$t - t_0 = \frac{C_0 - C}{V_m} + \frac{K_m}{V_m} \ln \frac{C_0}{C} \tag{7.9}$$

has been used to fit phenytoin levels in the plasma as a function of time 12 h after administration of the last of several oral doses to human subjects (see Fig. 7.2). In this case C_0 represents the phenytoin plasma concentration at 12 h after the last dose, $t_0 = 12$ h, and C is the phenytoin plasma concentration at time t, where $t > t_0$.

Conversion of (7.8) to common logarithms ($\ln x = 2.303 \log x$) and solving for log C yields

$$\log C = \frac{C_0 - C}{2.303 K_m} + \log C_0 - \frac{V_m}{2.303 K_m} t \tag{7.10}$$

Figure 7.3 shows the time course of elimination, as described by (7.10), of three different doses of a drug that is eliminated by a process with Michaelis-Menten kinetics. The lowest dose represents the case where $K_m \gg C$. At this dose the decline in plasma concentrations is first order with a slope of $-V_m/2.303K_m$. On the other hand, the highest dose yields initial concentrations which are considerably above K_m, so that drug levels decline initially at an essentially constant rate (see inset to Fig. 7.3). The curves show that the time required for an initial drug concentration to decrease by 50% is not independent of dose, but, in fact, increases with increasing dose. This particular pharmacokinetic property may present considerable clinical difficulty in the treatment of drug intoxications. Figure 7.3 also shows that regardless of the initial dose, when the plasma concentration becomes significantly less than K_m, elimination is describable by first-order kinetics and the slope of this linear portion of the curve is independent of dose. Semilogarithmic plots of plasma concentration or amount unexcreted versus time after administration of phenytoin (Fig. 7.2) or salicylate (Fig. 7.4) show characteristics that are remarkably similar to those described by the curves in Fig. 7.3.

To assess whether or not a drug possesses nonlinear kinetic properties, a series of single doses of varying size should be administered. If a plot of the resulting plasma concentrations divided by the administered dose are superimposable, the drug in question has linear kinetic properties over the concentration range examined. If, however, the resulting curves are not superimposable (see inset to Fig. 7.3), the drug behaves nonlinearly.

IN VIVO ESTIMATION OF K_m AND V_m

For a drug that is eliminated by a single capacity-limited process, there are a number of general methods which permit the initial estimation of apparent in vivo K_m and V_m values from plasma concentration-time data in the postabsorptive-postdistributive phase. Such estimates require the determination of the rate of change of the plasma concentration from one sampling time to the next, $\Delta C/\Delta t$, as a function of the plasma concentration C_m at the midpoint of the sampling interval (see Appendix F). The data are usually plotted according to one of the linearized forms of the Michaelis-Menten equation, such as the Lineweaver-Burk expression,

$$\frac{1}{\Delta C/\Delta t} = \frac{K_m}{V_m C_m} + \frac{1}{V_m} \qquad (7.11)$$

so that a plot of the reciprocal of $\Delta C/\Delta t$ versus the reciprocal of C_m yields a straight line with intercept $1/V_m$ and slope K_m/V_m. Two sometimes more reliable [11,12] plots are the Hanes-Woolf plot [13] and the Woolf-Augustinsson-Hofstee plot [13]. They are based on the relationships

$$\frac{C_m}{\Delta C / \Delta t} = \frac{K_m}{V_m} + \frac{C_m}{V_m} \tag{7.12}$$

and

$$\frac{\Delta C}{\Delta t} = V_m - \frac{(\Delta C / \Delta t) K_m}{C_m} \tag{7.13}$$

respectively. Based on (7.12), a plot of $C_m/(\Delta C / \Delta t)$ versus C_m should yield a straight line with a slope of $1/V_m$ and an intercept of K_m/V_m. Equation (7.13) indicates that a plot of $\Delta C / \Delta t$ versus $(\Delta C / \Delta t)/C_m$ gives a straight line with a slope of $-K_m$ and an intercept of V_m.

A method for estimating V_m and K_m directly from log C versus time data, obtained following the intravenous administration of a drug that can be adequately described by a one-compartment system, is also available [14]. Extrapolation of the terminal log-linear portion of the log C versus time plot, where the plot is described by (7.10), would yield a zero-time intercept of log C_0^* (see Fig. 7.5). The resulting straight line can be described by

$$\log C = \log C_0^* - \frac{V_m}{2.303 K_m} t \tag{7.14}$$

At low plasma concentrations (7.10) and (7.14) are identical. By setting the right-hand sides of these two equations equal to each other, the following expression is obtained:

$$\frac{C_0 - C}{2.303 K_m} + \log C_0 - \frac{V_m}{2.303 K_m} t = \log C_0^* - \frac{V_m}{2.303 K_m} \tag{7.15}$$

Cancellation of the common term, $V_m t/2.303 K_m$, and rearrangement yields

$$\frac{C_0 - C}{2.303 K_m} = \log \frac{C_0^*}{C_0} \tag{7.16}$$

Since the equality given by (7.15) is valid only at low concentrations, C_0 can be assumed to be significantly greater than C, and therefore $C_0 - C \simeq C_0$. Making this simplification in (7.16) and solving the resulting expression for K_m gives

$$K_m = \frac{C_0}{2.303 \log (C_0^*/C_0)} \tag{7.17}$$

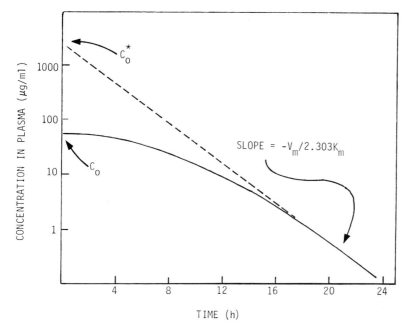

Fig. 7.5 Graphical method for estimating K_m and V_m after intravenous administration of a drug that is eliminated by a single Michaelis-Menten process. The solid line is described by Eq. (7.10). The terminal slope gives an estimate of the ratio of V_m to K_m, and the ratio of C_0^* to C_0 is used to estimate K_m [see Eq. (7.17)].

Since C_0^* and C_0 can be estimated from a log C versus time plot, an estimate of K_m is possible employing (7.17). V_m can be calculated from the slope of the terminal log-linear segment of the concentration versus time curve. Since slope $= -V_m/2.303K_m$, $V_m = -2.303(\text{slope})K_m$.

It is plausible to consider that drug elimination may involve a capacity-limited process in parallel with one or more first-order processes. Under these conditions, the foregoing methods for estimating V_m and K_m do not apply. When capacity-limited and first-order elimination occur in parallel, the rate of decline of drug levels in the plasma after intravenous administration in a one-compartment system is given by

$$-\frac{dC}{dt} = K'C + \frac{V_m C}{K_m + C} \tag{7.18}$$

where K' is the rate constant characterizing the various parallel first-order processes. The time course of drug levels under these conditions may be determined by integration of (7.18) as follows. Expansion of (7.18) yields

$$-\frac{dC}{dt} = \frac{K'C(K_m + C) + V_m C}{K_m + C} = \frac{K'K_m C + V_m C + K'C^2}{K_m + C} \tag{7.19}$$

Further simplification gives rise to

$$-\frac{dC}{dt} = \frac{C(K'K_m + KV_m + K'C)}{K_m + C} = \frac{C(a + K'C)}{K_m + C} \tag{7.20}$$

where $a = K'K_m + V_m$. Inversion and rearrangement of (7.20) yields

$$\frac{dt}{dC} = \frac{-(K_m + C)}{C(a + K'C)} = \frac{-K_m}{C(a + K'C)} - \frac{1}{a + K'C} \tag{7.21}$$

This equation is separable and can be rewritten as

$$dt = \frac{-K_m dC}{C(a + K'C)} - \frac{dC}{a + K'C} \tag{7.22}$$

The two terms in this equation are of the form $1/x(a + bx)$ and $1/(a + bx)$, respectively, the integrals of which are $(-1/a) \ln [(a + bx)/x]$ and $(1/b) \ln (a + bx)$ [15]. Therefore, integration of (7.22) gives

$$t = \frac{K_m}{a} \ln \frac{a + K'C}{C} - \frac{1}{K'} \ln (a + K'C) + i \tag{7.23}$$

Evaluating i at $t = 0$, where $C = C_0$, yields

$$i = -\frac{K_m}{a} \ln \frac{a + K'C_0}{C_0} + \frac{1}{K'} \ln (a + K'C_0) \tag{7.24}$$

Substituting this value of i in (7.23) and simplifying the resulting expression yields

$$at = K_m \ln \frac{C_0}{C} + \left(\frac{a}{K'} - K_m\right) \ln \frac{a + K'C_0}{a + K'C} \tag{7.25}$$

Since $a = K'K_m + V_m$,

$$(K'K_m + V_m)t = K_m \ln \frac{C_0}{C} + \left(\frac{K'K_m + V_m}{K'} - K_m\right) \ln \frac{K'K_m + V_m + K'C_0}{K'K_m + V_m + K'C} \tag{7.26}$$

or

$$t = \frac{1}{K'K_m + V_m}\left[K_m \ln \frac{C_0}{C} + \frac{V_m}{K'} \ln \frac{(C_0 + K_m)K' + V_m}{(C + K_m)K' + V_m}\right] \tag{7.27}$$

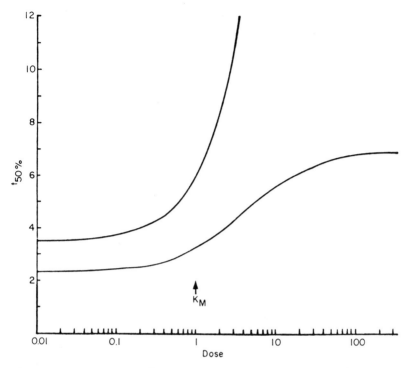

Fig. 7.6 Comparison of dose dependence of $t_{50\%}$ (time for elimination of 50% of the dose) after intravenous administration of a drug that is eliminated by a single Michaelis-Menten process (upper curve) or one that is eliminated by a single Michaelis-Menten process in parallel with a first-order process (lower curve). In each case, $K_m = 1.0$ and $V_m = 0.2$. The rate constant K' for the first-order process is equal to 0.1. (Data from Ref. 16.)

Equation (7.27), like (7.8), does not permit an explicit solution for C. Both (7.8) and (7.27) indicate that the time required to reduce an initial drug concentration by 50% is indeed dependent on the ad-ministered dose. Examples of this dependency are shown in Fig. 7.6.
Expanding (7.27) and solving for ln C gives

$$\ln C = \ln C_0 + \frac{V_m}{K'K_m} \ln \frac{(C_0 + K_m)K' + V_m}{(C + K_m)K' + V_m} - \left(K' + \frac{V_m}{K_m}\right) t \quad (7.28)$$

which in terms of common logarithms is

$$\log C = \log C_0 + \frac{V_m}{K'K_m} \log \frac{(C_0 + K_m)K' + V_m}{(C + K_m)K' + V_m} - \frac{K' + V_m/K_m}{2.303} t$$

$$(7.29)$$

At low concentrations (i.e., $K_m \gg C$), (7.29) becomes

$$\log C = \log C_0 + \frac{V_m}{K'K_m} \log \frac{(C_0 + K_m)K' + V_m}{K_m K' + V_m} - \frac{K' + V_m/K_m}{2.303} t$$

$$(7.30)$$

or

$$\log C = \log C_0^* - \frac{K' + V_m/K_m}{2.303} t \qquad (7.31)$$

where

$$\log C_0^* = \log C_0 + \frac{V_m}{K'K_m} \log \frac{(C_0 + K_m)K' + V_m}{K_m K' + V_m} \qquad (7.32)$$

As can be seen from (7.31), the slope of the terminal linear portion of a semilogrithmic plot of plasma concentration versus time at low plasma concentrations (i.e., $K_m \gg C$) will yield an estimate of the first-order elimination rate constant of a drug, $K' + V_m/K_m$ (see Fig. 7.7). The extrapolated intercept of this terminal linear phase will be log C_0^*.

For certain drugs that exhibit parallel capacity-limited and first-order elimination, it may be possible to administer sufficiently high doses intravenously so that initial drug concentrations are substantially larger than K_m. Under these conditions and where a one-compartment model applies, the initial segment of a semilogarithmic plot of plasma concentration versus time will be linear (see Fig. 7.7). The slope of this linear segment will be $-K'/2.303$ [14]. This can be demonstrated by assuming C to be much greater than K_m in (7.18) and solving for C. Therefore, estimates of both K' and $K' + V_m/K_m$ can be obtained directly from a semilogarithmic plot of plasma concentration versus time and the ratio V_m/K_m can be calculated for the case where there is one capacity-limited process in parallel with one or more first-order processes. The following approach can then be used to obtain initial estimates of K_m and V_m for this model. Expansion of the logarithmic term of (7.32) and rearrangement of this equation yields

$$\frac{K'K_m}{V_m} \log \frac{C_0^*}{C_0} = \log \left(1 + \frac{C_0 K'}{K_m K' + V_m} \right) \qquad (7.33)$$

Division of the numerator and denominator of this logarithmic term by K_m gives

$$\frac{K'K_m}{V_m} \log \frac{C_0^*}{C_0} = \log \left[1 + \frac{C_0 K'}{K_m (K' + V_m/K_m)} \right] \qquad (7.34)$$

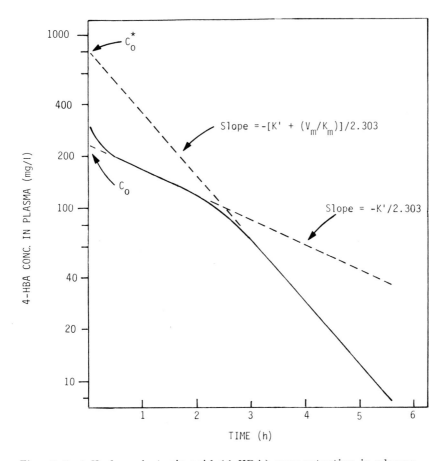

Fig. 7.7 4-Hydroxybutyric acid (4-HBA) concentration in plasma after intravenous administration. The compound appears to be eliminated by a Michaelis-Menten process in parallel with a first-order process. The initial slope gives an estimate of K' and the terminal slope provides an estimate of the ratio of V_m to K_m. K_m may be determined from Eq. (7.35). The deviation from theory for a short time after administration probably reflects drug distribution and the lack of strict adherence to a one-compartment model. (Data from Ref. 14.)

A solution for K_m based on this equation is

$$K_m = \frac{C_0 K'/(K' + V_m/K_m)}{(C_0^*/C_0)^{K'K_m/V_m} - 1} \qquad (7.35)$$

Since C_0 and C_0^* can be obtained directly from a semilogarithmic plasma concentration-time plot, and K' and V_m/K_m can be estimated as described above, an estimate of K_m is possible employing (7.35). Once K_m is known, V_m can be readily determined.

Although this is an interesting approach for the estimation of K', V_m, and K_m where there are parallel first-order and nonlinear elimination pathways, caution must be exercised. Initial plasma concentrations have to be sufficiently high (i.e., $C >> K_m$) to yield a semilogarithmic plasma concentration-time curve which is truly linear. If these con-

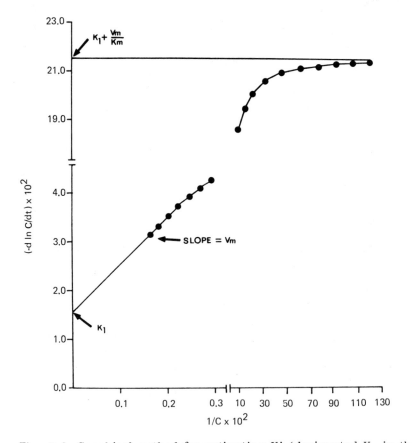

Fig. 7.8 Graphical method for estimating K' (designated K_1 in the plot), V_m and K_m based on Eqs. (7.36) to (7.39). At high concentrations, a plot of $-\Delta \ln C/\Delta t$ versus $1/C$ will be linear with a slope of V_m and an intercept equal to K' [see Eq. (7.38)], whereas at low concentrations the plot will asymptotically approach a limiting value equal to K' + (V_m/K_m) [see Eq. (7.39)]. (From Ref. 17, © 1973 Plenum Publishing Corp.)

centrations are not attained, an overestimate of K' will result. This, in turn, will produce errors in the estimates of V_m and K_m.

A different approach can also be used for the estimation of K_m and V_m where nonlinear and linear processes of drug elimination occur in parallel. At high plasma concentrations (i.e., $C \gg K_m$), (7.18) reduces to

$$- \frac{dC}{dt} = K'C + V_m \tag{7.36}$$

Division of both sides of (7.36) by C and recognition that $(-dC/dt)/C$ equals $-d \ln C/dt$ gives

$$- \frac{d \ln C}{dt} = K' + \frac{V_m}{C} \tag{7.37}$$

At low plasma concentrations (i.e., $K_m \gg C$), (7.18) becomes

$$- \frac{dC}{dt} = K'C + \frac{V_m}{K_m} C \tag{7.38}$$

and, therefore, the analogous expression to (7.37) is

$$- \frac{d \ln C}{dt} = K' + \frac{V_m}{K_m} \tag{7.39}$$

A plot of $- \Delta \ln C/\Delta t$ versus $1/C$ will consequently be linear with a slope of V_m and an intercept of K' at high plasma concentrations [Eq. (7.37)], but will reach an asymptotic value of $K' + V_m/K_m$ at low concentrations [Eq. (7.39)] from which K_m can be calculated (see Fig. 7.8).

This method for estimating K', V_m, and K_m has limitations which are similar to those noted for the previous approach. Sufficiently high plasma concentrations are required to yield a straight line from the $- \Delta \ln C/\Delta t$ versus $1/C$ plot to permit accurate estimates of V_m and K'.

Urine data can also be used to estimate V_m and K_m. Consider the following scheme:

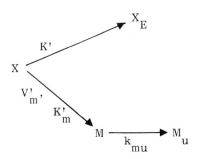

where X is the amount of drug in the body, X_E the amount of drug
eliminated by the linear or first-order processes, M the amount of
metabolite in the body which is formed by a capacity-limited process,
and M_u the amount of this metabolite present in the urine. All of
these amounts are time dependent. The constants K' and k_{mu} are
first-order rate constants, V_m' is the maximum rate of metabolite formation in units of amount per time, and K_m' is the Michaelis constant in
units of amount. Assuming that the urinary excretion rate of the
metabolite ($\Delta M_u / \Delta t$) is rate limited by its formation, and therefore
reflects the rate of formation, the following relationship for $\Delta M_u / \Delta t$
can be written:

$$\frac{\Delta M_u}{\Delta t} = \frac{V_m' X_m}{K_m' + X_m} \qquad\qquad (7.40)$$

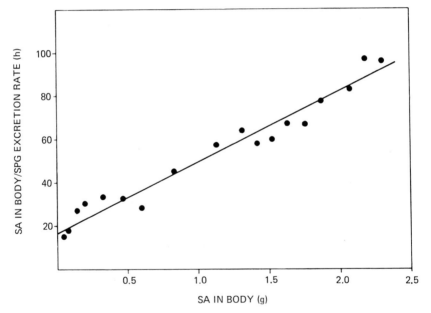

Fig. 7.9 Plot of linearized form of the Michaelis-Menten equation to
describe the formation of salicyl phenolic glucuronide (SPG) after a
single dose of salicylic acid (SA). According to Eq. (7.40) and the
corresponding form of Eq. (7.12), a plot of SA in the body divided
by the excretion rate of the metabolite (assuming that excretion of
SPG is rate limited by its formation) versus SA in the body should be
linear with slope equal to $1/V'_m$ and an intercept equal to K_m'. If the
formation of SPG followed first-order kinetics, the slope of the line
would be equal to zero. (From Ref. 23.)

where X_m is the amount of drug in the body at the midpoint of the urine collection interval. Division of the numerator and denominator by the apparent volume of distribution V yields

$$\frac{\Delta M_u}{\Delta t} = \frac{V'_m C_m}{K_m + C_m} \tag{7.41}$$

where K_m is as defined previously and equals K'_m/V, and C_m is the plasma concentration of drug at the midpoint of the collection interval. Equation (7.41) can be readily linearized [see Eqs. (7.11) to (7.13)] to yield estimates of V'_m and K_m. This approach has been used to evaluate the Michaelis-Menten parameters for two metabolites of salicylate, salicyl phenolic glucuronide, and salicyluric acid [6], and is illustrated in Fig. 7.9. The major limitation of this method is the assumption that the urinary excretion rate of the metabolite is rate limited by its formation. This situation certainly does not hold for all drugs and the assumption must be verified.

CLEARANCE, HALF-LIFE, AND VOLUME OF DISTRIBUTION

As with linear kinetics, the total body clearance Cl_s of a drug can be defined for the nonlinear situation as being equal to the rate of drug elimination dX_E/dt divided by the plasma concentration of drug C:

$$Cl_s = \frac{dX_E/dt}{C} \tag{7.42}$$

The rate of elimination for a drug eliminated by only one capacity-limited process is given by

$$\frac{1}{V} \frac{dX_E}{dt} = \frac{V_m C}{K_m + C} \tag{7.43}$$

or

$$\frac{dX_E}{dt} = \frac{V_m VC}{K_m + C} \tag{7.44}$$

Division of both sides of (7.44) by C yields

$$\frac{dX_E/dt}{C} = \frac{V_m V}{K_m + C} \tag{7.45}$$

Substitution of $V_m V/(K_m + C)$ for $(dX_E/dt)/C$ in (7.42) gives the following concentration-dependent expression for clearance:

$$Cl_s = \frac{V_m V}{K_m + C}$$ (7.46)

At low plasma concentrations, where $K_m \gg C$,

$$Cl_s = \frac{V_m}{K_m} V$$ (7.47)

whereas at high plasma concentrations, where $C \gg K_m$,

$$Cl_s = \frac{V_m}{C} V$$ (7.48)

Therefore, clearance is independent of concentration at very low concentrations, but decreases with increasing concentration; that is, the higher the plasma concentration of a drug, the slower the drug will be cleared from the plasma. The influence of nonlinear clearance on a drug's half-life ($t_{1/2}$) can be readily illustrated by recognizing that

$$t_{1/2} = \frac{0.693V}{Cl_s}$$ (7.49)

Substituting the value of Cl_s given in (7.46) for Cl_s in (7.49) and canceling common terms yields

$$t_{1/2} = \frac{0.693(K_m + C)}{V_m}$$ (7.50)

It is readily apparent from this relationship that the half-life of a drug is independent of plasma concentration at low concentrations, whereas at high concentrations the half-life, or $t_{50\%}$, will increase with an increase in the plasma concentration of drug (see Fig. 7.6).

For the case where there are linear pathways of elimination in parallel with a nonlinear process, the rate of drug elimination is given by

$$\frac{1}{V} \frac{dX_E}{dt} = \frac{V_m C}{K_m + C} + K'C$$ (7.51)

Multiplication of both sides of (7.51) by V/C yields

$$\frac{dX_E/dt}{C} = \frac{V_m V}{K_m + C} + K'V$$ (7.52)

Therefore, clearance is given by the relationship

$$Cl_s = \frac{V_m V}{K_m + C} + K'V \tag{7.53}$$

Substitution of this value for Cl_s in (7.49) gives the following relationship between half-life and plasma concentration:

$$t_{1/2} = \frac{0.693}{[V_m/(K_m + C)] + K'} \tag{7.54}$$

At low drug concentrations both clearance and half-life are independent of concentration. As the concentration increases clearance decreases; at very high concentrations, clearance attains a limiting value of $K'V$. On the other hand, the half-life increases with concentration, ultimately reaching a limiting value of 0.693/K' (see Fig. 7.6). A method for estimating the apparent volume of distribution of a drug eliminated *only* by Michaelis-Menten kinetics has been described [18]. This method was applied to ethanol in the cat and yielded an average value of 635 ml/kg, which is equivalent to total body water in this species.

DRUG CONCENTRATION AT STEADY STATE

The significance of a decrease in clearance with increasing plasma concentration of drug can be readily appreciated by considering chronic drug administration. The steady-state concentration C_{ss} of a drug is given by (see Chap. 3)

$$C_{ss} = \frac{DR}{Cl_s} \tag{7.55}$$

DR is the dose rate and equals infusion rate in the case of intravenous infusion and F dose/τ in the case of multiple oral dosing, where F is the systemic availability of the drug and τ is the dosing interval. As is illustrated in Fig. 7.10 and by Eq. (7.55), when Cl_s is given by (7.46) or (7.53), an increase in dose produces more than a proportional increase in steady-state concentration of a drug. The greater the contribution of the capacity-limited process to the overall elimination, the more dramatic is the increase in steady-state levels with increasing dose. This can be exemplified by salicylate where a twofold increase in the dose from 0.5 to 1.0 g every 8 h can result in a more than sixfold increase in steady-state salicylate body levels (Fig. 7.11). In addition, since half-life increases with concentration [see (7.50) and (7.54)], the time required to reach steady state will also increase with an increase in dose size. In the salicylate example cited above, the time to reach steady-state increased from 2 to 7 days.

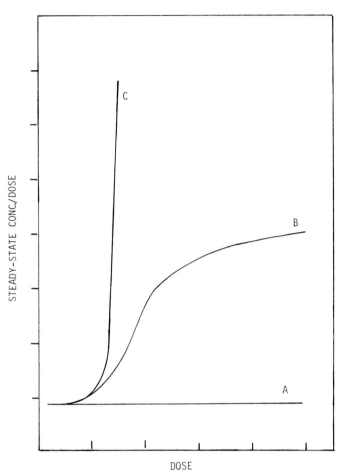

Fig. 7.10 Relationship between dose-adjusted steady-state concentrations and administered dose for drugs eliminated by first-order kinetics (A), parallel first-order and Michaelis-Menten kinetics (B), and Michaelis-Menten kinetics (C). (Data from Ref. 19.)

TIME TO STEADY STATE

The dependence in nonlinear systems of the time to reach steady state or some fraction thereof on the rate of drug administration can be demonstrated mathematically. If a drug is administered at a constant rate k_0 and is eliminated by a single pathway that is capacity limited, the following differential equation can be written:

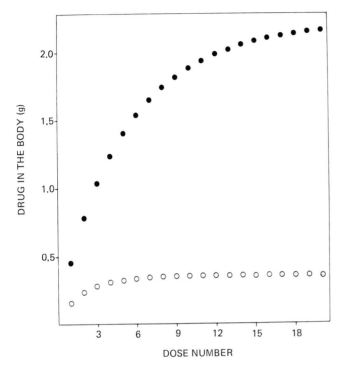

Fig. 7.11 Accumulation of salicylic acid in the body as a function of dose number when either 0.5 (O) or 1.0 (●) g doses are given every 8 h. (From Ref. 20, reprinted with permission.)

$$\frac{dC}{dt} = \frac{k_0}{V} - \frac{V_m C}{K_m + C} \qquad (7.56)$$

Expansion of (7.56) and collection of common terms yields

$$\frac{dC}{dt} = \frac{(k_0 K_m / V) + [(k_0/V) - V_m]C}{K_m + C} \qquad (7.57)$$

This equation is of the general form

$$\frac{dC}{dt} = \frac{x + yC}{z + C} \qquad (7.58)$$

which can be rearranged to give

$$\frac{z}{x + yC} \, dC + \frac{C}{x + yC} \, dC = dt \qquad (7.59)$$

The integral of (7.59) is [15]

$$\frac{z}{y} \ln (x + yC) + \frac{C}{y} - \frac{x}{y^2} \ln (x + yC) = t + i \qquad (7.60)$$

which can be simplified to

$$\frac{C}{y} + \frac{zy - x}{y^2} \ln (x + yC) = t + i \qquad (7.61)$$

At $t = 0$, $C = 0$ and

$$i = \frac{zy - x}{y^2} \ln x \qquad (7.62)$$

Substitution for i in (7.61) and rearrangement yields

$$t = \frac{C}{y} + \frac{zy - x}{y^2} \ln \left(1 + \frac{y}{x} C\right) \qquad (7.63)$$

Recognizing that $x = k_0 K_m / V$, $y = (k_0/V) - V_m$ and $z = K_m$ [(7.57) and (7.58)],

$$t = \frac{C}{(k_0/V) - V_m} + \frac{K_m [(k_0/V) - V_m] - k_0 K_m / V}{[(k_0/V) - V_m]^2}$$

$$\ln \left[1 + \frac{(k_0/V) - V_m}{k_0 K_m / V} C\right] \qquad (7.64)$$

Simplification gives the following:

$$t = \frac{C}{(k_0/V) - V_m} - \frac{K_m V_m}{[(k_0/V) - V_m]^2} \ln \left(1 + \frac{k_0 - VV_m}{k_0 K_m} C\right) \qquad (7.65)$$

The steady-state concentration C_{ss} of a drug that obeys the model above is given by

$$C_{ss} = \frac{k_0}{Cl_s} = \frac{k_0 (K_m + C_{ss})}{VV_m} \qquad (7.66)$$

where Cl_s at steady state is given by (7.46). Solving (7.66) for C_{ss} yields

$$-C_{ss} = \frac{k_0 K_m}{k_0 - VV_m} \qquad (7.67)$$

Substituting $-1/C_{ss}$ for $(k_0 - VV_m)/k_0 K_m$ in (7.65) and setting C/C_{ss} equal to f_{ss}, the fraction of the steady-state concentration, and

C equal to $f_{ss}C_{ss}$ gives the following expression for the time to reach a given fraction of steady state:

$$t = \frac{f_{ss}C_{ss}}{(k_0/V) - V_m} - \frac{K_m V_m}{[(k_0/V) - V_m]^2} \ln (1 - f_{ss})$$ (7.68)

The dependence of time to steady state on the rate of administration is clearly demonstrated. A relationship of the same form as (7.68) has been obtained from plasma concentration versus time data using numerical integration [21]. At a low administration rate (k_0 and $C_{ss} \to 0$), (7.68) reduces to

$$t = - \frac{1}{V_m/K_m} \ln (1 - f_{ss})$$ (7.69)

and hence time to steady state is independent of the rate of administration, while at a high infusion rate (k_0 and $C_{ss} \to \infty$)

$$t = \frac{f_{ss}C_{ss}}{k_0/V}$$ (7.70)

and the time to steady state is independent of drug elimination.

For the case where there is one or more first-order processes of elimination in parallel with a saturable process, the expression for time to reach a given fraction of steady state becomes relatively complex (see Appendix G). This expression is

$$t = \frac{1}{\sqrt{-q}} \left(K_m + \frac{b}{2K'} \right) \ln \frac{-2K'C + b - \sqrt{-q}}{b - \sqrt{-q}} \frac{1}{1 - f_{ss}}$$

$$- \frac{1}{2K'} \ln \frac{a + bC - K'C^2}{a}$$ (7.71)

where $a = k_0 K_m/V$, $b = (k_0/V) - K'K_m - Vm$, and $-q = b^2 + 4k_0 K_m K'/V$. When the rate of administration (i.e., k_0) is small, (7.71) simplifies to (see Appendix G)

$$t = \frac{-1}{K' + (V_m/K_m)} \ln (1 - f_{ss})$$ (7.72)

This relationship is identical in form to (7.69), illustrating that the time to achieve a certain fraction of steady state is dependent only on the rate constant or half-life of elimination under linear conditions. However, when the rate of administration becomes large, (7.71) reduces to (see Appendix G)

$$t = - \frac{1}{K'} \ln (1 - f_{ss})$$ (7.73)

Therefore, at high administration rates the time to steady state is dependent on the elimination rate constant for the first-order process.

AREA UNDER THE CURVE AND BIOAVAILABILITY

In theory, the area under the blood or plasma level versus time curve is proportional to the dose administered for drugs eliminated by first-order kinetics. However, for drugs that are eliminated by capacity-limited processes, area is not proportional to the administered dose. Rather, one finds that the area increases more than proportionally with an increase in dose. The total area under the drug level versus time curve ($\int_0^\infty C\,dt$) after the intravenous injection of a drug that is eliminated by a single capacity-limited process can be calculated for a one-compartment system as follows. Inversion of (7.1) and rearrangement of the resulting expression gives

$$C\,dt = -\frac{K_m + C}{V_m}\,dC \tag{7.74}$$

The expansion of (7.74) followed by integration over the limits $C = C_0$ at $t = 0$ and $C = 0$ at $t = \infty$ yields

$$\int_0^\infty C\,dt = -\int_{C_0}^0 \frac{K_m}{V_m}\,dC - \int_{C_0}^0 \frac{C}{V_m}\,dC \tag{7.75}$$

It follows that

$$\int_0^\infty C\,dt = -\frac{K_m}{V_m}\,C\,\Big|_{C_0}^0 - \frac{C^2}{2V_m}\,\Big|_{C_0}^0 \tag{7.76}$$

which when solved becomes

$$\int_0^\infty C\,dt = \frac{K_m}{V_m}\,C_0 + \frac{C_0^2}{2V_m} = \frac{C_0}{V_m}\left(K_m + \frac{C_0}{2}\right) \tag{7.77}$$

At sufficiently low doses such that $K_m \gg C_0/2$, (7.77) reduces to

$$\int_0^\infty C\,dt = \frac{K_m}{V_m}\,C_0 = \frac{K_m X_0}{V_m V} \tag{7.78}$$

where $C_0 = X_0/V$ and V is the apparent volume of distribution. Under these conditions the area under the curve is simply proportional to the dose X_0. Inspection of (7.77) readily indicates for the nonlinear situation that as the dose is increased, the area shows a stronger dependence on the dose. At sufficiently high dosage levels where $C_0/2 \gg K_m$, (7.77) reduces to

$$\int_0^\infty C \ dt = \frac{C_0^2}{2V_m} = \frac{X_0^2}{2V^2 V_m} \qquad (7.79)$$

which indicates that under these conditions the area is proportional
to the square of the dose and a relatively modest increase in the dose
may produce a dramatic increase in the total area under the drug
level in the plasma versus time curve.

The area under the curve after administration of a fixed dose of
a drug showing capacity-limited elimination may also vary with the
rate of absorption. The more rapidly a given dose is absorbed, the
more closely will the area approach that calculated by (7.77). In
other words, the area calculated from (7.77) for a given dose is a
maximum since it assumes that absorption is instantaneous. If absorption is sufficiently slow, the area will approach the minimum given by
(7.78). Figure 7.12 illustrates the effect of dose and absorption rate
on the area under the plasma concentration-time curve.

A nonlinear change in area with dose becomes important when
attempting to assess the bioavailability of a drug, since this parameter is generally determined by comparing the area under the curve
resulting from the administration of some test dosage form to the area
under the curve from the administration of a standard. Bioavailability
can be estimated for drugs eliminated by capacity-limited processes
in the following manner [17]. Integration of the term $-dC/dt$ yields

$$\int_0^\infty - \frac{dC}{dt} dt = \int_0^\infty -dC = -C \ \Big|_0^\infty = C_0 \qquad (7.80)$$

where C_0 is plasma concentration at time zero following intravenous
drug administration. For a one-compartment system, C_0 equals the
intravenous dose X_0 divided by the apparent volume of distribution
V. Therefore,

$$\int_0^\infty - \frac{dC}{dt} \ dt = C_0 = \frac{X_0}{V} \qquad (7.81)$$

From (7.81) it follows that a plot of $\int_0^\infty (-dC/dt) \ dt$ versus C_0 or
X_0/V will be linear and pass through the origin regardless of whether
or not the model is linear. The value of C_0 or X_0/V can be determined
by numerical differentiation of intravenous plasma concentration versus
time data, and measurement of the area under the curve resulting from
a plot of $-dC/dt$ versus time.

After oral administration the rate of drug elimination from the body
dX_E/dt, is given by

$$\frac{1}{V} \frac{dX_E}{dt} = K'C + \frac{V_m C}{K_m + C} \qquad (7.82)$$

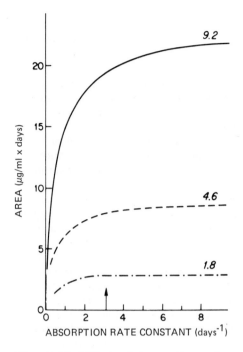

Fig. 7.12 Effect of absorption rate and dose on the area under the drug concentration in serum versus time curve after single doses of phenytoin. The curves reflect doses of 1.8, 4.6, and 9.2 mg/kg. The arrow marks the approximate absorption rate constant in a typical patient with the dosage form studied. (From Ref. 22, © 1976 Plenum Publishing Corp.)

where X_E is the amount eliminated to time t. If the amount ultimately eliminated is equal to the amount absorbed [i.e., $(X_E)_\infty = FX_0$, where F is the fraction of the orally administered dose absorbed], then

$$\frac{1}{V} \int_0^\infty \frac{dX_E}{dt} \, dt = \int_0^\infty \left(K'C + \frac{V_m C}{K_m + C} \right) dt = \frac{FX_0}{V} \qquad (7.83)$$

since $\int_0^\infty (dX_E/dt) \, dt$ equals $(X_E)_\infty$. The bioavailability or fraction absorbed of an orally administered dose can be determined by dividing Eq. (7.83) by Eq. (7.81). This yields

$$\frac{FX_0/V}{X_0/V} = \frac{[(1/V) \int_0^\infty (dX_E/dt)]_{oral}}{[\int_0^\infty - (dC/dt) dt]_{i.v.}} \qquad (7.84)$$

If equal doses are administered intravenously and orally, and it is assumed that volume of distribution remains constant,

$$F = \frac{[(1/V) \int_0^\infty (dX_E/dt)dt]_{oral}}{[\int_0^\infty - (dC/dt)dt]_{i.v.}} \tag{7.85}$$

Therefore, the absolute bioavailability of an oral dosage form can be determined by measuring the area under a $-dC/dt$ versus time plot using intravenous data, and generating values of $(dX_E/dt)/V$ from oral plasma concentration versus time data using (7.82). The latter determination requires K', V_m, and K_m, which can be obtained from the intravenous data by methods discussed previously in this chapter. Once the $(dX_E/dt)/V$ data are calculated, the area under a plot of $(dX_E/dt)/V$ versus time provides an estimate of the numerator of (7.85). This method has been applied to the determination of phenytoin bioavailability. It was demonstrated that the use of the nonlinear approach yielded a bioavailability estimate of 0.98 as compared to 0.87 when linear kinetics were assumed [22].

COMPOSITION OF URINARY EXCRETION PRODUCTS

For a drug eliminated from the body by multiple pathways, one of which is nonlinear, the composition of urinary excretion products will vary with dose. We illustrate this with the following scheme:

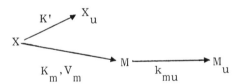

It is assumed that there are two pathways of elimination for the parent drug, a capacity-limited pathway for the formation of metabolite M and a first-order pathway for the urinary excretion of unchanged drug. X_u and M_u are the cumulative amounts of unchanged drug and metabolite in the urine at time t, and K' and k_{mu} are the first-order rate constants for urinary excretion of unchanged drug and metabolite, respectively. X is the amount of unchanged drug in the body at time t, and K_m and V_m are the Michaelis-Menten parameters for the capacity-limited formation of M. The rate of appearance of unchanged drug in the urine is given by the differential equation

$$\frac{dX_u}{dt} = K'X \tag{7.86}$$

or

$$\frac{dX_u}{dt} = K'VC \tag{7.87}$$

since the amount of drug in the body X equals the product of the
volume of distribution and the plasma concentration. Integration of
Eq. (7.87) from time zero to infinity yields

$$X_u^\infty = K'V \int_0^\infty C\, dt \tag{7.88}$$

where X_u^∞ is the total amount of unchanged drug eliminated in the urine
following the administration of a given dose, and $\int_0^\infty C\, dt$ is the area
under the resulting plasma concentration versus time curve.

Equation (7.18) is the differential equation for plasma concentration for the model above. Factoring out C and expanding (7.18)
gives

$$\frac{dC}{dt} = -C\, \frac{K'K_m + V_m + K'C}{K_m + C} \tag{7.89}$$

which when inverted and rearranged becomes

$$C\, dt = -\frac{K_m + C}{K'K_m + V_m + K'C}\, dC \tag{7.90}$$

By expanding (7.90) and taking the integral over the limits $C = C_0$ at
$t = 0$ and $C = 0$ at $t = \infty$, the following is obtained:

$$\int_0^\infty C\, dt = \int_{C_0}^0 \frac{K_m}{K'K_m + V_m + K'C}\, dC - \int_{C_0}^0 \frac{C}{K'K_m + V_m + K'C}\, dC \tag{7.91}$$

The two terms to be integrated are of the general forms $dx/(a + bx)$
and $x\, dx/(a + bx)$, respectively, the integrals of which are $(1/b)\ln$
$(a + bx)$ and $(x/b) - (a/b^2)\ln(a + bx)$ [15]. Therefore, (7.91)
when integrated becomes

$$\int_0^\infty C\, dt = -\frac{K_m}{K'}\ln(K'K_m + V_m + K'C)\,\Big|_{C_0}^0 - \frac{C}{K'}\Big|_{C_0}^0$$

$$+ \frac{K'K_m + V_m}{(K')^2}\ln(K'K_m + V_m + K'C)\,\Big|_{C_0}^0 \tag{7.92}$$

Collecting common terms and simplifying provides

$$\int_0^\infty C\, dt = -\frac{C}{K'}\Big|_{C_0}^0 + \frac{V_m}{(K')^2}\ln(K'K_m + V_m + K'C)\,\Big|_{C_0}^0 \tag{7.93}$$

Solving (7.93) gives the following expression for the area under the curve:

$$\int_0^\infty C \, dt = \frac{C_0}{K'} - \frac{V_m}{(K')^2} \ln \left(\frac{K'C_0}{K'K_m + V_m} + 1 \right) \tag{7.94}$$

By substituting this value of $\int_0^\infty C \, dt$ for $\int_0^\infty C \, dt$ in (7.88), the following expression for X_u^∞ is obtained:

$$X_u^\infty = C_0 V - \frac{VV_m}{K'} \ln \left(\frac{K'C_0}{K'K_m + V_m} + 1 \right) \tag{7.95}$$

At very low plasma concentrations the natural log term becomes approximately equal to $K'C_0/(K'K_m + V_m)$ since for very small numbers $\ln (1 + x)$ becomes approximately equal to x [15]. Therefore, at low concentrations, (7.95) becomes

$$X_u^\infty = C_0 V - \frac{VV_m}{K'} \frac{K'C_0}{K'K_m + V_m} = C_0 V - \frac{C_0 VV_m}{K'K_m + V_m} = C_0 V \frac{K'K_m}{K'K_m + V_m} \tag{7.96}$$

Recognizing that $C_0 V$ equals the dose X_0 and dividing the numerator and denominator by K_m yields

$$X_u^\infty = X_0 \frac{K'}{K' + V_m/K_m} \tag{7.97}$$

This illustrates that at low doses the amount of unchanged drug in the urine is directly proportional to the administered dose. As the dose is increased and the capacity of the enzyme system becomes limited, the amount of unchanged drug appearing in the urine will increase more than proportionally to the increase in dose as illustrated by (7.95).

According to the scheme above, at time infinity

$$X_u^\infty + M_u^\infty = X_0 \tag{7.98}$$

where M_u^∞ is the total amount of metabolite in the urine at time infinity. Solving (7.98) for M_u^∞ and substituting the value of X_u^∞ in (7.95) yields

$$M_u^\infty = X_0 - C_0 V + \frac{VV_m}{K'} \ln \left(\frac{K'C_0}{K'K_m + V_m} + 1 \right) = \frac{VV_m}{K'}$$

$$\ln \left(\frac{K'C_0}{K'K_m + V_m} + 1 \right) \tag{7.99}$$

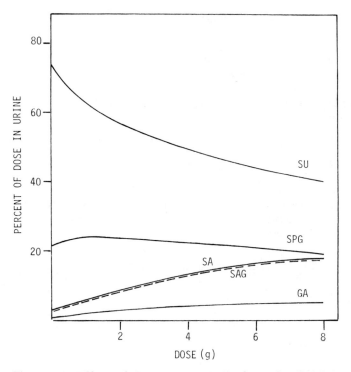

Fig. 7.13 Effect of dose on metabolic fate of salicylic acid in humans. The curves are based on urinary excretion data from four healthy subjects. SU is salicyluric acid, SPG is salicyl phenolic glucuronide, SA is salicylic acid, SAG is salicyl acyl glucuronide (dashed line), and GA is gentisic acid. (Data from Ref. 23.)

This equation indicates that M_u^{∞} will increase less than proportionally with an increase in dose. At low doses (7.99) reduces to

$$M_u^{\infty} = \frac{VV_m}{K'} \frac{K'C_0}{K'K_m + V_m} = \frac{C_0 VV_m}{K'K_m + V_m} \qquad (7.100)$$

Substituting X_0 for $C_0 V$ and dividing the numerator and denominator by K_m gives

$$M_u^{\infty} = X_0 \frac{V_m/K_m}{K' + V_m/K_m} \qquad (7.101)$$

As is evident from (7.101), at low doses M_u^{∞} is directly proportional to dose.

The influence of dose on excretion patterns is readily demonstrated with salicylate. As can be seen in Fig. 7.13, the fraction of the dose

eliminated as salicyluric acid, SU, a metabolite formed by a capacity-
limited process, decreases with dose. For those excretion products
formed or eliminated by first-order kinetics, the fraction of the dose
eliminated as such increases with dose (see SA, SAG, and GA). The
enzyme system responsible for the formation of the phenolic glucuronide
is capacity limited but has a higher capacity than the system responsible
for the formation of salicyluric acid. Consequently, the fraction eliminated as this metabolite initially increases with dose, and then decreases with dose as this enzyme system becomes saturated.

The composition of excretion products will also be dependent on
the rate of drug absorption when the drug is subject to capacity-
limited metabolism. The more rapid the absorption, the higher the
drug level in the body and the lower the fraction of the dose converted
to the metabolite formed by capacity-limited metabolism. This phenomenon has been demonstrated in humans with p-aminobenzoic acid,
which is eliminated by capacity-limited acetylation as well as excreted
unchanged [24]. When 55 µmoles/kg was given at once, 56% of the
dose was acetylated, whereas when 10 consecutive 5.5 µmoles/kg doses
were administered at 30 min intervals, 91% of the dose was acetylated.
After administration of 110 µmoles/kg to fasted subjects, which should
result in rapid absorption, 51% of the dose was acetylated. However,
when the same dose was administered to subjects after a high-fat
meal, which is known to reduce gastric emptying and the absorption
rate of many drugs, 90% of the dose was acetylated.

OTHER NONLINEAR ELIMINATION PROCESSES

Dose-dependent elimination kinetics may be due to effects other than a
limited capacity of biotransformation or excretion processes. If a drug
is partly reabsorbed from renal tubules by a capacity-limited process,
the elimination (urinary excretion) of large doses proceeds more rapidly than the elimination of smaller doses. Capacity-limited reabsorption
has been demonstrated for several compounds, including riboflavin [25],
bethanidine [26], cephapirin [27], and cephaloridine [27]. There is
evidence to suggest that some drug metabolites can inhibit their own
metabolism [28,29]. This process of product inhibition can also cause
dose-dependent effects, with large doses being relatively more slowly
eliminated than small doses [30]. However, whereas the rate of decline
of drug concentrations in the postdistributive phase at any given concentration of drug in the body will be independent of dose in the case
of simple Michaelis-Menten kinetics [see (7.1)], this rate will tend to
decrease with increasing dose in the case of product inhibition. Moreover, drug elimination may appear to be first order but with half-lives
increasing with increasing dose provided that the initial drug levels
(i.e., the intravenous doses) are lower than K_m and elimination of the
inhibiting metabolite is relatively slow (see Fig. 7.14). These obser-

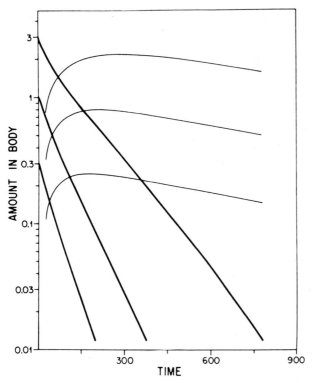

Fig. 7.14 Effect of competitive inhibition by a metabolite (light lines) on the time course of parent drug (heavy lines) after intravenous administration of different doses of the drug. Although the semilogarithmic plots of amount of drug in the body are apparently linear, the half-life increases with dose. (From Ref. 31, © 1973 Plenum Publishing Corp.)

vations can be explained by the following relationship, which describes the rate of change in plasma concentrations for a drug with one pathway of elimination that is subject to competitive product inhibition [13]:

$$-\frac{dC}{dt} = \frac{V_m C}{K_m (1 + C_m/K_p) + C} \qquad (7.102)$$

where C_m is the concentration of inhibiting metabolite and K_p is the equilibrium constant for the enzyme-metabolite (product) complex. Dose dependence with similar characteristics has been observed in humans with dicumarol [32] (see Fig. 7.15) and in dogs with phenytoin [33].

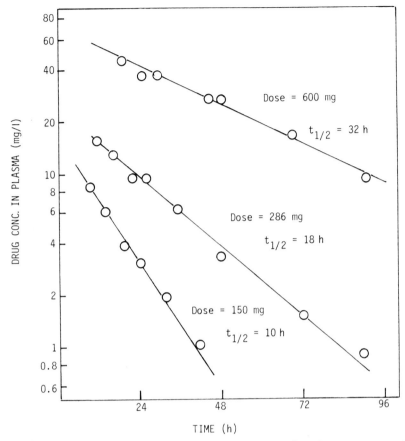

Fig. 7.15 Dicumarol concentration in plasma after intravenous administration of different doses. (Data from Ref. 32.)

ENZYME INDUCTION

Another type of nonlinear kinetics is seen when a drug induces its own metabolism. It has been suggested that enzyme induction is a result of new protein synthesis and not a change in substrate affinity [34]. Based on this premise, a model to describe the change in enzyme concentration following induction has been described by Berlin and Schimke [35]. Prior to induction the rate of change of enzyme levels, dE/dt, is a function of the rate of synthesis and rate of degradation of the enzyme; that is,

$$\frac{dE}{dt} = S - kE \qquad (7.103)$$

where S is the rate of enzyme synthesis and is assumed to be zero order and k is the first-order rate constant for enzyme degradation. Assuming that a steady state for the enzyme exists prior to induction (i.e., $dE/dt = 0$), it follows that

$$E = \frac{S}{k} \tag{7.104}$$

Following induction, a new steady-state enzyme level, E', will be determined by the new ratio S'/k'; that is,

$$E' = \frac{S'}{k'} \tag{7.105}$$

The rate at which E approaches E' can be given by the differential equation

$$\frac{dE}{dt} = S' - k'E \tag{7.106}$$

Rearrangement of (7.106) yields

$$\frac{dE}{S' - k'E} = dt \tag{7.107}$$

which when integrated becomes

$$-\frac{1}{k'} \ln (S' - k'E_t) = t + i \tag{7.108}$$

where E_t is the concentration of enzyme at some time t after the start of administration of the drug. At $t = 0$, $E_t = E_0$, the enzyme level prior to induction, and therefore

$$i = -\frac{1}{k'} \ln (S' - k'E_0) \tag{7.109}$$

Substitution for i in (7.108) according to (7.109) and rearrangement gives

$$\ln \frac{S' - k'E_t}{S' - k'E_0} = -k't \tag{7.110}$$

which in exponential terms becomes

$$\frac{S' - k'E_t}{S' - k'E_0} = e^{-k't} \tag{7.111}$$

Solving (7.111) for E_t yields

$$E_t = \frac{S'}{k'} - \frac{S' - k'E_0}{k'} e^{-k't} \tag{7.112}$$

Substitution of S/k for E_0 according to (7.104) and further simplification produces the following expression for E_t:

$$E_t = \frac{S'}{k'} - \left(\frac{S'}{k'} - \frac{S}{k} \right) e^{-k't} \tag{7.113}$$

Therefore, the enzyme level during induction is dependent on the preinduction and induced steady-state enzyme concentrations, S/k and S'/k', respectively, and the first-order rate constant for enzyme degradation, k'.

An expression similar to (7.113) can be obtained to describe the change in maximum velocity V_{m_t} during induction. V_m is equal to k_2E [see Appendix G, Eq. (G.8)] prior to induction, while at steady state after induction $V_m' = k_2E'$, where k_2 is the rate constant for the formation of metabolite. Substitution of S/k for E and S'/k' for E' according to (7.104) and (7.105), respectively, yields the expressions

$$\frac{S}{k} = \frac{V_m}{k_2} \tag{7.114}$$

and

$$\frac{S'}{k'} = \frac{V_m'}{k_2} \tag{7.115}$$

Further, substitution for S/k and S'/k', according to (7.114) and (7.115), as well as substitution of V_{m_t}/k_2 for E_t in (7.113) and cancelation of common terms yields

$$V_{m_t} = V_m' - (V_m' - V_m)e^{-k't} \tag{7.116}$$

The time course of the change in the systemic clearance Cl_{s_t} of a drug following self-induction can be given by a similar expression,

$$Cl_{s_t} = Cl_s' - (Cl_s' - Cl_s)e^{-k't} \tag{7.117}$$

where Cl_s is the preinduction clearance and Cl_s' is the clearance at steady-state postinduction. Equation (7.117) can be obtained from (7.116) by recognizing that clearance equals the sum of the clearance of the inducible Cl_{s_i} and noninducible Cl_{s_n} pathways, and that

$$Cl_{s_i} = Vk_i = V \frac{V_m}{K_m} \tag{7.118}$$

where k_i is the first-order rate constant for elimination by the inducible pathway.

Of interest is the plasma concentration-time course of a drug that is subject to self-induction. In a one-compartment system where a drug is administered at a constant rate DR and is eliminated by first-order processes,

$$C = \frac{DR}{Cl_s} [1 - e^{-(Cl_s/V)t}]$$
(7.119)

where Cl_s and V are as defined previously. Once self-induction begins, Cl_s will become time dependent and will be given by (7.117). Therefore, substitution of Cl_{s_t}, according to (7.117), for Cl_s in (7.119) will yield an expression that describes the plasma concentration as a function of time for a drug that is subject to self-induction. If there is a time delay between drug administration and the beginning of the self-induction, t in (7.117) should be replaced by $t - t_0$, where t_0 is the time at which induction began. The kinetic properties of carbamazepine appear to behave in a nonlinear manner as a result of self-induction (see Fig. 7.16) [36].

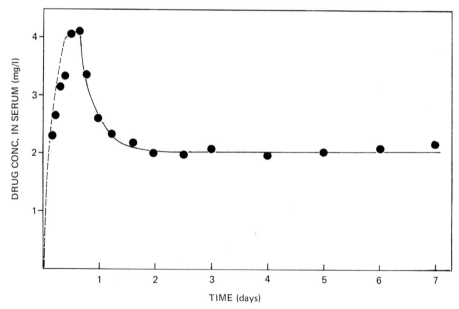

Fig. 7.16 Carbamazepine concentration in serum during continuous constant rate intravenous infusion of the drug for 7 days to a monkey. The data suggest pronounced autoinduction of carbamazepine metabolism. The continuous line corresponds to the following equation: $C = 2.04 + 2.06 \exp [-0.693/5.8(t - t_0)]$, where $t_0 = 16$ h. (Data from Ref. 36.)

Enzyme induction has been cited as an example of time-dependent rather than dose-dependent or concentration-dependent pharmaco-kinetics. The reason for this is that the changes in clearance one observes are not obviously related to drug concentration or dose but may be described as a function of time [see Eq. (7.117)]. Levy [37], in a comprehensive discussion of time-dependent pharmacokinetics, has noted the following: "A major distinguishing feature between dose and time dependency is that the latter involves an actual physio-logical or biochemical change in the organ(s) of the body associated with the drug disposition parameters in question. For example, in time dependence of the auto- or heteroinduction type, the increase in drug intrinsic clearance results from an increase in amount of en-zyme (in protein synthesis). However, in a typical Michaelis-Menten dose-dependency, drug clearance changes with concentration and such a system should not be considered time-dependent simply because the values of pharmacokinetic parameters also change with time." Other examples of time-dependent pharmacokinetics are circadian rhythms in drug absorption, distribution, and elimination.

NONLINEAR BINDING

In discussions of nonlinear pharmacokinetics, capacity-limited elimina-tion generally receives greatest attention because it is the most common and best understood. Although it is recognized that drugs are re-versibly bound to proteins in the vascular space and to proteins and other materials in the "tissues," it is generally assumed that the frac-tion bound is essentially constant and independent of the drug concen-tration at the site of binding. However, it is obvious that there is a finite amount of each tissue which can bind a given drug and that the amount of drug which can be taken up per gram of given tissue will be related to the number of available binding sites and to some type of affinity constant. Accordingly, at sufficiently high concentrations of drug, one may find that the fraction bound decreases with increasing concentration. This will result in an alteration in the kinetics of a drug.

The following model will serve as a basis for considering the effect of nonlinear vascular protein and tissue binding on drug plasma con-centration versus time profiles, and on the resultant pharmacokinetic parameters derived from such profiles:

Vascular Space	Nonvascular Space
Plasma-bound drug	Tissue-bound drug
$\Uparrow\Downarrow$	$\Uparrow\Downarrow$
Free drug $\rightleftharpoons$	Free drug

k

The parameter k is the first-order elimination rate constant. In the vascular compartment, drug will interact with protein to form a drug-protein complex according to the scheme

$$C_f + P_f \underset{k_1}{\overset{k_2}{\rightleftharpoons}} C_b$$

where C_f and C_b are the molar concentrations of free and bound drug in the vascular space, respectively. C_b is equal to the concentration of occupied protein binding sites. P_f is the molar concentration of free protein binding sites, and the parameters k_2 and k_1 are rate constants. From the scheme it follows that

$$\frac{dC_f}{dt} = k_2 C_b - k_1 C_f P_f \tag{7.120}$$

Based on the steady-state assumption (i.e., $dC_f/dt = 0$),

$$\frac{k_2}{k_1} = \frac{C_f P_f}{C_b} \tag{7.121}$$

The total concentration of vascular protein binding sites, nP, where n is the number of binding sites per protein molecule and P is the molar concentration of protein, is given by

$$nP = P_f + C_b \tag{7.122}$$

Solving (7.122) for P_f, substituting this value for P_f in (7.121), and recognizing that k_2/k_1 is equal to the dissociation constant for the drug-protein complex, K_d, yields

$$K_d = \frac{C_f(nP - C_b)}{C_b} \tag{7.123}$$

which when solved for C_b becomes

$$C_b = \frac{C_f nP}{K_d + C_f} \tag{7.124}$$

The total concentration of drug in the vascular space, C_t, is equal to the sum of the concentrations of free and bound drug:

$$C_t = C_f + C_b \tag{7.125}$$

Substitution for C_b according to (7.124) gives

$$C_t = C_f + \frac{C_f nP}{K_d + C_f} \tag{7.126}$$

An expression for the total drug concentration in the tissues, C_t^T, which includes everything but the vascular space, can be obtained in an analogous manner. The resulting equation is given by

$$C_t^T = C_f + \frac{C_f A}{K_d^T + C_f} \tag{7.127}$$

where K_d^T is the dissociation constant for the drug tissue complex and A is a constant similar to nP. When the binding to vascular protein or tissue is linear, total drug concentrations in the vascular space and tissue are given by

$$C_t = \frac{C_f}{f_B} \tag{7.128}$$

and

$$C_t^T = \frac{C_f}{f_T} \tag{7.129}$$

respectively, where f_B is the fraction free in the vascular space and f_T is the fraction free in the tissues.

Expansion followed by differentiation of (7.126) and (7.127) and collection of common terms yields

$$\frac{dC_t}{dt} = \frac{(dC_f/dt)\{(K_d + C_f)(2C_f + K_d + nP) - [C_f^2 + (K_d + nP)C_f]\}}{(K_d + C_f)^2} \tag{7.130}$$

and

$$\frac{dC_t^T}{dt} = \frac{(dC_f/dt)\{(K_d^T + C_f)(2C_f + K_d^T + A) - [C_f^2 + (K_d^T + A)C_f]\}}{(K_d^T + C_f)^2} \tag{7.131}$$

These equations can be further simplified to give

$$\frac{dC_t}{dt} = \frac{(dC_f/dt)(C_f^2 + 2C_f K_d + nPK_d + K_d^2)}{(K_d + C_f)^2} \tag{7.132}$$

and

$$\frac{dC_t^T}{dt} = \frac{(dC_f/dt)[C_f^2 + 2C_f K_d^T + AK_d^T + (K_d^T)^2]}{(K_d^T + C_f)^2} \tag{7.133}$$

When there is linear binding, differentiation of (7.128) and (7.129) results in the following two equations:

$$\frac{dC_t}{dt} = \frac{dC_f/dt}{f_B} \tag{7.134}$$

and

$$\frac{dC_t^T}{dt} = \frac{dC_f/dt}{f_T} \tag{7.135}$$

respectively. When a dose D of a drug is given, the following mass balance can be written:

$$X_B + X_T + X_E = D \tag{7.136}$$

where X_B and X_T are the amounts of drug in the vascular space and tissue, respectively, and X_E is the amount of drug eliminated from the body by all routes of elimination. Differentiation of (7.136) yields

$$\frac{dX_B}{dt} + \frac{dX_T}{dt} + \frac{dX_E}{dt} = 0 \tag{7.137}$$

The rate of elimination, dX_E/dt, is given by

$$\frac{dX_E}{dt} = kV_B C_t \tag{7.138}$$

where V_B is intravascular volume. Recognizing that $X_B = V_B C_t$ and $X_T = V_T C_t^T$, where V_T is the tissue volume, (7.137) may be written as

$$V_B = \frac{dC_t}{dt} + V_T \frac{dC_t^T}{dt} + \frac{dX_E}{dt} = 0 \tag{7.139}$$

where dX_E/dt is given by (7.138). To evaluate the influence of linear or nonlinear vascular protein and/or tissue binding on drug disposition, the appropriate expressions for dX_E/dt, dC_t/dt, and dC_t^T/dt as given by (7.138) and (7.132) to (7.135) can be substituted into (7.139). Numerical analysis of the resulting equation will provide insight into the influence of nonlinear binding to vascular protein and/or tissue protein on drug disposition [38].

The effect of nonlinear binding can be illustrated by the following relationships:

$$V = V_B + \frac{f_B}{f_T} V_T \qquad (5.49)$$

and

$$Cl = Q \frac{f_B Cl_I'}{Q + f_B Cl_I'} \qquad (8.27)$$

where V_B, V_T, f_B, and f_T are defined above, and V is the apparent volume of distribution. Cl and Cl_I' are clearance and intrinsic clearance of free drug from the blood, respectively, and Q is blood flow to the eliminating organ. The influence of nonlinear binding on the shape of a log plasma concentration versus time can be illustrated by recognizing that half-life $(t_{1/2})$ equals $0.693V/Cl$ [Eq. (2.217)], and that if half-life increases or decreases with time, a concave or convex curve will result. For drugs with a low intrinsic clearance (i.e., $Q \gg f_B Cl_I'$), where nonlinear binding occurs in the vascular space, a decrease in volume of distribution and clearance should be observed as a function of time after an intravenous bolus dose because of the decrease in free fraction as drug concentration in the vascular space decreases. Under the conditions noted above, the log plasma concentration versus time curve may appear curved even when a one-compartment model with first-order elimination is extant. The effect of binding on clearance will tend to make the curves concave, whereas the effect of binding on volume of distribution will tend to make the curves convex (see Fig. 7.17). As linear tissue binding increases, there is a general tendency to straighten the concave log plasma concentration-time curves resulting from nonlinear protein binding in the vascular space. Nonlinear tissue binding with linear protein binding in the vascular space will result in no net change in clearance with time, but will result in an increase in volume of distribution with time. This becomes readily apparent by considering Eqs. (5.49) and (8.27). The consequence will be a concave log plasma concentration versus time curve even though a single compartment is extant.

Nonlinear protein binding in the vascular space or nonlinear tissue binding will have the same effect on volume of distribution of drugs with a high clearance as they do on drugs with a low clearance. However, changes in protein binding in the vascular space should have little if any effect on the clearance of highly cleared drugs (i.e., $f_B Cl_I' \gg Q$), and the total area under a plasma concentration versus time curve should be a simple linear function of dose or amount absorbed. This lack of dependence of clearance on binding can be readily appreciated by considering (8.27). Therefore, the shape of log plasma concentra-

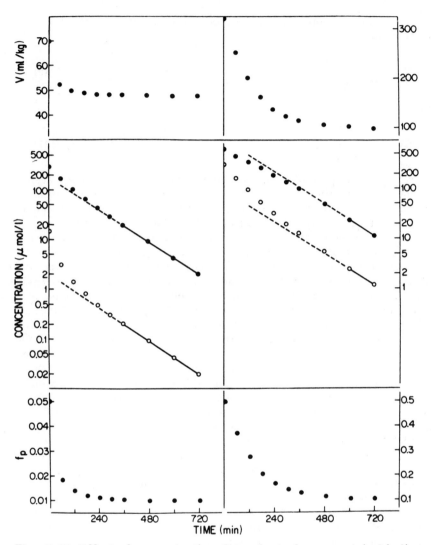

Fig. 7.17 Effect of concentration-dependent plasma protein binding (assuming no tissue binding) on the time course of free (O) and total (●) drug concentration in the plasma. Also shown are the instantaneous apparent volume of distribution V and the free fraction in the plasma f_p. In the panel on the left, the effect of plasma protein binding on clearance predominates and the total drug concentration in plasma curve is concave, whereas in the panel on the right, the effect of binding on volume of distribution predominates and the curve describing total drug concentration in plasma is convex. (From Ref. 38, © 1979 Plenum Publishing Corp.)

tion versus time curves will appear convex since the effect of protein binding in the vascular space on volume of distribution will be the primary factor influencing this shape. Such curves may be interpreted incorrectly as indicating nonlinear or Michaelis-Menten drug elimination.

SOME PROBLEMS IN QUANTIFYING NONLINEAR PHARMACOKINETICS

Because of the possible effects of nonlinear binding on log plasma concentration versus time profiles, it is simplistic always to interpret log plasma concentration times curves on the basis of multicompartment pharmacokinetic models or to simply assume nonlinear elimination. Interpretation is complicated by the fact that tissue binding is difficult to characterize since tissue represents such an heterogeneous phase. Whether or not a multiexponential plasma concentration versus time curve is a consequence of the distribution characteristics of a drug or a result of nonlinear binding in the vascular or extravascular space can be evaluated by giving an intravenous bolus dose and an intravenous infusion of a drug such that drug concentrations immediately after the bolus dose and upon termination of the infusion are equal. If the drug does in fact confer multiexponential characteristics on the body as a result of its distribution properties, the distribution phase postinfusion will be less pronounced than that after the intravenous bolus dose. However, if the multiexponential characteristics are a result of nonlinear binding, the distributive phases postinfusion and postbolus will be equivalent (see Fig. 7.18) [39].

Although the equations developed in previous sections of this chapter have been based on a one-compartment system, the principles discussed apply regardless of the compartmental characteristics of the drug. However, in the case of capacity-limited elimination, errors do occur in the estimation of K_m and V_m if a one-compartment system is assumed when in fact a multicompartment system is more appropriate. This can be readily appreciated by considering that in a multicompartment system, the ratio V_m/K_m equals k_{10}, the elimination rate constant, not the smallest exponent (typically β). If data are incorrectly assumed to obey a one-compartment system, the estimate of V_m/K_m will approximate β, the terminal disposition rate constant, rather than approximating k_{10}.

As would be expected, V_m/K_m estimated assuming a one-compartment system will always be less than the value obtained when the data are analyzed according to the appropriate multicompartment system. In addition, the value of V_m obtained by one-compartment analysis will always be less than the V_m of a multicompartment system, while K_m may be overestimated or underestimated when multicompartment data are analyzed assuming a one-compartment system [40]. Therefore, V_m

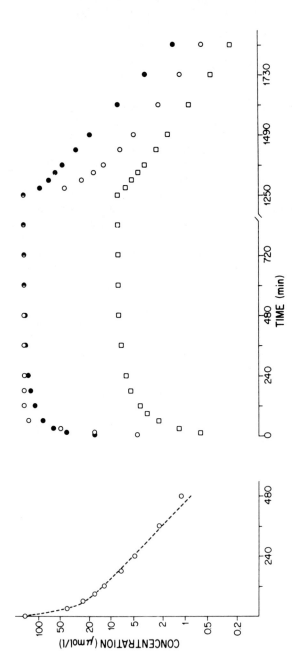

Fig. 7.18 Time course of drug concentration in plasma (O) following a single intravenous dose (panel on left), and during and after constant rate intravenous infusion (panel on right) of drug with nonlinear tissue binding in a one-compartment system. Drug concentrations after the bolus and upon cessation of the infusion are superimposable. Infusion at a lower rate yields proportionately lower steady-state concentrations (□), but the time required to reach steady state is longer than during the higher rate infusion. Drug concentrations in plasma (●), predicted by incorrectly assuming that the data after intravenous bolus administration could be described by a linear biexponential model, take longer to reach steady state and have a much less pronounced postinfusion distribution phase. (From Ref. 39, © 1979 Plenum Publishing Corp.)

and K_m values obtained assuming an incorrect model must be interpreted and used with caution.

Another problem is encountered when a drug is eliminated by more than one capacity-limited pathway. In linear models, first-order elimination rate constants for parallel pathways can be summed as a means of simplifying the model. It would be advantageous if data described by parallel Michaelis-Menten equations could be approximated over several orders of magnitude by a single Michaelis-Menten equation with constants V_m and K_m insensitive to large changes in dose. Approximation of data by a single Michaelis-Menten equation appears reasonable when values of K_m for parallel pathways are within a factor of 3 of each other [41]. The constants obtained, however, are generally not characteristic of any one enzyme system. When values of K_m are separated by a factor of 5 or more, data cannot be well represented over several orders of magnitude by a single Michaelis-Menten equation, and therefore, simplification of such a system is inappropriate. In this case V_m and K_m increase markedly with dose. To determine whether a system can be adequately described by a single Michaelis-Menten equation requires that the parameters V_m and K_m be relatively constant over the extremes of the dose range of interest.

A final point to consider is that some drugs exert dose-dependent effects on blood circulation, urine pH, and on other physiologic processes that may affect drug disposition. For example, it is well known that the elimination of certain drugs is influenced largely by the rate of hepatic blood flow. Some of these drugs may actually reduce hepatic blood flow either directly or indirectly via an effect on cardiac index. In such cases one may observe a decrease in the half-life and/or clearance of the drug with increasing dose.

REFERENCES

1. M. Mayersohn. Ascorbic acid absorption in man. *Eur. J. Pharmacol.* *19*:140 (1972).
2. R. Runkel, E. Forchielli, H. Sevelius, M. Chaplin, and E. Segre. Nonlinear plasma level response to high doses of naproxen. *Clin. Pharmacol. Ther.* *15*:261 (1974).
3. R. Runkel, M. D. Chaplin, H. Sevelius, E. Ortega, and E. Segre. Pharmacokinetics of naproxen overdoses. *Clin. Pharmacol. Ther.* *20*:269 (1976).
4. F. Lundquist and H. Wolthers. The kinetics of alcohol elimination in man. *Acta Pharmacol. Toxicol.* *14*:265 (1958).
5. G. Levy. Pharmacokinetics of salicylate elimination in man. *J. Pharm. Sci.* *54*:959 (1965).
6. G. Levy, T. Tsuchiya, and L. P. Amsel. Limited capacity for salicyl phenolic glucuronide formation and its effect on the kinetics of salicylate elimination in man. *Clin. Pharmacol. Ther.* *13*:258 (1972).

7.   K. Arnold and N. Gerber. The rate of decline of diphenyl-
     hydantoin in human plasma. *Clin. Pharmacol. Ther.* *11*:121
     (1970).
8.   E. Martin, T. N. Tozer, L. B. Sheiner, and S. Riegelman.
     The clinical pharmacokinetics of phenytoin. *J. Pharmacokinet.*
     Biopharm. *5*:579 (1977).
9.   P. K. Wilkinson, A. J. Sedman, E. Sakmar, R. H. Earhart,
     D. J. Weidler, and J. G. Wagner. Blood ethanol concentrations
     during and following constant-rate intravenous infusion of
     alcohol. *Clin. Pharmacol. Ther.* *19*:213 (1976).
10. N. Gerber and J. G. Wagner. Explanation of dose-dependent
     decline of diphenylhydantoin plasma levels by fitting to the
     integrated form of Michaelis-Menten equation. *Res. Commun.*
     Chem. Pathol. Pharmacol. *3*:455 (1972).
11. J. E. Dowd and D. S. Riggs. A comparison of estimates of
     Michaelis-Menten kinetic constants from various linear transforma-
     tions. *J. Biol. Chem.* *240*:863 (1965).
12. P. W. Mullen and R. W. Foster. Comparative evaluation of six
     techniques for determining the Michaelis-Menten parameters
     relating phenytoin dose and steady-state serum concentrations.
     J. Pharm. Pharmacol. *31*:100 (1979).
13. I. H. Segel. *Enzyme Kinetics.* Wiley, New York, 1975, pp.
     208–214.
14. C. A. M. van Ginnekan, J. M. Van Rossum, and H. L. J. M.
     Fleuren. Linear and nonlinear kinetics of drug elimination:
     I. Kinetics on the basis of a single capacity-limited pathway
     of elimination with or without simultaneous supply-limited
     elimination. *J. Pharmacokinet. Biopharm.* *2*:395 (1974).
15. W. H. Beyer (Ed.). *CRC Standard Mathematical Tables.*
     CRC Press, West Palm Beach, Fla., 1978.
16. G. Levy. Dose-dependent effects in pharmacokinetics. In
     Importance of Fundamental Principles in Drug Evaluation,
     D. H. Tedeschi and R. E. Tedeschi (Eds.). Raven Press,
     New York, 1968, pp. 141–172.
17. L. Martis and R. H. Levy. Bioavailability calculations for
     drugs showing simultaneous first-order and capacity-limited
     elimination kinetics. *J. Pharmacokinet. Biopharm.* *1*:283
     (1973).
18. Y. J. Lin, D. J. Weidler, D. C. Garg, and J. G. Wagner.
     Novel method for estimating volume of distribution of a drug
     obeying Michaelis-Menten elimination kinetics. *J. Pharmacokinet.*
     Biopharm. *6*:197 (1978).
19. T. Tsuchiya and G. Levy. Relationship between dose and
     plateau levels of drugs eliminated by parallel first-order and
     capacity-limited kinetics. *J. Pharm. Sci.* *61*:541 (1972).

20. G. Levy and T. Tsuchiya. Salicylate accumulation kinetics in man. *N. Engl. J. Med.* *287*:430 (1972).

21. J. G. Wagner. Time to reach steady-state and prediction of steady-state concentrations for drugs obeying Michaelis-Menten elimination kinetics. *J. Pharmacokinet. Biopharm.* *6*:209 (1978).

22. W. J. Jusko, J. R. Koup, and G. Alvan. Nonlinear assessment of phenytoin bioavailability. *J. Pharmacokinet. Biopharm.* *4*:327 (1976).

23. T. Tsuchiya and G. Levy. Biotransformation of salicylic acid to its acyl and phenolic glucuronides in man. *J. Pharm. Sci.* *61*:800 (1972).

24. M. M. Drucker, S. H. Blondheim, and L. Wislicki. Factors affecting acetylation in vivo of para-aminobenzoic acid by human subjects. *Clin. Sci.* *27*:133 (1964).

25. W. J. Jusko and G. Levy. Pharmacokinetic evidence for saturable renal tubular reabsorption of riboflavin. *J. Pharm. Sci.* *59*:765 (1970).

26. A. N. Chremos, D. Shen, M. Gibaldi, J. D. Proctor, and J. H. Newman. Time dependent changes in renal clearance of bethanidine in humans. *J. Pharm. Sci.* *65*:140 (1976).

27. A. Arvidsson, O. Borga, and G. Alvan. Renal excretion of cephapirin and cephaloridine: Evidence for saturable tubular reabsorption. *Clin. Pharmacol. Ther.* *25*:870 (1979).

28. E. Jahnchen and G. Levy. Inhibition of phenylbutazone elimination by its metabolite oxyphenbutazone. *Proc. Soc. Exp. Biol.* *141*:963 (1972).

29. J. J. Ashley and G. Levy. Inhibition of diphenylhydantoin elimination by its major metabolite. *Res. Commun. Chem. Pathol. Pharmacol.* *4*:297 (1972).

30. J. J. Ashley and G. Levy. Kinetics of diphenylhydantoin elimination in rats. *J. Pharmacokinet. Biopharm.* *1*:99 (1973).

31. D. Perrier, J. J. Ashley, and G. Levy. Effect of product inhibition on kinetics of drug elimination. *J. Pharmacokinet. Biopharm.* *1*:231 (1973).

32. R. A. O'Reilly, P. M. Aggeler, and L. S. Leong. Studies on the coumarin anticoagulant drugs: A comparison of the pharmacodynamics of dicumarol and warfarin in man. *Thromb. Diath. Haemorrh.* *11*:1 (1964).

33. P. G. Dayton, S. A. Cucinell, M. Weiss, and J. M. Perel. Dose-dependence of drug plasma level decline in dogs. *J. Pharmacol. Exp. Ther.* *158*:305 (1967).

34. A. Goldstein, L. Aronow, and S. M. Kalman (Eds.). *Principles of Drug Action: The Basis of Pharmacology*. Wiley, New York, 1974, pp. 273--283.

35. C. M. Berlin and R. T. Schimke. Influence of turnover rates on the responses of enzymes to cortisone. *Mol. Pharmacol.* *1*:149 (1965).

36. W. H. Pitlick and R. H. Levy. Time-dependent kinetics: I. Exponential autoinduction of carbamazepine in monkeys. *J. Pharm. Sci.* *66*:647 (1977).

37. R. Levy. Time-dependent pharmacokinetics. In "Pharmacokinetics: Theory and Methods," M. Rowland and G. Tucker (Subject Eds.), in *The International Encyclopedia of Pharmacology and Therapeutics.* Pergamon Press, Oxford, 1982.

38. P. J. McNamara, G. Levy, and M. Gibaldi. Effect of plasma protein and tissue binding on the time course of drug concentration in plasma. *J. Pharmacokinet. Biopharm.* *7*:195 (1979).

39. P. J. McNamara, J. T. Slattery, M. Gibaldi, and G. Levy. Accumulation kinetics of drugs with nonlinear plasma protein and tissue binding characteristics. *J. Pharmacokinet. Biopharm.* *7*:397 (1979).

40. A. J. Sedman and J. G. Wagner. Importance of the use of the appropriate pharmacokinetic model to analyze in vivo enzyme constants. *J. Pharmacokinet. Biopharm.* *2*:161 (1974).

41. A. J. Sedman and J. G. Wagner. Quantitative pooling of Michaelis-Menten equations in models with parallel metabolite formation paths. *J. Pharmacokinet. Biopharm.* *2*:149 (1974).

8

Clearance Concepts

Pharmacokinetic theory of drug elimination has traditionally been based on rate concepts, and the apparent efficiency of elimination processes has usually been described in terms of first-order rate constants or half-lives. This approach has certainly been appropriate and useful for many applications but leads to rather serious problems when one wishes to apply pharmacokinetics in an anatomical/physiological context and to examine drug elimination in a mechanistic sense. An alternative approach that has been found to be much more valuable for such applications is the use of *clearance* parameters to characterize drug disposition.

ORGAN CLEARANCE

The best way to understand *clearance* is to consider the situation in a single, well-perfused organ that is capable of drug elimination (see Fig. 8.1). Blood flow through the organ is denoted as Q (ml/min). The drug concentration in the arterial blood entering the organ is C_A, whereas that in the venous blood leaving the organ is C_V. If the organ metabolizes or excretes some of the drug, $C_V < C_A$.

The rate at which drug enters the organ is given by the product of C_A and Q, whereas the rate at which drug leaves the organ is given by the product of C_V and Q. Mass-balance considerations dictate that the rate of drug elimination by the organ is equal to the difference between the rate in and the rate out:

$$\text{Rate of elimination} = C_A Q - C_V Q = Q(C_A - C_V) \qquad (8.1)$$

If one compares the rate of drug elimination with the rate at which drug enters the organ, one obtains a dimensionless quantity that is termed the extraction ratio, ER:

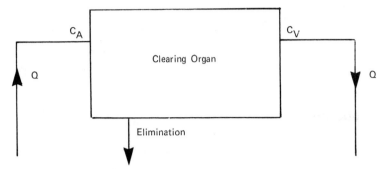

Fig. 8.1 Flow model for drug clearance by an organ. The term Q denotes blood flow rate through the organ and the terms C_A and C_V denote drug concentrations in arterial and venous blood, respectively. If the organ is a site of drug elimination, $C_V < C_A$.

$$ER = \frac{Q(C_A - C_V)}{QC_A} = \frac{C_A - C_V}{C_A} \tag{8.2}$$

The extraction ratio quantifies the efficiency of the organ with respect to drug elimination under fixed conditions of flow. If the organ is incapable of eliminating the drug, $C_A = C_V$ and the extraction ratio is zero. On the other hand, if the organ is so efficient in metabolizing or excreting the drug that $C_V \simeq 0$ the extraction ratio approaches unity.

We can also think of the extraction ratio as an index of how efficiently the organ clears the blood flowing through it of drug. For example, an extraction ratio of 0.8 tells us that 80% of the blood flowing through the organ will be completely cleared of drug. Following this line of reasoning, we can define the organ clearance of a drug as the product of extraction ratio and flow:

$$Cl = \frac{Q(C_A - C_V)}{C_A} = Q \cdot ER \tag{8.3}$$

It follows that the ratio of clearance to flow is equal to the extraction ratio.

We can also infer from Eq. (8.3) that clearance is the ratio of elimination rate to the drug concentration in blood entering the organ. This relationship makes it relatively easy to determine the renal clearance of any drug that is excreted, to some measurable extent, unmetabolized in the urine. The excretion rate of a drug can be estimated by determining the drug concentration in a volume of urine collected for relatively short, known periods of time after administration. By dividing the excretion rate by the drug concentration in plasma or blood at the midpoint of the urine collection period, one can estimate renal clearance. The same method can also be used under certain conditions to estimate biliary clearance.

TOTAL CLEARANCE

The total clearance of drug from the body almost always involves more than one organ. By definition, total or systemic clearance is the sum of all individual organ clearances that contribute to the overall elimination of a drug. However, the only organ clearance that can be routinely determined independently in humans is renal clearance because, for all practical purposes, this is the only organ for which we can easily determine an elimination rate. Therefore, a different approach is required to estimate the systemic or total clearance of most drugs.

We can state, by analogy to Eq. (8.3), that total or systemic clearance Cl_s is equal to the ratio of overall elimination rate dX/dt to drug concentration in blood or plasma C:

$$Cl_s = \frac{dX/dt}{C} \tag{8.4}$$

Integrating the right-hand side of Eq. (8.4) with respect to time from $t = 0$ to $t = \infty$, we obtain

$$Cl_s = \frac{\int_0^\infty (dX/dt)\ dt}{\int_0^\infty C\ dt} \tag{8.5}$$

The term $\int_0^\infty (dX/dt)\ dt$ is equal to the total amount of drug ultimately eliminated, or the administered dose D in the case of intravenous administration. The term $\int_0^\infty C\ dt$ is equivalent to the total area under the drug concentration in blood or plasma versus time curve, AUC. Therefore,

$$Cl_s = \frac{D}{AUC} \tag{8.6}$$

We can also show that the systemic clearance of a drug is equal to the infusion rate k_0 divided by the steady-state concentration C_{ss} of drug in blood or plasma after prolonged constant rate intravenous infusion:

$$Cl_s = \frac{k_0}{C_{ss}} \tag{8.7}$$

and that Cl_s is equal to the dosing rate divided by the average drug concentration in blood or plasma during a dosing interval at steady state after repetitive intravenous administration of fixed doses at fixed intervals, $\overline{C}_{ss}$:

$$Cl_s = \frac{\text{dosing rate}}{\bar{C}_{ss}} \qquad (8.8)$$

Dosing rate is usually expressed in terms of mg/h (i.e., dose/τ), where τ is the fixed dosing interval. Equation (8.8) may be used for oral repetitive administration when complete systemic availability can be assumed. Hence for any drug we can determine renal clearance and systemic clearance.

HEPATIC CLEARANCE

The difference between systemic clearance and renal clearance is often termed nonrenal clearance. For certain drugs we can assume that nonrenal clearance is equal to hepatic clearance (i.e., the clearance of drug from the blood by the liver). For drugs that are virtually completely metabolized (i.e., renal clearance is negligible), we can sometimes assume that systemic clearance is equal to hepatic clearance. Under these conditions, it follows from Eq. (8.3) that hepatic clearance (Cl_H) is given by

$$Cl_H = Q_H \cdot ER \qquad (8.9)$$

where Q_H is hepatic blood flow (about 1.5 liters/min in humans) and ER is the hepatic extraction ratio (which can range from 0 to 1).

The maximum value of Cl_H is hepatic blood flow. If the nonrenal clearance of a drug exceeds hepatic blood flow, it is evident that nonhepatic metabolism or other nonhepatic elimination processes (other than renal excretion) are taking place and that nonrenal clearance is not equal to hepatic clearance.

A cursory examination of Eq. (8.9) suggests that hepatic clearance is directly proportional to hepatic blood flow. This is not the case, however, because the extraction ratio is also dependent on hepatic blood flow. In principle, the larger the blood flow, the smaller is the extraction ratio [1]. The relationship between hepatic blood flow and extraction ratio has been derived using compartmental models [2] and using a perfusion model [3]. The latter approach is presented in this chapter.

Consider the model in Fig. 8.2 and assume that a bolus of drug is introduced into the reservoir, yielding an initial concentration C_i^o. The principles of mass balance require the following relationships to exist:

$$-V_R \frac{dC_i}{dt} = Q(C_i - C_o) \qquad (8.10)$$

and

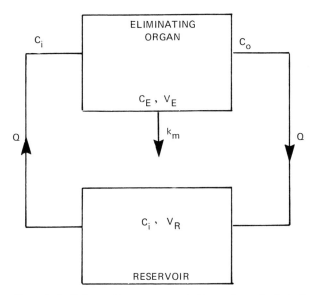

Fig. 8.2 Schematic representation of an isolated perfused organ system consisting of a reservoir and an eliminating organ. The terms are defined as follows: Q is perfusate (blood) flow rate, C_i is drug concentration in the reservoir and in the arterial blood entering the organ, C_o is drug concentration in emergent venous blood, V_E and V_R are the volumes of the eliminating organ and reservoir, respectively, and k_m is the first-order rate constant for drug elimination. C_E is the drug concentration in the eliminating organ and, in this case, is equivalent to $K_P C_o$, where K_P is a partition coefficient.

$$K_P V_E \frac{dC_o}{dt} = Q(C_i - C_o) - k_m K_P V_E C_o \qquad (8.11)$$

where C_i is the drug concentration in the reservoir and entering the eliminating organ; C_o is the drug concentration leaving the eliminating organ and entering the reservoir; V_E and V_R are the volumes of the eliminating organ and reservoir, respectively; Q is blood flow; k_m is the intrinsic first-order rate constant for drug elimination; and K_P is the apparent partition coefficient of drug between the eliminating organ and the emergent blood (i.e., $K_P = C_E/C_o$, where C_E is the drug concentration in the eliminating organ). Equation (8.10) tells us that the net rate of loss of drug from the reservoir is equal to the difference between the rate into and the rate out of the organ and Eq. (8.11) tells us that the rate of change of the amount ($V_E C_E$ or $K_P V_E C_o$) of drug in the eliminating organ is equal to the difference between the rate in QC_i and the sum of the rate out and the rate of elimination (i.e., the sum of QC_o and $k_m V_E C_E$ or $k_m K_P V_E C_o$).

Solving Eqs. (8.10) and (8.11) for C_i and C_o in the usual manner, we obtain [3]

$$C_i = C_i^o \frac{(Q/K_pV_E) + k_m - \alpha}{\beta - \alpha} e^{-\alpha t} + C_i^o \frac{(Q/K_pV_E) + k_m - \beta}{\alpha - \beta} e^{-\beta t}$$

(8.12)

and

$$C_o = \frac{C_i^o Q(e^{-\alpha t} - e^{-\beta t})}{K_pV_E(\beta - \alpha)}$$

(8.13)

where

$$\alpha + \beta = \frac{Q}{V_R} + \frac{Q}{K_pV_E} + k_m$$

(8.14)

and

$$\alpha\beta = \frac{Qk_m}{V_R}$$

(8.15)

Since clearance is equal to the ratio of dose to area [see Eq. (8.6)], it follows that

$$Cl = \frac{V_R C_i^o}{\int_0^\infty C_i \, dt}$$

(8.16)

Integrating Eq. (8.12) from $t = 0$ to $t = \infty$, and substituting this expression into Eq. (8.16), we obtain [3]

$$Cl = Q \frac{k_m K_pV_E}{Q + k_m K_pV_E}$$

(8.17)

It follows from Eq. (8.9) that

$$ER = \frac{k_m K_pV_E}{Q + k_m K_pV_E}$$

(8.18)

Equation (8.18) shows that the extraction ratio of a drug is a function of both the intrinsic ability of the organ to eliminate the drug, $k_m K_pV_E$, and the blood flow to the organ.

Equation (8.17) may also be derived by assuming that drug is infused into the reservoir at a constant rate k_o until steady state is achieved, rather than administered as a single bolus. The net rate of loss of drug from the reservoir is now given by

$$-V_R \frac{dC_i}{dt} = Q(C_i - C_o) - k_0 \tag{8.19}$$

Equation (8.11) still describes the rate of change of the amount of drug in the eliminating organ. At steady state C_i and C_o are constant (i.e., $C_{i,ss}$ and $C_{o,ss}$, respectively). Therefore, $dC_{i,ss}/dt$ and $dC_{o,ss}/dt$ are equal to zero. It follows from Eqs. (8.19) and (8.11) that

$$k_o = Q(C_{i,ss} - C_{o,ss}) = k_m K_P V_E C_{o,ss} \tag{8.20}$$

and that

$$C_{i,ss} = \frac{k_m K_P V_E C_{o,ss} + QC_{o,ss}}{Q} \tag{8.21}$$

According to Eq. (8.3), clearance may be obtained by measurements across the eliminating organ:

$$Cl = \frac{Q(C_{i,ss} - C_{o,ss})}{C_{i,ss}} \tag{8.22}$$

Substituting for the numerator according to Eq. (8.20) and for $C_{i,ss}$ according to Eq. (8.21), and rearranging terms, we obtain

$$Cl = \frac{Qk_m K_P V_E C_{o,ss}}{k_m K_P V_E C_{o,ss} + QC_{o,ss}} \tag{8.23}$$

which simplifies to Eq. (8.17).

The term $k_m K_P V_E$ in Eq. (8.17) or (8.18) is equivalent to the clearance capacity or intrinsic clearance Cl_I of the organ for the specific drug. Thus we may write that

$$Cl = Q \frac{Cl_I}{Q + Cl_I} = Q \cdot ER \tag{8.24}$$

If Cl_I reflects solely hepatic metabolism of the drug by a single enzyme system, consideration of classical enzyme kinetics indicates that Cl is equivalent to the ratio of V_m (the maximum rate of metabolism) to K_m (the Michaelis constant) [4]. Experimental verification of this hypothesis has been provided for several drugs [4,5]. Examples are shown in Fig. 8.3.

Equation (8.24) tells us that the systemic clearance of a drug that is eliminated solely by metabolism in the liver is a function of both hepatic blood flow Q and the intrinsic ability of the liver to metabolize the drug, Cl_I. For many drugs, including antipyrine, most barbiturates, anticonvulsants, hypoglycemic agents, and

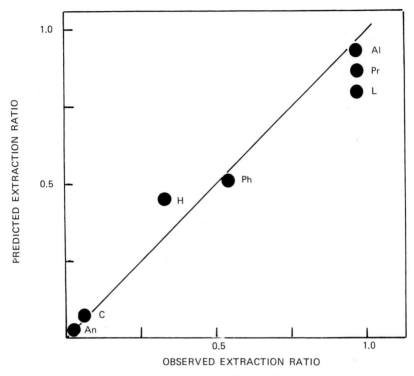

Fig. 8.3 Correlation between extraction ratios observed in an isolated perfused rat liver and those predicted from liver homogenate estimates of V_m and K_m. The drugs studied were alprenolol (Al), antipyrine (An), carbamazepine (C), hexobarbital (H), lidocaine (L), phenytoin (Ph), and propranolol (Pr). [From Ref. 4, © 1971 American Society for Pharmacology and Experimental Therapeutics. The Williams and Wilkins Company (agent).]

coumarin anticoagulants, we find that the intrinsic clearance in humans is considerably smaller than hepatic blood flow. If $Q >> Cl_I$, it follows that Eq. (8.24) reduces to

$$Cl \simeq Cl_I \qquad\qquad\qquad (8.25)$$

Equation (8.25) was developed without taking plasma protein binding into consideration and is, therefore, an oversimplification for most drugs. It does, however, apply directly to antipyrine, because this drug is virtually unbound in body water and is essentially completely metabolized by the liver. In humans, the systemic clearance of antipyrine appears to be a direct measure of the liver's ability to metabolize the drug. Certain diseases, administration of drugs or chemicals that inhibit or induce enzymes in the liver, or other perturbations that affect the quality or quantity of hepatic microsomal enzymes or cellular access to these enzymes will proportionately affect the systemic clearance of antipyrine or similar drugs. For this reason it has been proposed that antipyrine clearance be used as an index of liver function [6].

In recent years it has come to light that some drugs, including many analgesics, tricyclic antidepressants, and beta blockers, have intrinsic clearance values in humans that significantly exceed hepatic blood flow. The systemic clearance of such drugs shows a strong dependence on hepatic blood flow. The reason for this is easily demonstrated by considering a second limiting case for Eq. (8.24). If $Cl_I \gg Q$, then

$$Cl \sim Q \tag{8.26}$$

Although this exact case is rare, Eq. (8.26) does approximate the situation for drugs such as propranolol or lidocaine. The systemic clearance of drugs that show hepatic blood flow-dependent elimination is affected by various factors that affect blood flow to the liver, including heart disease and liver disease or the administration of certain drugs that affect the cardiovascular system. On the other hand, the systemic clearance of such drugs is rather independent of factors that affect the drug-metabolizing enzymes in the liver, such as the administration of enzyme-inducing drugs or chemicals.

HEPATIC CLEARANCE AND DRUG BINDING IN BLOOD

As we have noted, the preceding discussion applies strictly to drugs that are unbound in the vascular space. However, it is well recognized that most drugs are bound to blood constituents, particularly to plasma proteins. Moreover, it has been generally believed that this binding retards hepatic metabolism or renal excretion since the availability of drug to the metabolic or excretory sites is limited to the fraction of drug in the circulating blood which is free or unbound. Although this restriction is true for many drugs, there are exceptions. It is apparent that the elimination of certain drugs is not limited to the free drug delivered to the liver or kidneys because their extraction ratio is greater than their free fraction [1]. In fact, there are examples, such as the elimination of propranolol in humans (see Fig. 8.4), where clearance is essentially independent of binding in the blood [7].

It is evident that Eq. (8.24) must be modified to take blood binding into account. The following relationship has been proposed [1] and experimentally verified [8]:

$$Cl = Q \frac{f_B Cl_I'}{Q + f_B Cl_I'} \tag{8.27}$$

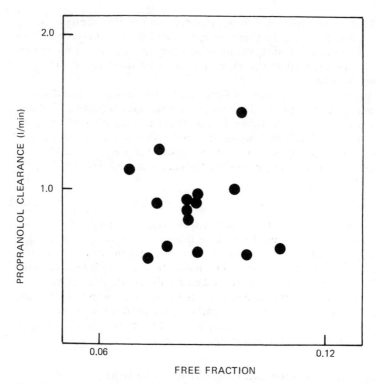

Fig. 8.4 Lack of correlation between the systemic clearance of propranolol and fraction of drug in the blood that is unbound. Because of propranolol's high hepatic extraction ratio, its clearance is largely dependent on hepatic blood flow and relatively independent of drug binding in blood or intrinsic hepatic clearance. (Data from Ref. 7.)

where f_B is the fraction free in blood [i.e., the ratio of free drug concentration in blood to total (bound and unbound) drug concentration in blood] and Cl_I' is the intrinsic clearance of free (unbound) drug. The relationship between clearance and drug binding for warfarin, phenytoin, and propranolol is shown in Fig. 8.5. Since most investigators measure the fraction free in plasma f_p rather than in blood, it is important to recognize that

$$f_B = \frac{f_p C_P}{C_B} \tag{8.28}$$

where C_P is the total drug concentration in plasma and C_B is the total drug concentration in blood. The drug concentration in blood may be calculated from the drug concentration in plasma by means of the following relationship:

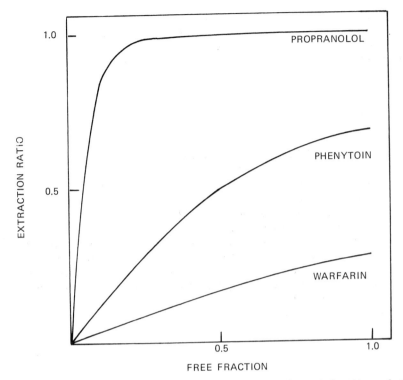

FREE FRACTION

Fig. 8.5 Relationship between extraction ratio and fraction of drug in the blood that is unbound, for a drug (under physiological conditions) with a high extraction ratio (propranolol), one that has a low extraction ratio (warfarin), and a third that has an intermediate extraction ratio (phenytoin), in the isolated perfused rat liver. Throughout most of the range of free fraction values the extraction ratio of propranolol is virtually independent of drug binding, whereas that of warfarin shows an almost linear dependence on drug binding. (From Ref. 8.)

$$C_B = C_{RBC} \cdot HCT + C_P(1 - HCT) \qquad (8.29)$$

where C_{RBC} is the drug concentration in the red blood cells and HCT is the hematocrit.

For drugs that show a low extraction ratio (i.e., $f_B Cl_I' \ll Q$), Eq. (8.27) reduces to

$$Cl = f_B Cl_I' \qquad (8.30)$$

These drugs are said to be *restricted* in their hepatic metabolism. Systemic clearance is a function of both binding in the blood and the intrinsic ability of the liver to eliminate the drug. Perturbations that affect plasma protein binding will have a direct effect on the clearance of such drugs (see warfarin and phenytoin in Fig. 8.5).

On the other hand, for drugs that show a high extraction ratio (i.e., $f_B Cl_I' \gg Q$), Eq. (8.27) reduces to Eq. (8.26) (i.e., the systemic clearance approximates hepatic blood flow). The clearance of these so-called *nonrestricted* drugs is largely independent of changes in plasma protein binding (see propranolol in Fig. 8.5).

DRUG BINDING AND FREE DRUG CONCENTRATION

Since the steady-state concentration of a drug in plasma or blood is a function of clearance, it follows that a change in binding can markedly affect total drug levels at steady state of a restricted (low extraction ratio) drug, whereas the total levels at steady state of a nonrestricted (high extraction ratio) drug would be relatively unaffected. However, it is also important to consider the effect of binding on the steady-state concentration of free (unbound) drug since this is usually considered to be the pharmacologically active component. Total drug levels in blood after continuous constant rate intravenous infusion to steady state are given by

$$C_{ss} = \frac{k_0}{Cl} \tag{8.31}$$

and free drug levels are given by

$$C_{ss,free} = \frac{f_B k_0}{Cl} \tag{8.32}$$

For a restricted drug, $Cl \sim f_B Cl_I'$. Therefore,

$$C_{ss} = \frac{k_0}{f_B Cl_I'} \tag{8.33}$$

and

$$C_{ss,free} = \frac{k_0}{Cl_I'} \tag{8.34}$$

On the other hand, for a totally nonrestricted drug, $Cl \sim Q$. It follows that

$$C_{ss} = \frac{k_0}{Q} \tag{8.35}$$

and that

$$C_{ss,free} = \frac{f_B k_0}{Q} \qquad (8.36)$$

Thus, for a poorly extracted drug, an increase in f_B can markedly affect systemic clearance and total drug levels but has little effect on free drug concentrations [see Eq. (8.34)]. Conversely, for a very well extracted drug, an increase in f_B will have little effect on systemic clearance and total drug levels but can substantially affect free drug concentrations [see Eq. (8.36)].

HALF-LIFE, INTRINSIC CLEARANCE, AND BINDING

The half-life of a drug is related to its apparent volume of distribution and its systemic clearance:

$$t_{1/2} = 0.693 \frac{V}{Cl_s} \qquad (8.37)$$

In any case, we may substitute Eq. (5.48) for V, and in the case of a drug eliminated solely by hepatic metabolism, we may substitute Eq. (8.27) for Cl_s, to obtain

$$t_{1/2} = \frac{V_B + V_T(f_B/f_T)}{Q(f_B Cl_I')/(Q + f_B Cl_I')} (0.693) \qquad (8.38)$$

where V_B and f_B are the volume and free fraction of drug in the vascular space, V_T and f_T are the volume and free fraction of drug in the extravascular space, and Q is the hepatic blood flow.

It follows that for a drug with a high extraction ratio

$$t_{1/2} = \frac{V_B + V_T(f_B/f_T)}{Q} (0.693) \qquad (8.39)$$

whereas for a drug with a low extraction ratio

$$t_{1/2} = \frac{V_B + V_T(f_B/f_T)}{f_B Cl_I'} (0.693) \qquad (8.40)$$

or

$$t_{1/2} = \left(\frac{V_B}{f_B Cl_I'} + \frac{V_T}{f_T Cl_I'} \right) 0.693 \qquad (8.41)$$

Inspection of Eq. (8.39) indicates that the half-life of an unrestricted drug is a function of blood and tissue binding as well as hepatic blood flow. A change in intrinsic clearance is expected to have little effect on the half-life of a high-extraction-ratio drug. In support of this hypothesis, the half-life of alprenolol in healthy volunteers was found to be 2.3 h before and 1.8 h during treatment with pentobarbital, an enzyme-inducing agent that increased the intrinsic clearance of the drug by more than fourfold [9]. On the other hand, a decrease in the plasma protein binding (i.e., an increase in f_B) of a drug with a high extraction ratio will increase the half-life of the drug, whereas an increase in binding results in a decrease in half-life [1]. Thus the response of such drugs to changes in binding appears to run counter to the conventional thinking that plasma protein binding protects a drug from elimination.

A similar evaluation of Eq. (8.41), which applies to a drug with a low extraction ratio, leads to more conventional conclusions. An increase in intrinsic clearance should produce a proportional decrease in half-life. An increase in plasma protein binding is predicted to produce a decrease in half-life, but the extent of the change in half-life depends on the relative magnitude of $V_B/f_B Cl_I'$ compared to $V_T/f_T Cl_I'$. If the first term predominates, an increase in binding should yield a proportional decrease in half-life. If the second term predominates, an increase in blood binding would have little effect on half-life. The latter situation appears to be the more common.

FIRST-PASS EFFECT

A particularly important characteristic of drugs that show a high hepatic extraction ratio, typified by propranolol or lidocaine, is that on oral administration *presystemic* or *first-pass* metabolism is significant and the amount of drug reaching the systemic circulation may be considerably less than the dose administered. Since the entire blood supply draining the upper gastrointestinal tract passes through the liver before reaching the general circulation, the fraction F of an oral dose that reaches the systemic circulation, assuming complete absorption, is given by

$$F = 1 - ER \qquad (8.42)$$

where ER is the extraction ratio. Thus the area under the drug concentration in blood or plasma versus time curve after an oral dose of propranolol, which has a hepatic extraction ratio of 0.64 in humans [7], is only about one-third of that found on intravenous administration of the same dose.

The area under the drug concentration in blood or plasma versus time curve after oral administration of a drug that is completely absorbed and eliminated only by hepatic metabolism is, in fact, related to intrinsic hepatic clearance. Recognizing that F is simply the ratio of area under the curve after oral adminstration to that after intravenous administration and that ER is a function of intrinsic clearance and blood flow [see Eq. (8.24)], we may rewrite Eq. (8.24) as

$$\frac{AUC_{oral}}{AUC_{i.v.}} = 1 - \frac{Cl_I}{Q + Cl_I} \tag{8.43}$$

Rearranging terms and multiplying both sides of the equation by the administered dose D, we obtain

$$\frac{D(Q + Cl_I)}{(Q)AUC_{i.v.}} = \frac{D}{AUC_{oral}} = Cl_{oral} \tag{8.44}$$

The ratio of dose to AUC_{oral} has been termed the apparent oral clearance. Recognizing that $D/AUC_{i.v.}$ is the systemic clearance Cl and substituting for Cl according to Eq. (8.24), we obtain

$$Cl_{oral} = \frac{Q(Cl_I)(Q + Cl_I)}{Q(Q + Cl_I)} \tag{8.45}$$

On canceling terms we find that

$$Cl_{oral} = Cl_I = f_B Cl_I' \tag{8.46}$$

Thus, under the stated condition, we can obtain an estimate of the intrinsic hepatic clearance of total drug Cl_I by measuring the area under the curve after oral administration [2]. Furthermore, by determining the fraction free in blood, we can estimate the intrinsic clearance of free drug Cl_I'.

Equation (8.46) applies in principle to all drugs that are solely eliminated by the liver and that can be described by linear pharmacokinetics, irrespective of hepatic extraction ratio. Hence, for a drug with a low extraction ratio, the apparent clearance after oral administration (assuming complete absorption) is identical to its systemic clearance [see Eq. (8.30)]. This is not true for a drug with a high hepatic extraction ratio. The systemic clearance of such a drug is independent of Cl_I' [see Eq. (8.26)], whereas its oral clearance and the AUC resulting from oral administration are a direct function of Cl_I'. Thus various perturbations that affect liver enzyme activity may have little effect on the pharmacokinetics of a high clearance drug after intravenous administration but substantial effect after oral administration. For example, treatment with an enzyme inducer may have little effect on the systemic clearance of drugs such as propranolol, lidocaine, or imipramine but may substantially increase the first-pass effect to which the drug is subjected after oral administration, resulting in a far smaller systemic availability. In support of this hypothesis, Alvan et al. [9] report a ratio of AUC values on intravenous administration of alprenolol before and during treatment with an enzyme-inducing agent of 1.2, compared to a ratio of 4.6 on oral administration under the same conditions.

The equations presented above indicate that the area under the drug concentration in blood versus time curve after oral administration (AUC_{oral}) under conditions of constant hepatic blood flow is a function of administered dose (assuming complete absorption) and intrinsic clearance but is independent of blood flow. This is somewhat puzzling since we know that for a drug with a high extraction ratio, systemic clearance increases, extraction ratio decreases, and therefore $AUC_{i.v.}$ decreases and F increases with increasing blood flow [see Eqs. (8.18), (8.24), and (8.42)]. However, AUC_{oral} (assuming complete absorption) is given by

$$AUC_{oral} = \frac{FD}{Cl} \tag{8.47}$$

where F is the fraction of the dose escaping first-pass metabolism, and we find that an increase or decrease in hepatic blood flow from one administration to another produces exactly the same increase or decrease in both F and Cl so that there is no net effect on AUC_{oral}.

On the other hand, fluctuations in hepatic blood flow during a dosing interval may affect AUC_{oral}. For example, a higher than average hepatic blood flow during the gastrointestinal absorption of a drug with a high extraction ratio, followed by a return to normal when absorption is essentially complete but most of the drug is still in the body, will cause an increase in AUC_{oral} (see Fig. 8.6). The reason for this is that the transient increase in hepatic blood flow during absorption will have a much greater effect on the first-pass metabolism than on overall systemic clearance (i.e., F is increased more than is Cl). This phenomenon may explain why the administration of propranolol or metoprolol with a meal results in a larger AUC_{oral} than is found when the drug is given to fasted subjects [10].

Determination of the areas under the curves after intravenous and oral administration of a high extraction ratio drug permits one to estimate hepatic blood flow Q. The ratio of areas after administration of equal doses gives the systemic availability F. Assuming that absorption is complete and elimination occurs solely by hepatic metabolism, the extraction ratio is given by

$$ER = 1 - F \tag{8.48}$$

Rearranging Eq. (8.24), we obtain

$$Q = \frac{Cl}{ER} \tag{8.49}$$

where systemic clearance Cl is estimated from the ratio of intravenous dose to $AUC_{i.v.}$.

The extent to which a drug is subject to first-pass metabolism may be estimated from area-under-the-curve data obtained after oral *or* intravenous administration of a high extraction ratio drug [11]. Since the systemic availability of a drug is given by (8.42) and since systemic clearance is the product of Q and ER, we can show that

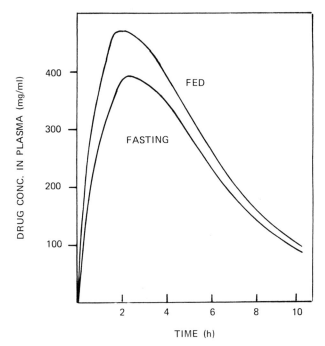

Fig. 8.6 Drug concentration in plasma after oral administration of a drug with a high hepatic extraction ratio under fasting and nonfasting conditions. The lower curve (labeled fasting) was simulated by maintaining hepatic blood flow constant at 1.5 liters/min throughout. The upper curve (labeled fed) was simulated assuming that, for the first 2 h after drug administration, hepatic blood flow was elevated to a value of 2.5 liters/min, then reduced to a value of 1.5 liters/min for the remainder of the observation period. (From Ref. 10.)

$$F = 1 - ER = 1 - \frac{Q \cdot ER}{Q} = 1 - \frac{Cl}{Q} = 1 - \frac{D}{Q \cdot AUC_{i.v.}} \qquad (8.50)$$

Thus the systemic availability of a drug subject to first-pass metabolism may be estimated from Eq. (8.50) by determining $AUC_{i.v.}$ and substituting an appropriate average value for Q (e.g., 1.5 liters/min in humans). Equation (8.50) tells us that drugs with low systemic clearances relative to hepatic blood flow will be subject to a negligible first-pass effect and will have a systemic availability after oral administration that approaches unity provided that gastrointestinal absorption is complete and chemical or enzymatic conversions in the gut are negligible. On the other hand, as systemic clearance approaches hepatic blood flow, systemic availability approaches zero.

If we multiply Eq. (8.50) by AUC_{oral}, we obtain

$$F \cdot AUC_{oral} = AUC_{oral} - \frac{D \cdot AUC_{oral}}{Q \cdot AUC_{i.v.}} \tag{8.51}$$

or

$$F \cdot AUC_{oral} = AUC_{oral} - \frac{FD}{Q} \tag{8.52}$$

Rearranging terms to solve for F, we obtain

$$F = \frac{Q}{Q + (D/AUC_{oral})} = \frac{Q}{Q + Cl_I} \tag{8.53}$$

Thus the systemic availability of a drug subject to first-pass metabolism may also be estimated from Eq. (8.53) by determining AUC_{oral} and substituting an appropriate average value for hepatic blood flow. Equation (8.53) tells that the higher the intrinsic hepatic clearance, the lower is the systemic availability of a drug.

Equations (8.50) and (8.53) apply exactly only to drugs with linear pharmacokinetic characteristics, which are absorbed completely after oral administration and are eliminated only by hepatic metabolism. Equation (8.50) may be applied to drugs that are partially excreted unchanged if Cl is replaced by hepatic clearance Cl_H. Hepatic clearance may be estimated from

$$Cl_H = Cl - Cl_r \tag{8.54}$$

where Cl is systemic or total clearance and Cl_r is renal clearance. Equation (8.54) assumes that all nonrenal clearance may be assigned to the liver.

The actual systemic availability of a drug may be less than or greater than the value predicted by Eq. (8.50). Less-than-predicted values will be observed if the drug is incompletely absorbed because of dosage form or permeability factors or if the drug is subject to chemical or metabolic breakdown in the gut. Greater-than-predicted values may be found if hepatic metabolism is capacity limited or if nonhepatic systemic metabolism is significant.

GUT WALL CLEARANCE

The systemic availability F of drugs subject to both first-pass hepatic and intestinal mucosa metabolism has also been considered [12,13]. Under certain conditions (see the model in Fig. 8.7), it can be shown that F is given by

$$F = \frac{Q_{HV}Q_{PV}}{(Q_{HV} + Cl_{HI})(Q_{PV} + Cl_{GI})} \tag{8.55}$$

where $F = (AUC)_{oral}/(AUC)_{i.v.}$, Q_{HV} is total hepatic blood flow, (i.e., the sum of hepatic arterial flow Q_{HA} and portal venous flow

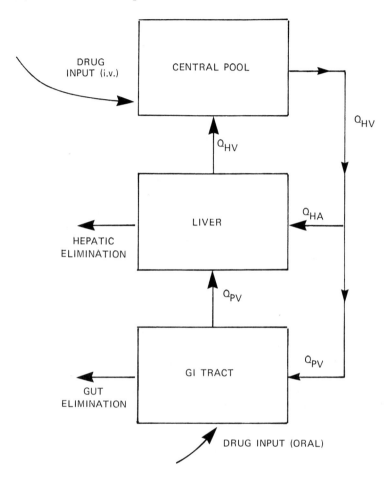

Fig. 8.7 Flow model describing the perfusion of the gastrointestinal tract and liver and showing the course of drug given orally and intravenously. After oral administration the drug is potentially subject to first-pass effects in the gut wall and in the liver. Blood flow terms are defined as follows: Q_{HV} is total hepatic blood flow, Q_{HA} is hepatic artery blood flow, and Q_{PV} is portal vein blood flow.

Q_{PV}, which is equal to the flow in the hepatic vein), Cl_{HI} is intrinsic hepatic clearance, and Cl_{GI} is intrinsic intestinal mucosal clearance. The ratio of Q_{PV} to Q_{HV} is about 0.8 in the rat, 0.75 in the dog, and 0.7 in humans.

In the absence of gut wall metabolism, Eq. (8.55) reduces to Eq. (8.53), whch can be rearranged to give Eq. (8.50), where $Q = Q_{HV}$. In the absence of significant first-pass hepatic metabolism (i.e., $Cl_{HI} \ll Q_{HV}$), Eq. (8.55) reduces to

$$F = \frac{Q_{PV}}{Q_{PV} + Cl_{GI}} \qquad (8.56)$$

which can be rearranged to give

$$F = 1 - \frac{D}{AUC_{i.v.} \cdot Q_{PV}} \qquad (8.57)$$

When a drug is subject to both first-pass hepatic metabolism and gut wall metabolism, it has been shown that the actual systemic availability is always intermediate between the value predicted by Eq. (8.57) (underestimate) and that predicted by Eq. (8.50) (overestimate) [12].

The Pang-Gillette model [13] for first-pass metabolism is more complex than that proposed by Colburn and Gibaldi [12] in that it incorporates biliary excretion of drug and metabolite as well as enterohepatic cycling of parent drug, and considers both oral and intraperitoneal administration of the drug.

LUNG CLEARANCE

It is well known that the liver is not the only site of drug metabolism. Several extrahepatic tissues, including the intestinal mucosa, kidney, and lung, contain drug-metabolizing enzymes. Because of the lung's unique anatomical position in the circulatory system (see Fig. 8.8), drug metabolism by this organ presents some interesting implications for the evaluation of first-pass effects and systemic availability.

In the absence of drug metabolism by the lung, the systemic availability of a drug is given by the well-known equation

$$F_{oral} = \frac{AUC_{oral}}{AUC_{i.v.}} \qquad (8.58)$$

where F_{oral} is the fraction of the administered dose reaching the systemic circulation, and AUC_{oral} and $AUC_{i.v.}$ represent the total areas under the drug concentration in blood versus time curves after oral and intravenous administration, respectively, assuming venous blood sampling. A value of F_{oral} of less than 1 may be the result of one or more of the following factors: (1) physical-chemical properties of the drug and/or dosage form; (2) gut and/or gut wall metabolism of the drug, and (3) hepatic first-pass metabolism of the drug. Under these conditions Eq. (8.58) is assumed to provide an absolute estimate of the availability of the orally administered drug to the target organ(s) since a compound given intravenously may be regarded as 100% available.

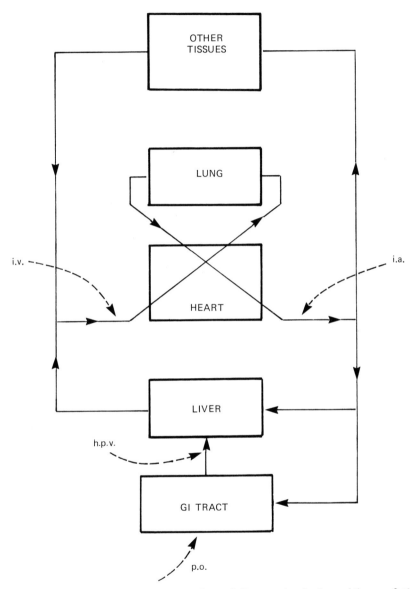

Fig. 8.8 Schematic representation of the anatomical positions of the potential sites of drug elimination (i.e., the gastrointestinal tract, the liver, and the lung) and of several routes of administration, including oral (p.o.), hepatic portal vein (h.p.v.), intravenous (i.v.), and intra-arterial (i.a.).

Strictly speaking, this is not correct when drug clearance by the lung is significant. Under these conditions a more appropriate expression for absolute availability is

$$F_{oral} = \frac{AUC_{oral}}{AUC_{i.a.}} \qquad (8.59)$$

where $AUC_{i.a.}$ is the total area under the curve after intra-arterial administration, assuming arterial blood sampling. The AUC in arterial blood will be larger after intra-arterial administration of a drug than after intravenous administration of the same dose, if lung clearance is significant.

As shown in Fig. 8.8, there are three potential sites for metabolism across which an orally administered drug must pass before reaching the systemic circulation: the gastrointestinal mucosa, the liver, and the lung. Since these organs are arranged in series, it can be seen, if one assumes complete absorption, that F_{oral} is equal to the product of the fractions of dose escaping first-pass metabolism by the gastrointestinal mucosa f_G, liver f_H, and lung f_L:

$$F_{oral} = f_G f_H f_L \qquad (8.60)$$

Similarly, the absolute systemic availability of a drug given by injection into the hepatic portal vein $F_{h.p.v.}$, or by intraperitoneal injection, may be represented as

$$F_{h.p.v.} = f_H f_L \qquad (8.61)$$

whereas that of a drug given intravenously is simply

$$F_{i.v.} = f_L \qquad (8.62)$$

It follows that

$$f_G = \frac{AUC_{oral}}{AUC_{h.p.v.}} \qquad (8.63)$$

$$f_H = \frac{AUC_{hpv}}{AUC_{i.v.}} \qquad (8.64)$$

and

$$f_L = \frac{AUC_{i.v.}}{AUC_{i.a.}} \qquad (8.65)$$

where the subscripts on the right-hand side of each equation refer to route of administration and the AUC terms relate to drug concentrations in arterial blood.

Table 8.1 Effect of Route of Administration on the Area Under the Drug Concentration in Blood Versus Time Curve, AUC, After a Single 1.5 mg/kg Dose of Phenol.

Route	AUC	Relative Bioavailability (%)
Intra-arterial (i.a.)	6.13	100
Intravenous (i.v.)	2.53	41
Hepatic portal vein (h.p.v.)	2.22	36
Oral (p.o.)	0.18	3

Notes: The values represent the means of five to seven rats. The difference between p.o. and h.p.v. administration reflects a first-pass effect in the gut; the difference between i.v. and i.a. adminstration reflects a first-pass effect in the lung.
Source: From Ref. 14.

Cassidy and Houston [14] have used the equations outlined above to evaluate the relative contributions of intestinal mucosa, liver, and lung in the elimination of phenol in the rat. The AUC values (carotid artery blood) resulting from a single 1.5 mg/kg dose of phenol, using different routes of administration, are shown in Table 8.1. The results indicate that phenol undergoes a very large first-pass effect in the rat when given orally. Only 3% of the dose appears as parent drug in the systemic circulation. Application of Eqs. (8.63), to (8.65) to the data suggest that gut and/or gut wall metabolism is the major cause of the low systemic availability ($f_G = 0.08$), but pronounced lung metabolism is also evident ($f_L = 0.38$). The role of hepatic enzymes appears small ($f_H = 0.94$).

RENAL CLEARANCE

The theoretical concepts presented above concerning hepatic clearance and the relationship between drug binding in blood and hepatic clearance are well defined and largely experimentally verified. Corresponding theory and experimental data concerning renal clearance are much more limited. Because the net renal excretion of a drug is determined by filtration, active secretion, and reabsorption, the model for renal clearance is more complicated than that described for hepatic clearance. Renal clearance Cl_r can be described by the following equation [15]:

$$Cl_r = (Cl_{rf} + Cl_{rs})(1 - FR) \qquad (8.66)$$

wher Cl_{rf} is renal filtration clearance, Cl_{rs} is renal secretion clearance, and FR is the fraction of drug filtered and secreted that is reabsorbed. The rate of filtration depends on the volume of fluid that is filtered in the glomerulus and the unbound concentration of drug in the blood since plasma proteins and drug bound to these proteins are not filtered. The volume filtered is usually estimated from creatinine clearance Cl_{cr}. The renal filtration clearance may therefore be expressed as

$$Cl_{rf} = f_B Cl_{cr} \tag{8.67}$$

where f_B is the free fraction of drug in the blood.

Drug secretion in the kidney depends on the affinity of drug to active transport carrier proteins relative to plasma proteins, the rate of transfer of drug across the tubular membrane, and the rate of delivery of the drug to the secretory site. A relationship similar to Eq. (8.27) that incorporates these factors is the following.

$$Cl_{rs} = \frac{Q_K f_B Cl'_{I(K)}}{Q_K + f_B Cl'_{I(K)}} \tag{8.68}$$

where Q_K is blood flow to the kidney and $Cl'_{I(K)}$ is the intrinsic renal tubular secretion clearance with respect to unbound drug. Combining Eqs. (8.67) and (8.68) and making the appropriate substitutions in Eq. (8.66), we find that renal clearance is given by

$$Cl_r = f_B \left(Cl_{cr} + \frac{Q_K Cl'_{I(K)}}{Q_K + f_B Cl'_{I(K)}} \right) (1 - FR) \tag{8.69}$$

If $Q_K \gg f_B Cl'_{I(K)}$, Eq. (8.69) reduces to

$$Cl_r = f_B (Cl_{cr} + Cl'_{I(K)})(1 - FR) \tag{8.70}$$

Under these conditions a plot of renal clearance versus f_B should be linear and intersect the origin [16].

If tubular reabsorption is prevented (which may be possible with certain acids or bases by changing urine pH), FR = 0 and Eq. (8.70) may be rearranged to yield

$$Cl'_{I(K)} = \frac{Cl_r}{f_B} - Cl_{cr} \tag{8.71}$$

On the other hand, if tubular secretion is blocked (which may be possible for certain acid drugs by administering probenecid), $Cl'_{I(K)} = 0$ and Eq. (8.70) may be rearranged to yield [16]

$$FR = 1 - \frac{Cl_r}{f_B Cl_{cr}} \tag{8.72}$$

With FR determined by means of Eq. (8.72), $Cl'_{I(K)}$ can be calculated by rearranging Eq. (8.70) [16]:

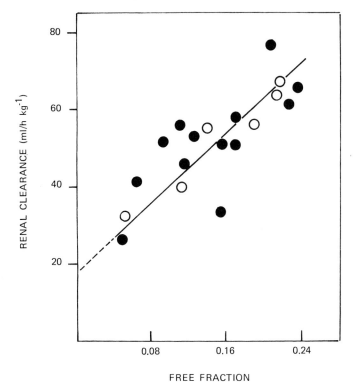

FREE FRACTION

Fig. 8.9 Relationship between renal clearance and free fraction of sulfisoxazole in serum in 13 rats (●) and in six of these rats retested 1 week later (○). The regression line and correlation coefficient (r) are based on data from the first experiment; r = 0.79. According to Eq. (8.75), the slope of the regression line is related to the product of creatinine clearance and the fraction of drug evading tubular reabsorption and the intercept value is related to the product of renal blood flow and the fraction of drug evading reabsorption. (From Ref. 17, reprinted with permission.)

$$Cl'_{I(K)} = \frac{Cl_r}{f_B(1 - FR)} - Cl_{cr} \tag{8.73}$$

Thus under certain experimental conditions we may be able to estimate FR and intrinsic secretion clearance for some drugs.

Considering the other limiting case for Eq. (8.69) [i.e., $f_B Cl'_{I(K)} >> Q_K$], we find that this expression reduces to

$$Cl_r = f_B\left(Cl_{cr} + \frac{Q_K}{f_B}\right)(1 - FR) \tag{8.74}$$

or

$$Cl_r = f_B Cl_{cr}(1 - FR) + Q_K(1 - FR) \qquad (8.75)$$

In this case a plot of renal clearance versus f_B should be linear and have a positive intercept. Such a relationship has been observed with respect to the renal clearance of sulfisoxazole in rats (see Fig. 8.9).

Dividing the slope of a plot of Cl_r versus f_B by its intercept yields

$$\frac{\text{Slope}}{\text{Intercept}} = \frac{Cl_{cr}}{Q_K} \qquad (8.76)$$

By substituting experimental values for Cl_{cr} in this equation, we can calculate Q_K, the blood flow or effective blood flow to the kidney [16].

CLEARANCE CONCEPTS APPLIED TO METABOLITES

There is increasing interest in the contribution of drug metabolites to drug efficacy or adverse effects and we frequently wish to know the relative concentrations of metabolite and parent drug on chronic dosing. At steady state, the rate of formation of a metabolite must equal its rate of elimination. We may express this relationship for a one-compartment model as follows:

$$k_f V_p C_{p,ss} = k_m V_m C_{m,ss} \qquad (8.77)$$

where k_f is the first-order formation rate constant, k_m is the metabolite elimination rate constant, and V_p and $C_{p,ss}$ and V_m and $C_{m,ss}$ denote the apparent volumes of distribution and steady-state concentrations of parent drug and metabolite, respectively. Recognizing that k_f is equal to $f_m K$, where f_m is the fraction of parent drug converted to this metabolite and K is the overall elimination rate constant of the drug, and that the product of a rate constant and a volume is clear-ance, we find that on rearranging Eq. (8.77),

$$\frac{C_{m,ss}}{C_{p,ss}} = \frac{f_m Cl_p}{Cl_m} \qquad (8.78)$$

where Cl_p and Cl_m represent the total systemic clearances of parent drug and metabolite, respectively.

Equation (8.78) suggests that administration of the metabolite is required to calculate this ratio. However, Lane and Levy [18] have shown that this ratio, as well as the actual value of $C_{m,ss}$, can be estimated from data obtained after a single dose of the parent drug without the need for metabolite administration.

The clearance of parent drug after intravenous administration is given by

$$Cl_p = \frac{D_p}{(AUC_p)_p} \tag{8.79}$$

Kaplan et. al. [19] have shown that f_m is equal to the ratio of AUC for the metabolite after administration of a dose D_p of the parent drug to that after administration of an equimolar dose D_m of the metabolite. That is,

$$f_m = \frac{(AUC_m)_p}{D_p} \frac{D_m}{(AUC_m)_m} = \frac{(AUC_m)_p}{D_p} Cl_m \tag{8.80}$$

where $(AUC_a)_b$ refers to the total area under the concentration of a in blood versus time curve after a single intravenous dose of b; the subscripts m and p refer to metabolite and parent drug, respectively. The ratio of dose of metabolite to $(AUC_m)_m$ is metabolite clearance Cl_m.

Substituting for Cl_p and f_m in Eq. (8.78) according to Eqs. (8.79) and (8.80), respectively, and canceling common terms yields

$$\frac{C_{m,ss}}{C_{p,ss}} = \frac{(AUC_m)_p}{(AUC_p)_p} \tag{8.81}$$

Equation (8.81) shows that the ratio of steady-state concentrations of metabolite and parent drug can be estimated by determining drug and metabolite concentrations in blood after a single intravenous dose of parent drug. Equation (8.81) also applies to the oral administration of any drug, irrespective of extraction ratio, if absorption is complete. It does not apply to intravenous administration of drugs with medium to high hepatic extraction ratios [20].

Clearance concepts have also been useful in understanding the effects of changes in plasma protein binding on the metabolic fate of a drug [21]. Consider a drug that is excreted in the urine and metabolized in the liver to a single product, which is excreted in the urine as such. The fraction metabolized f_m after intravenous administration is given by

$$f_m = \frac{Cl_H}{Cl_s} = \frac{Cl_H}{Cl_H + Cl_r} \tag{8.82}$$

where Cl_H is hepatic clearance, Cl_s is total or systemic clearance, and Cl_r is renal clearance. If the drug has a low hepatic extraction ratio and is excreted solely by glomerular filtration, then according to Eqs. (8.30), (8.66), and (8.67), we may rewrite Eq. (8.82) as follows:

$$f_m = \frac{f_B Cl'_{I(H)}}{f_B Cl'_{I(H)} + f_B Cl_{cr}(1 - FR)} \tag{8.83}$$

or

$$f_m = \frac{Cl'_{I(H)}}{Cl'_{I(H)} + Cl_{cr}(1 - FR)} \tag{8.84}$$

where f_B is the fraction unbound in blood, $Cl'_{I(H)}$ the intrinsic hepatic clearance of unbound drug, FR the fraction of drug filtered that is reabsorbed, and Cl_{cr} is creatinine clearance. Under these conditions the fraction metabolized is independent of plasma protein binding.

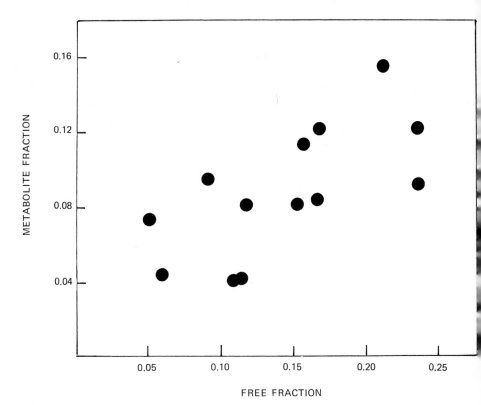

Fig. 8.10 Relationship between the fraction of a 20 mg/kg intravenous dose of sulfisoxazole excreted in the urine as metabolites and the free fraction of sulfisoxazole in serum in 13 rats. There is a distinct trend toward an increasing metabolite fraction with increases in free fraction as predicted by Eq. (8.86); the correlation coefficient is 0.68. (From Ref. 21, reprinted with permission.)

On the other hand, if the drug has a low extraction ratio but is excreted by filtration as well as tubular secretion, then according to Eqs. (8.30) and (8.69), we must express Eq. (8.82) as follows:

$$f_m = \frac{f_B Cl'_{I(H)}}{f_B Cl'_{I(H)} + f_B Cl_{cr}(1 - FR) + \dfrac{Q_K f_B Cl'_{I(K)}}{Q_K + f_B Cl'_{I(K)}}(1 - FR)}$$

(8.85)

or

$$f_m = \frac{Cl'_{I(H)}}{Cl'_{I(H)} + Cl_{cr}(1 - FR) + \dfrac{Q_K Cl'_{I(K)}}{Q_K + f_B Cl'_{I(K)}}(1 - FR)}$$

(8.86)

where Q_K denotes renal blood flow and $Cl'_{I(K)}$ denotes intrinsic secretory clearance with respect to unbound drug. In the case where $f_B Cl'_{I(K)} \gg Q_K$, Eq. (8.86) reduces to [21]

$$f_m = \frac{Cl'_{I(H)}}{Cl'_{I(H)} + Cl_{cr}(1 - FR) + (Q_K/f_B)(1 - FR)}$$

(8.87)

Equations (8.86) and (8.87) indicate that under these conditions, the fraction metabolized increases as the binding of drug in blood decreases. This relationship has been observed with sulfisoxazole in the rat (see Fig. 8.10).

PHYSICAL MODELS OF ORGAN CLEARANCE

All of the equations and relationship developed thus far in this chapter are based on the assumption that the eliminating organ is a single (homogeneous) well-stirred compartment and that distribution occurs so rapidly that drug in the emergent venous blood is in equilibrium with that throughout the liver, so that, assuming passive diffusion, the concentrations of unbound drug in venous blood and in the clearing organ are equal. An alternative to the "well-stirred" model [3] is the "parallel tube" model [22−24], which envisions that the eliminating organ is composed of a number of identical and parallel tubes with enzymes distributed uniformly along the tubes. The parallel tube model probably provides a realistic description of the liver, at least from an anatomic point of view. Contrary to the assumptions of the well-stirred model, the parallel tube model suggests that the concentration of unbound drug in emergent venous blood will be less than the average

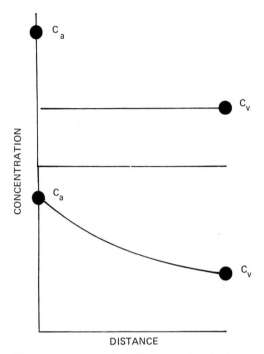

Fig. 8.11 Concentration gradient of a drug across an eliminating organ as envisioned by the well-stirred model (above) and the parallel tube model (below). C_a and C_v denote drug concentrations in arterial and emergent venous blood.

free drug concentration in the liver, which is given by $(C_a' - C_v')/\ln (C_a'/C_v')$, where C' denotes unbound drug concentration, and the subscripts a and v denote arterial and venous blood, respectively. The difference between the two models in terms of concentration gradient across the clearing organ can be seen in Fig. 8.11.

Each model gives rise to a unique set of equations to describe particular pharmacokinetic parameters [24]. For example, in the well-stirred model we have defined clearance by Eq. (8.27). The corresponding equation for clearance according to the parallel tube model is

$$Cl = Q(1 - e^{-f_B Cl_I'/Q}) \tag{8.88}$$

where the term in parentheses is equal to the extraction ratio ER.

It is difficult to prove the validity of either one of these models or even to differentiate experimentally between them because although the relationships among parameters such as blood flow, intrinsic clearance, clearance, and unbound fraction of drug are mathematically distinct, they are quantitatively similar in most instances. In fact, for drugs with very high or very low extraction ratios, both models predict the same limiting equations for clearance [i.e., Eqs. (8.26) and (8.30)]. This is readily seen by considering Eq. (8.88) when $f_B Cl'_I \gg Q$ or when $Q \gg f_B Cl'_I$. In the former situation, $\exp(-f_B Cl'_I/Q) \to 0$ and $Cl \to Q$ [Eq. (8.26)], whereas in the latter situation, $\exp(-f_B Cl'_I/Q) \to 1 - (f_B Cl'_I/Q)$ and $Cl \to f_B Cl'_I$ [Eq. (8.30)] [24].

Theoretical analysis [24] of the two models of organ clearance has revealed that the most powerful discriminator between them is the effect of blood flow on either the emergent drug concentration in venous blood (C_{out} or C_V) of a drug with a very high extraction ratio [which is given by $C_{in}(1 - ER)$ or $C_a(1 - ER)$] or, in the case of hepatic clearance, the systemic availability F after oral administration of a drug with a very high extraction ratio (which is given by $1 - ER$). The reason for this discrimination is that the systemic availability of a drug with a high hepatic extraction ratio changes linearly with blood flow for the well-stirred model ($F = Q/f_B Cl'_I$) but changes exponentially with blood flow for the parallel tube model [$F = \exp(-f_B Cl'_I/Q)$] [24]. For a drug with an extraction ratio of 0.95, systemic availability would be expected to increase from 5% to 9.5% upon doubling of hepatic blood flow from 1 to 2 ml/min per gram of liver for the well-stirred model. An increase from 5% to 22.4% would be expected under the same circumstances for the parallel tube model [24].

The effect of changes in blood flow rate on the hepatic clearance of lidocaine (extraction ratio > 0.99) has been examined in the perfused rat liver [25,26]. Concentrations of lidocaine and its metabolite monoethyl glycine xylidide (MEGX) in the emergent venous blood were better predicted by the well-stirred model than by the parallel tube model. Despite these interesting findings, it is probably premature at this time to conclude which of the physical models for organ clearance is the more generally appropriate.

BLOOD CLEARANCE VERSUS PLASMA CLEARANCE

The various equations and relationships discussed throughout most of this chapter have not only been based on the well-stirred model, they have also assumed that blood rather than plasma is the perfusion medium which flows through and bathes the clearing organs. This conceptual approach is, at first glance, at variance with common experimental procedures which call for determining drug binding and drug concentrations in plasma rather than blood. However, this difficulty is easily overcome since relatively little more laboratory work need be done to express drug binding and drug concentration in terms of blood rather than plasma [see Eqs. (8.28) and (8.29)].

Unfortunately, most pharmacokinetic studies that have been published to date do not provide enough data to express drug binding and drug concentration in terms of blood. Moreover, most of the values of systemic clearance for individual drugs that have been reported are in fact plasma clearance rather than blood clearance values. It is appropriate, therefore, to consider under what circumstances plasma clearance is a reasonable approximation of blood clearance and under what circumstances it is not.

It is evident from Eq. (8.29) that when a drug is uniformly distributed throughout the blood (i.e., when drug binding is similar in plasma and red blood cells), $C_B \simeq C_p$ since $f_B \simeq f_p$. When this condition prevails, plasma clearance Cl_p will approximate blood clearance Cl_B.

In the more usual case, we find that drug binding in plasma exceeds that in red blood cells, so that $C_B < C_p$, AUC(blood) < AUC(plasma) and [according to Eq. (8.6)], $Cl_B > Cl_p$. Hence under these conditions plasma clearance will underestimate blood clearance. According to Eq. (8.29), the maximum error will occur when C_{RBC} is negligible, so that $C_B/C_p = 1 - HCT$ and $Cl_B/Cl_p = 1/(1 - HCT)$, or about 1.67 in humans.

Much larger errors may be encountered when drug binding to red blood cells exceeds binding in plasma. In this case $C_B > C_p$, AUC(blood) > AUC(plasma), and $Cl_p > Cl_B$. The ratio of C_B to C_p will depend on the relative binding to RBC and plasma; Cl_p can substantially overestimate Cl_B and, in fact, exceed hepatic blood flow.

It is also of interest to consider whether or not plasma parameters (i.e., C_p, f_p, and plasma flow rate Q_p) can be used to approximate intrinsic clearance (i.e., Cl_I'). We may rewrite Eq. (8.27) in terms of plasma parameters as follows:

$$Cl_p = Q_p \frac{f_p (Cl_I')_{pl}}{Q_p + f_p (Cl_I')_{pl}} \tag{8.89}$$

where $(Cl_I')_{pl}$ is the intrinsic clearance of unbound drug referenced to plasma. We can now solve Eq. (8.89) for $(Cl_I')_{pl}$ and compare this value with Cl_I' obtained from Eq. (8.27), which assumes blood parameters. Rearrangement of Eq. (8.89) yields

$$(Cl_I')_{pl} = \frac{Q_p Cl_p}{f_p (Q_p - Cl_p)} \tag{8.90}$$

Therefore, the ratio of intrinsic clearance using plasma data to that from blood data is

$$\frac{(Cl_I')_{pl}}{Cl_I'} = \frac{f_B}{f_p} \frac{Q_p Cl_p}{Q_B Cl_B} \frac{Q_B - Cl_B}{Q_p - Cl_p} \tag{8.91}$$

which may be simplified to

$$\frac{(Cl'_I)_{pl}}{Cl'_I} = \frac{Q_p(Q_B - Cl_B)}{Q_B(Q_p - Cl_p)} \qquad (8.92)$$

since $f_B/f_p = C_p/C_B$ and $Cl_p/Cl_B = C_B/C_p$.

For drugs that bind preferentially in plasma (i.e., $Cl_B > Cl_p$) and have a low extraction ratio (i.e., $Q_B \gg Cl_B$ and $Q_p \gg Cl_p$), we find that the ratio of intrinsic clearance values [Eq. (8.92)] approximates unity and conclude that $(Cl'_I)_{pl} \sim Cl'_I$. This case holds for any drug, irrespective of extraction ratio, that is negligibly bound to red blood cells and is essentially restricted to the plasma, since under these conditions $(Q_B - Cl_B)/(Q_p - Cl_p) \sim Q_B/Q_p$. However, as the extraction ratio of a drug increases, any binding to red blood cells will cause $(Cl'_I)_{pl}$ to increasingly overestimate Cl'_I. Very large errors are encountered with drugs that have high extraction ratios and are uniformly distributed in blood (i.e., when $C_p \rightarrow C_B$ and $Cl_p \rightarrow Q_p$).

The situation is still more complicated when blood binding is greater than plasma binding (i.e., when $f_B < f_p$ and $Cl_B < Cl_p$). Even under these conditions, drugs with very low extraction ratios present few problems since $Q_B \gg Cl_B$ and $Q_p \gg Cl_p$, and $(Cl'_I)_{pl} \sim Cl'_I$. However, the ratio of $(Cl'_I)_{pl}$ to Cl'_I increases substantially in response to small changes in extraction ratio, so that even for drugs with medium extraction ratio values, $(Cl'_I)_{pl}$ may seriously overestimate Cl'_I.

In summary, plasma clearance will reasonably approximate blood clearance when plasma binding equals or exceeds blood binding. Maximum errors are on the order of 40%. On the other hand, when blood binding exceeds plasma binding, very large errors may be introduced. The incorrect use of plasma parameters to calculate the intrinsic clearance of a drug [see Eq. (8.90)] yields reasonably accurate answers for drugs with low extraction ratios. Although this information is useful for evaluating literature data, it should be evident that all pharmacokinetic studies should be designed to yield information regarding blood-related parameters.

REFERENCES

1. G. R. Wilkinson and D. G. Shand. A physiological approach to hepatic drug clearance. *Clin. Pharmacol. Ther.* 18:377 (1975).

2. D. Perrier and M. Gibaldi. Clearance and biologic half-life as indices of intrinsic hepatic metabolism. *J. Pharmacol. Exp. Ther.* 191:17 (1974).

3. M. Rowland, L. Z. Benet, and G. G. Graham. Clearance concepts in pharmacokinetics. *J. Pharmacokinet. Biopharm.* 1:123 (1973).

4. A. Rane, G. R. Wilkinson, and D. G. Shand. Prediction of hepatic extraction ratio from in vitro measurement of intrinsic clearance. *J. Pharmacol. Exp. Ther.* *200*:420 (1977).

5. D. A. Wiersma and R. A. Roth. Clearance of 5-hydroxytryptamine by rat lung and liver: The importance of relative perfusion and intrinsic clearance. *J. Pharmacol. Exp. Ther.* *212*:97 (1980).

6. P. B. Andreasen and L. Ranek. Liver failure and drug metabolism. *Scand. J. Gastroenterol.* *10*:293 (1975).

7. D. M. Kornhauser, A. J. J. Wood, R. E. Vestal, G. R. Wilkinson, R. A. Branch, and D. G. Shand. Biological determinants of propranolol disposition in man. *Clin. Pharmacol. Ther.* *23*:165 (1978).

8. D. G. Shand, R. H. Cotham, and G. R. Wilkinson. Perfusion-limited effects of plasma drug binding on hepatic drug extraction. *Life Sci.* *19*:125 (1976).

9. G. Alvan, K. Piafsky, M. Lind, and C. von Bahr. Effect of pentobarbital on the disposition of alprenolol. *Clin. Pharmacol. Ther.* *22*:316 (1977).

10. A. J. McLean, P. J. McNamara, P. du Souich, M. Gibaldi, and D. Lalka. Food, splanchnic blood flow, and bioavailability of drugs subject to first-pass metabolism. *Clin. Pharmacol. Ther.* *24*:5 (1978).

11. M. Gibaldi, R. N. Boyes, and S. Feldman. Influence of first-pass effect on availability of drug on oral administration. *J. Pharm. Sci.* *60*:1330 (1971).

12. W. A. Colburn and M. Gibaldi. Pharmacokinetic model of pre-systemic metabolism. *Drug Metab. Dispos.* *6*:193 (1978).

13. K. S. Pang and J. R. Gillette. A theoretical examination of the effects of gut wall metabolism, hepatic elimination, and enterohepatic recycling on estimates of bioavailability and of hepatic blood flow. *J. Pharmacokinet. Biopharm.* *6*:355 (1978).

14. M. K. Cassidy and J. B. Houston. In vivo assessment of extra-hepatic conjugative metabolism in first pass effects using the model compound phenol. *J. Pharm. Pharmacol.* *32*:57 (1980).

15. S. Øie and L. Z. Benet. Altered drug disposition in disease states. *Annu. Rep. Med. Chem.* *15*:277 (1980).

16. G. Levy. Effect of plasma protein binding on renal clearance of drugs. *J. Pharm. Sci.* *69*:482 (1980).

17. A. Yacobi and G. Levy. Effect of serum protein binding on sulfisoxazole distribution, metabolism and excretion in rats. *J. Pharm. Sci.* *68*:742 (1979).

18. E. A. Lane and R. Levy. Prediction of steady-state behavior of metabolite from dosing of parent drug. *J. Pharm. Sci.* *69*:610 (1980).

19. S. A. Kaplan, M. L. Jack, S. Cotler, and K. Alexander. Utilization of area under the curve to elucidate the disposition of an extensively biotransformed drug. *J. Pharmacokinet. Biopharm.* *1*:201 (1973).

20. E. A. Lane and R. Levy. Metabolite to parent drug concen-
    tration ratio as a function of parent drug extraction ratio:
    Cases of nonportal route of administration. *J. Pharmacokinet.
    Biopharm.* 9:489 (1981).
21. G. Levy. Quantitative change in metabolic fate of drug related
    to serum protein binding. *J. Pharm. Sci.* 69:746 (1980).
22. K. Winkler, S. Keiding, and N. Tygstrup. Clearance as a
    quantitative measure of liver function. In *The Liver: Quanti-
    tative Aspects of Structure and Functions*, P. Baumgartner and
    R. Presig (Eds.). Karger, Basel; 1973, pp. 144–155.
23. K. Winkler, L. Bass, S. Keiding, and N. Tygstrup. The effect
    of hepatic perfusion on assessment of kinetic constants. In
    Alfred Benson Symposium VI: Regulation of Hepatic Metabolism,
    F. Lundquist and N. Tygstrup (Eds.). Munksgaard, Copenhagen;
    1974, pp. 797–807.
24. K. S. Pang and M. Rowland. Hepatic clearance of drugs: I.
    Theoretical considerations of a "well-stirred" model and a
    "parallel tube" model. Influence of hepatic blood flow, plasma
    and blood cell binding, and the hepatocellular enzymatic activity
    on hepatic drug clearance. *J. Pharmacokinet. Biopharm.*
    5:625 (1977).
25. K. S. Pang and M. Rowland. Hepatic clearance of drugs: II.
    Experimental evidence for acceptance of the "well-stirred"
    model over the "parallel tube" model using lidocaine in the per-
    fused rat liver in situ preparation. *J. Pharmacokinet. Biopharm.*
    5:655 (1977).
26. K. S. Pang and M. Rowland. Hepatic clearance of drugs: III.
    Additional experimental evidence supporting the "well-stirred"
    model, using metabolite (MEGX) generated from lidocaine under
    varying hepatic blood flow rates and linear conditions in the
    perfused rat liver in situ preparation. *J. Pharmacokinet.
    Biopharm.* 5:681 (1977).

9
Physiological Pharmacokinetic Models

Pharmacokinetic models are developed to describe and predict the time course of drugs and/or related chemicals throughout the body. The classical approaches, introduced in Chaps. 1 and 2, lead to the elaboration of compartmental models which often have important clinical applications, particularly in the development of dosage regimens. However, these models are inherently limited in the amount of information they provide because, in the usual case, the compartments and the parameters have no obvious relationship to anatomical structure or physiological function of the species under study. The introduction of clearance concepts (outlined in Chap. 8) to pharmacokinetic models represents an enormous step toward bridging the gap between mathematical description and physiological reality but still results in an incomplete picture.

In recent years efforts have been directed toward the development of physiologically realistic pharmacokinetic models. These detailed models are elaborated on the basis of the known anatomy and physiology of humans or other animals and incorporate physiological, anatomical, and physiochemical data. The history of this development and the applications have recently been reviewed by Himmelstein and Lutz [1].

In principle, these comprehensive models are superior to classical compartment models in several respects. Ideally, they provide an exact description of the time course of drug concentration in any organ or tissue and are therefore able to provide greater insight to drug distribution in the body. Also, since the parameters of these models correspond to actual physiological and anatomical measures, such as organ blood flows and volumes, changes in the disposition kinetics of drug because of physiological or pathological alterations in body function may be predicted by perturbation of the appropriate parameter(s) [2]. Finally, these models introduce the possibility of animal scale-up which would provide a rational basis for the correlation of drug data among animal species [3].

A physiological pharmacokinetic model is composed of a series of lumped compartments (body regions) representing organs or tissue spaces whose drug concentrations are assumed to be uniform. The compartments are arranged in a flow diagram as illustrated by the general example in Fig. 9.1. The first step in the development of a physiological pharmacokinetic model is the selection of compartments to be included. An excellent discussion of this selection process has been presented by Bischoff [4], who notes that there is no simple way

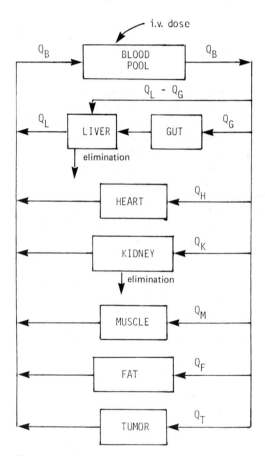

Fig. 9.1 Schematic representation of different regions of the body arranged in a flow diagram which constitutes a physiological pharma-cokinetic model. The term Q denotes blood flow rate to a region. Sub-scripts are as follows: B, blood; L, liver; G, gut; H, heart; K, kidney; M, muscle; F, fat; T, tumor. In this particular model the liver and kidney are eliminating compartments.

to describe which body regions should be included and which might
be excluded, since judgment is required as to the important aspects
of the drug distribution events. An initial choice is made based on
the pharmacodynamic, pharmacokinetic, and physiochemical characteristics of the drug as well as the anatomy and physiology of the
body. Clearly, we wish to include body regions in which the drug
exerts a pharmacologic or toxicologic effect. We must include organs
that are involved in the elimination of the drug. It makes sense to
include tissues or fluids that are easily sampled and tissue spaces
that contain relatively large amounts of the drug.

Once the selection has been made, the kinds of information required by the model can be classified as (1) anatomical (e.g., organ
and tissue volumes), (2) physiological (e.g., blood flow rates and
enzyme reaction parameters), (3) thermodynamic (e.g., drug-protein
binding isotherms), and (4) transport (e.g., membrane permeabilities).
Rarely will all this information be needed for a specific model. We can
often ignore transport and we can frequently express enzyme reaction
and binding parameters in simple terms.

Body regions can usually be viewed as consisting of a large number
of a single type of cell randomly distributed in the interstitial fluid
and supplied with blood by a capillary. This representation is often
further simplified, as shown in Fig. 9.2, by subdividing the region
into three homogeneous fluid compartments: the capillary blood volume,
the interstitial water, and the intracellular space. Most physiological
pharmacokinetic models developed to data are based on the assumption
that drug movement within a body region is much more rapid than the
rate of delivery of drug to the region by the perfusing blood. In other
words, exchange of drug between capillary blood and interstitial water

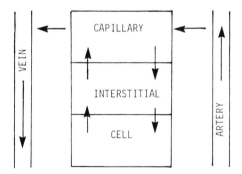

Fig. 9.2 Model for blood perfusion of local tissue region. Often,
drug transport between capillary blood and interstitial space and between interstitial space and intracellular space is a very fast process
compared to the rate of blood perfusion. Under these conditions the
entire region may be considered as a lumped compartment (see Fig.
9.1).

is considered to be very rapid and the cell membrane is considered
to be very permeable to the drug. In this case the concentration of
a drug in the emergent (venous) blood from a tissue region is in
equilibrium with that in the tissue. In effect, drug distribution into
various body regions is rate limited by blood flow and specific regions
can be represented by a single compartment as shown in Fig. 9.1.
The assumption of perfusion-limited transport is applicable to relatively
low molecular weight, weakly ionized, lipid-soluble drugs for which
diffusion and movement across lipoidal membranes should be relatively
rapid. On the other hand, membrane transport can be a slow step in
the overall uptake of very polar, highly ionized, or charged drugs.

BLOOD FLOW RATE-LIMITED MODELS

All blood flow rate-limited physiological pharmacokinetic models are
basically similar to the one shown in Fig. 9.1. Differential mass balance
equations are written for each compartment to describe the inflow,
outflow, accumulation, and disappearance of drug, and are solved
simultaneously with the aid of a computer. The equations for this
model can be derived using an approach suggested by Rowland et al.
[5]. However, it is convenient to first examine a simpler model
(Fig. 9.3A) and to consider separately drug distribution to a noneliminating region such as the muscle (Fig. 9.3B) and to an eliminating
region such as the liver (Fig. 9.3C).

The rates of change of *total concentration* of drug in the blood C_B
and in the muscle C_M as a function of time for the model shown in
Fig. 9.3B are

$$V_B \frac{dC_B}{dt} = Q_M C_o - Q_M C_i \tag{9.1}$$

and

$$V_M \frac{dC_M}{dt} = Q_M C_i - Q_M C_o \tag{9.2}$$

where V_B and V_M are volumes of the blood and muscle compartments,
respectively; Q_M is blood flow to the muscle; and C_i and C_o are drug
concentrations in blood entering and leaving the muscle compartment,
respectively. The drug concentration in afferent blood C_i is equivalent
to arterial blood concentration C_B. The drug concentration in efferent
blood C_o, however, is equivalent to C_M only if there is no drug binding
in the system or if binding is the same in blood and muscle. If this
is not the case, then

$$C_o = \frac{C_M}{R_M} \tag{9.3}$$

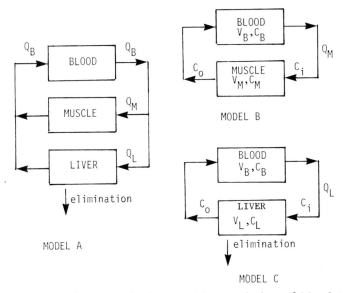

MODEL B

MODEL A

MODEL C

Fig. 9.3 Some simple flow models consisting of blood pool, noneliminating compartment, and eliminating compartment (model A), blood pool and noneliminating compartment (model B), and blood pool and eliminating compartment (model C). The terms Q, V, and C denote blood flow rate to a given region, anatomical volume of a region, and drug concentration, respectively. Subscripts indicate blood (B), muscle (M), and liver (L). The terms C_i and C_o signify drug concentrations in afferent (arterial) and efferent (venous) blood, respectively. In model A, $Q_B = Q_M + Q_L$.

where R_M is a partition coefficient relating total drug concentration in the tissue to total drug concentration in the venous blood at equilibrium. Since the total drug concentration in a compartment is equal to the free concentration divided by the fraction free, and since the concentration of free drug is assumed to be the same in all compartments, R_M is also given by

$$R_M = \frac{f_B}{f_M} \tag{9.4}$$

where f_B is the fraction free (unbound) of drug in the blood and f_M is the fraction free in the muscle.

It follows that (9.1) and (9.2) may be expressed as

$$V_B \frac{dC_B}{dt} = Q_M \frac{C_M}{R_M} - Q_M C_B \tag{9.5}$$

and

$$V_M \frac{dC_M}{dt} = Q_M \left(C_B - \frac{C_M}{R_M} \right) \tag{9.6}$$

The differential equations applying to drug distribution to an eliminating compartment (Fig. 9.3C), assuming that elimination rate is a function of free drug concentration in the compartment, are

$$V_B \frac{dC_B}{dt} = Q_L C_o - Q_L C_i \tag{9.7}$$

and

$$V_L \frac{dC_L}{dt} = Q_L C_i - Q_L C_o - Cl'_L C'_L \tag{9.8}$$

where C_L and C'_L are total and free drug concentrations in the liver, respectively, and Cl'_L is the intrinsic clearance with respect to free drug concentration in the liver.

Expressing C_i and C_o in (9.7) and (9.8) in terms of total drug concentrations in the respective compartments, we obtain

$$V_B = \frac{dC_B}{dt} = Q_L \frac{C_L}{R_L} - Q_L C_B \tag{9.9}$$

and

$$V_L \frac{dC_L}{dt} = Q_L \left(C_B - \frac{C_L}{R_L} \right) - Cl'_L C'_L \tag{9.10}$$

where R_L is the equilibrium distribution ratio of drug between the liver and the emergent venous blood.

The free drug concentration in the liver is given by

$$C'_L = f_L C_L \tag{9.11}$$

where f_L is the free fraction of drug in the liver. The free fraction in the liver can be expressed in terms of the free fraction in the blood as follows [see Eq. (9.4)]:

$$f_L = \frac{f_B}{R_L} \tag{9.12}$$

Thus we may write (9.10) as

$$V_L \left(\frac{dC_L}{dt} \right) = Q_L \left(C_B - \frac{C_L}{R_L} \right) - \frac{f_B Cl'_L C_L}{R_L} \tag{9.13}$$

The elimination rate term on the right hand side of (9.10) or (9.13) results from the assumption that the rate of elimination is a function of free drug concentration in the elimination compartment. Most reports concerning blood flow rate-limited physiologically based pharmacokinetic models [3,4] have expressed this term as $Cl_L C_L / R_L$; this condition prevails when either $f_B = 1$ or the rate of drug elimination is a function of total drug concentration in the emergent venous blood (C_0 or C_L / R_L). Rowland et al. [5] express this term as $Cl_L C_L$; this condition prevails when either $f_L = 1$ or the elimination rate is a function of total drug concentration in the eliminating compartment.

The appropriate differential equations describing the more complete model in Fig. 9.3A may be deduced by considering Eqs. (9.5), (9.6), (9.9), and (9.10). It follows that

$$V_B \frac{dC_B}{dt} = Q_M \frac{C_M}{R_M} + Q_L \frac{C_L}{R_L} - Q_B C_B \qquad (9.14)$$

$$V_M \frac{dC_M}{dt} = Q_M \left(C_B - \frac{C_M}{R_M} \right) \qquad (9.15)$$

and

$$V_L \frac{dC_L}{dt} = Q_L \left(C_B - \frac{C_L}{R_L} \right) - Cl_L' C_L' \qquad (9.16)$$

or

$$V_L \frac{dC_L}{dt} = Q_L \left(C_B - \frac{C_L}{R_L} \right) - \frac{f_B Cl_L' C_L}{R_L} \qquad (9.17)$$

It can now be appreciated that the task of writing the differential equations for a model as complex as that in Fig. 9.1 is relatively straightforward. The mass-balance rate equation for total drug concentration in a noneliminating compartment such as the heart, muscle, fat, or tumor region is given by an equation similar to (9.15). The mass-balance rate equation for a compartment that metabolizes, excretes, or otherwise eliminates the drug must also contain a term to account for elimination [see (9.16)]. The liver compartment of the model shown in Fig. 9.1 is a more accurate representation of the mammalian anatomy. Total drug concentration as a function of time for this model is given by

$$V_L \frac{dC_L}{dt} = (Q_L - Q_G) C_B + Q_G \frac{C_G}{R_G} - Q_L \frac{C_L}{R_L} - Cl_L' C_L' \qquad (9.18)$$

where it is assumed that elimination is a first-order (linear) process and is a function of free drug concentration in the liver (i.e., C_L'). The subscripts denote liver (L), gastrointestinal tract (G), and blood (B). The mass-balance rate equation for drug in the blood pool is given by

$$V_B \frac{dC_B}{dt} = Q_L \frac{C_L}{R_L} + Q_H \frac{C_H}{R_H} + Q_K \frac{C_K}{R_K} + Q_M \frac{C_M}{R_M}$$

$$+ Q_F \frac{C_F}{R_F} + Q_T \frac{C_T}{R_T} - Q_B C_B \tag{9.19}$$

where the subscripts denote heart (H), kidney (K), muscle (M), fat (F), and tumor (T).

The addition of other body regions to the model usually presents few difficulties. For each new compartment, we must add an additional mass-balance rate equation [such as (9.15) or (9.16)] to the series as well as an additional term [i.e., $Q_t(C_t/R_t)$, where t refers to the new compartment] to the equation describing drug concentration in the blood pool [e.g., (9.19)]. The incorporation of the lung in a physiological pharmacokinetic model is somewhat more complicated because of its anatomical position (see Fig. 9.4). In this case the mass-balance rate equation for drug in the blood pool is given by

$$V_B \frac{dC_B}{dt} = Q_{Lu} \frac{C_{Lu}}{R_{Lu}} - Q_B C_B \tag{9.20}$$

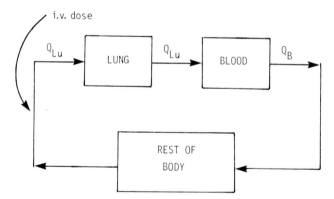

Fig. 9.4 Blood flow model showing the anatomical position of the lung relative to the site of intravenous drug administration. Q denotes blood flow rate. The subscripts refer to the lung (Lu) and blood (B). $Q_{Lu} = Q_B$. (Data from Ref. 14.)

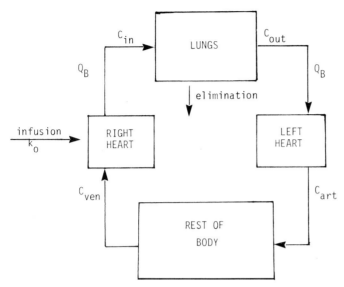

Fig. 9.5 Blood flow model showing the anatomical position of the lung relative to the site of intravenous drug administration, venous blood, and arterial blood. The model assumes that drug is given by intravenous infusion at a constant rate equal to k_0. C_{in} and C_{out} are drug concentrations in afferent and efferent blood perfusing the lung. Q_B denotes total blood flow rate (cardiac output). C_{art} and C_{ven} are drug concentrations in the arterial and venous blood pool. (Data from Ref. 18.)

and that for drug in the lung is given by

$$V_{Lu} \frac{dC_{Lu}}{dt} = \sum \left(Q_t \frac{C_t}{R_t} \right) - Q_{Lu} \frac{C_{Lu}}{R_{Lu}} \qquad (9.21)$$

where the subscript Lu denotes the lung and the summation term applies to all other compartments (except the blood pool) in the model. As indicated in Fig. 9.4, $Q_{Lu} = Q_B$.

The input function (dosing) for the model is usually handled by a programming step. For example, an intravenous bolus dose or relatively short intravenous infusion is introduced as an initial condition for the blood pool, while the initial condition for the amount of drug in all other compartments is set at zero. This approach works well in most situations. An exception is the case where drug is eliminated by the lung, particularly when lung clearance is significant compared to blood flow rate. In this situation one should probably split the blood pool into a venous pool and arterial pool (see Fig. 9.5) and program the initial condition for the venous pool. Since this model is different from that shown in Fig. 9.1 or 9.4, a different set of differential equations is required.

EXPERIMENTAL CONSIDERATIONS

The blood flow rates and tissue volumes required to solve the differential equations may be determined experimentally, but this is rarely done. Typically, one employs average values that are appropriate for size and animal species. A listing of volumes and blood flow rates of different body regions for a standard man (70 kg body weight, 1.83 m^2 surface area, 30 to 39 years) is presented in Table 9.1. Values for other species, including the dog [6—8], the rat [9—11], the mouse [7,11,12], and the monkey [7,11,13], are available in the biomedical literature. Some investigators have developed scaling relations for organ volumes as a function of mammal body weight [11].

Although there is general agreement that R values must be determined experimentally for a specific drug, a value determined in one species may not apply to a second species. There is also some

Table 9.1 Volumes and Blood Flow Rates of Different Body Regions for a Standard Man

Tissue	Volume (liters)	Blood Flow Rate (ml/min)
Blood	5.4	—
Arterial	1.4	—
Venous	4.0	—
Plasma	3.0	—
Muscle	30.0	1200
Kidneys	0.3	1250
Liver	1.5	1500
Heart	0.3	240
Gastrointestinal tract	2.4	1200
Fat	10.0	200
Lung	0.6	—
Brain	1.5	750

Note: Characteristics of the standard man are: 70 kg body weight, 1.83 m^2 surface area, 30 to 39 years of age, and cardiac output of , 5600 ml/min.

confusion as to the appropriate method of determining the tissue-to-blood partition coefficient of a drug. Some investigators have made measurements after a single bolus dose of a drug, whereas others have determined the distribution ratio only after infusing the drug to steady state. Chen and Gross [14] have discussed the difficulty in relating R values to partition coefficients determined after a single dose. They clearly show that, in general, R values for both eliminating and noneliminating tissues should be calculated from distribution ratios determined at steady state. A distribution ratio determined some time after a single bolus dose of a drug will approximate the R value in a noneliminating tissue only for drugs with relatively long half-lives [14]. The same may not be true in an eliminating tissue.

The tissue-to-blood distribution ratio determined at steady state is equivalent to the R value for any noneliminating tissue or compartment. This may be seen by considering Eq. (9.15) at steady state. Under these conditions the differential term is equal to zero and the equation may be rearranged to yield

$$R_M = \frac{C_M^{ss}}{C_B^{ss}} \tag{9.22}$$

where the superscript ss denotes steady state.

The situation is more complex in an eliminating compartment. The steady-state ratio of drug concentration in tissue to that in blood for a tissue that eliminates the drug will always underestimate the R value. This may be seen by considering Eq. (9.16) at steady state. Under these conditions the equation reduces to

$$Q_L C_B^{ss} - Q_L \frac{C_L^{ss}}{R_L} - Cl'_L C_L'^{ss} = 0 \tag{9.23}$$

or [according to Eq. (9.17)]

$$Q_L C_B^{ss} - Q_L \frac{C_L^{ss}}{R_L} - \frac{f_B Cl'_L C_L^{ss}}{R_L} = 0 \tag{9.24}$$

Rearranging terms and solving for R_L yields

$$R_L = \frac{C_L^{ss}}{C_B^{ss}} \frac{Q_L + f_B Cl'_L}{Q_L} \tag{9.25}$$

If the effective intrinsic clearance is much smaller than organ blood flow rate, the steady-state distribution ratio will approximate the R value. If this is not the case, $R_L > C_L^{ss}/C_B^{ss}$. Large errors are

encountered for drugs with high effective intrinsic clearances relative to organ blood flow rate. In these cases R values must be calculated based on both steady-state distribution ratios and estimates
of organ blood flow rates, as indicated by Eq. (9.25).

BLOOD CLEARANCE

Drug clearance from the blood is defined as the intravenous dose divided by the total area under the drug concentration in blood versus
time curve. Consider the model shown in Fig. 9.3A. Solving Eqs.
(9.14), (9.15), and (9.17) simultaneously for C_B, integrating the resulting triexponential equations from $t = 0$ to $t = \infty$, and dividing the
dose by this area yields

$$Cl_B = \frac{Q_L f_B Cl'_L}{Q_L + f_B Cl'_L} \tag{9.26}$$

which is the familiar expression for clearance proposed by Wilkinson
and Shand [15]. Equation (9.26) indicates for a drug such as indocyanine green with a relatively high effective intrinsic clearance (i.e.,
$f_B Cl'_L \gg Q_L$) that drug clearance from the blood approximates liver
blood flow, whereas for a drug with a relatively low effective intrinsic
clearance (i.e., $Q_L \gg f_B Cl'_L$), drug clearance from the blood approximates effective intrinsic clearance and is proportional to the fraction
free in the blood, f_B.

If we were to assume that the elimination rate was a function of
the total drug concentration in the emergent venous blood of the
eliminating orgen, Eq. (9.26), which defines blood clearance, would
take the form

$$Cl_B = \frac{Q_L Cl_L}{Q_L + Cl_L} \tag{9.27}$$

This equation indicates that drug clearance from the blood is independent of drug binding in the blood, which is inconsistent with considerable evidence from various systems that demonstrates, for drugs
with relatively low effective intrinsic clearance, a marked dependence
of Cl_B on plasma protein binding.

On the other hand, if we assume that elimination rate is a function
of total drug concentration in the liver, we must redefine (9.26) as
follows:

$$Cl_B = \frac{Q_L R_L Cl_L}{Q_L + R_L Cl_L} \tag{9.28}$$

For a drug with a low effective intrinsic clearance,

$$Cl_B \simeq R_L Cl_L = \frac{f_B Cl_L}{f_L} \qquad (9.29)$$

Equation (9.28) differs from (9.26) by indicating for drugs with a low effective intrinsic clearance, a dependence of blood clearance on liver binding as well as blood binding. If, in fact, for a given drug liver binding varied much less than plasma protein or blood binding, or if a perturbation that affected blood binding had little or no effect on liver binding, R_L would be approximately proportional to f_B and (9.28) or (9.29) would be consistent with experimental evidence. Not surprisingly, there have been few studies examining the relationship between partition coefficient and clearance. Yacobi and Levy [16] studied the distribution of warfarin between serum and liver in intact rats and found that R_L averaged about 2.5, varying about twofold. However, serum protein binding in the same animals varied about ten-fold and drug clearance from the serum was strongly correlated with serum protein binding (r = 0.95) but did not correlate with R_L (r = 0.16). A similar but less clear-cut situation is found with di-cumarol [17], which showed an average R_L value of 0.5. Although there is a significant correlation between clearance and free fraction in serum (r = 0.88), there is also a significant albeit weaker correla-tion between clearance and R_L (r = 0.72).

The differentiation of (9.28), which assumes elimination rate to be a function of *total* drug concentration, from (9.26), which assumes elimination rate to be a function of *free* drug concentration, presents an unresolved dilemma because of the limited experimental work carried out to date. A conceptual dilemma also exists in that one can ev-vision drug binding to specific proteins in the liver such as ligandin which would promote metabolism and thereby create a situation where elimination rate is a function of total drug concentration. The evidence available at this time suggests that Eq. (9.26), which is based on free drug concentration in the eliminating organ, is the more general one.

Estimates of the clearance terms required to solve the series of differential equations that characterize the physiologic pharmacokinetic model are obtained from experimental data in the species of interest. For drugs with relatively low effective intrinsic clearances, renal or biliary clearance may be measured directly by simultaneously sampling blood and urine or bile, whereas metabolic clearance may be estimated inferentially by assuming that metabolic clearance represents the dif-ference between total clearance and the sum of renal and biliary clearances. If renal, biliary, or metabolic clearance (assuming that it occurs in a single compartment) is flow rate dependent, one must estimate the intrinsic clearance by means of an equation similar to (9.26), using experimentally determined or literature estimates of organ blood flow.

LUNG CLEARANCE

The model shown in Fig. 9.5 suggests that when the lung contributes substantially to the overall elimination of a drug, there may be difficulty in interpreting experimentally determined estimates of clearance. For example, there are examples where the total blood clearance of a drug exceeds cardiac output. This situation would appear to be prohibited by the equations developed in this chapter. One plausible explanation for this phenomenon is drug elimination in the blood itself. However, in most instances these drugs have been found to be chemically and metabolically stable in fresh whole blood or plasma. Collins et al. [18] have recently shown that clearance of a drug by the lung could result in blood clearance values that exceed total blood flow rate.

If we assume constant rate drug infusion into the right ventricle (see Fig. 9.5), at steady state the pulmonary extraction ratio E_p is given by

$$E_p = \frac{C_{in} - C_{out}}{C_{in}} \tag{9.30}$$

and

$$C_{out} = (1 - E_p)C_{in} \tag{9.31}$$

If drug were cleared only by the lung, the lung input concentration would represent a mixing of the lung output with the infused drug:

$$C_{in} = C_{out} + \frac{k_0}{Q_B} \tag{9.32}$$

where k_0 is the drug infusion rate and Q_B is equal to cardiac output. Combining Eqs. (9.31) and (9.32) and solving for C_{out}, we obtain

$$C_{out} = \frac{k_0(1 - E_p)}{Q_B E_p} \tag{9.33}$$

Drug clearance from the blood is given by the ratio of infusion rate to drug concentration in the blood at steady state. Therefore, drug clearance from arterial blood is given by

$$Cl_{art} = \frac{k_0}{C_{art}} = \frac{k_0}{C_{out}} \tag{9.34}$$

or, according to Eq. (9.33),

$$Cl_{art} = \frac{Q_B E_p}{1 - E_p} \tag{9.35}$$

It is evident from Eq. (9.35) that Cl_{art} exceeds Q_B whenever E_p exceeds 0.5, even if the lung is the sole site of drug elimination. A more general expression which takes into consideration drug elimination by other organs and tissues is as follows:

$$Cl_{art} = \frac{k_0}{C_{out}} = \frac{Q_B E_p}{1 - E_p} + \sum Q_t E_t \qquad (9.36)$$

where Q_t is the blood flow rate to an eliminating tissue and E_t is the drug extraction ratio for that tissue.

The preceding analysis applies strictly only when drug concentration is measured in arterial blood or plasma [18]. Drug concentration in venous blood may be substituted only if there is no elimination in tissues drained by the vein that is sampled. Although this substitution may be valid for many drugs, uncertainty must prevail for any drug that is subject to extrahepatic nonrenal elimination. For the case of sampling from a vein that drains eliminating tissue, the steady-state drug concentration is given by

$$C_{ven} = (1 - E_t) C_{art} \qquad (9.37)$$

where E_t is the drug extraction ratio of the eliminating tissue. It follows from Eq. (9.34) that

$$C_{ven} = \frac{(1 - E_t) k_0}{Cl_{art}} \qquad (9.38)$$

Since drug clearance from venous blood is given by k_0/C_{ven}, it follows that

$$Cl_{ven} = \frac{Cl_{art}}{1 - E_t} \qquad (9.39)$$

Thus in the absence of elimination by the local tissue which is drained by the sampling vein, $Cl_{ven} = Cl_{art}$. In any case, Cl_{ven} will always be greater than or equal to Cl_{art}. Therefore, whether blood is sampled from the venous or arterial side, clearance can exceed cardiac output if pulmonary elimination is significant.

APPARENT VOLUME OF DISTRIBUTION

The apparent volume of distribution at steady state for a drug is a function of the anatomical volume into which it distributes as well as the degree of binding in blood and extravascular tissues. For the model shown in Fig. 9.3A, the apparent volume of distribution is given by

$$V = V_B + R_L V_L + R_M V_M \qquad (9.40)$$

or

$$V = V_B + \frac{f_B V_L}{f_L} + \frac{f_B V_M}{f_M} \qquad (9.41)$$

For the general case

$$V = V_B + \sum R_t V_t \qquad (9.42)$$

or

$$V = V_B + f_B \left(\sum \frac{V_t}{f_t} \right) \qquad (9.43)$$

Benowitz et al. [13] have demonstrated for lidocaine in the monkey that the pharmacokinetically derived volume of distribution at steady state V_{ss} (see Chap. 5) is equivalent to the sum of the products of tissue masses (volumes) and equilibrium distribution ratios (R values) as indicated in Eq. (9.42).

NONLINEAR DISPOSITION

In the absence of specific information to the contrary, we usually assume that drug elimination is a linear process and introduce a single clearance term in the mass-balance rate equation for the body regions capable of elimination [see Eq. (9.16) or (9.18)]. However, at sufficiently high doses, enzyme-mediated processes such as drug metabolism, renal tubular secretion, or biliary secretion may require concentration-dependent clearance terms to describe the time course of drug in each body region. Assuming that drug metabolism in the liver is described by Michaelis-Menten kinetics, one must rewrite (9.16) as follows:

$$V_L \frac{dC_L}{dt} = Q_L \left(C_B - \frac{C_L}{R_L} \right) - \frac{V_m C_L'}{K_m' + C_L'} \qquad (9.44)$$

where C_L and C_L' are the total and free drug concentrations in liver, respectively; V_m is the maximum rate of elimination (mass units/time units) from the liver; and K_m' is the Michaelis constant (concentration units) with respect to free drug. The ratio of V_m to K_m' is equal to Cl_L', the intrinsic clearance with respect to free drug concentration in the liver.

Estimates of V_m and K_m may be obtained from in vivo pharmacokinetic data (see Chap. 7). Some investigators have successfully estimated values for V_m and K_m from in vitro enzyme kinetic data [19–21].

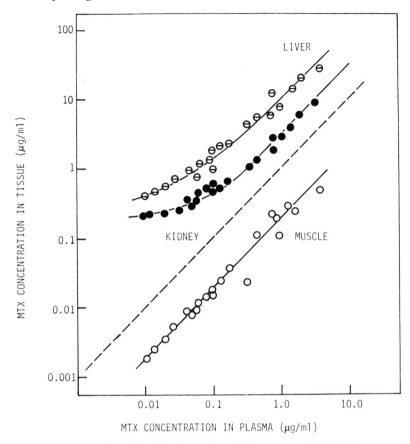

MTX CONCENTRATION IN PLASMA (µg/ml)

Fig. 9.6 Relative distribution of methotrexate (MTX) between plasma
and muscle, kidney, or liver in the mouse following intravenous doses
of 0.1, 0.3, and 3 mg/kg. Drug concentrations were determined at
times ranging from 5 to 120 min following injection. During the period
of observation a unique relationship exists between drug concentration
in the plasma and the concentration in each of these three tissues.
Distribution into the muscle is linear and apparently limited to the
extracellular space. At high drug concentrations in plasma, distribution into both kidney and liver is linear, but the drug is concentrated
in these organs to the extent of about 3:1 and 10:1, respectively. At
low drug concentrations in plasma, concentrations in these tissues
appear to approach constant values presumed to be associated with
strong binding of methotrexate to dihydrofolate reductase. (From
Ref. 22, reprinted with permission of the author.)

Drug binding to plasma proteins and tissue components is usually assumed to be linear and effectively accounted for by introducing an R value in the mass-balance rate equation. This simplification, however, may not always be appropriate. In the case of methotrexate [22], tissue-to-blood partition coefficients show a marked concentration dependence, at least in some tissues (see Fig. 9.6). This is believed to be the result of strong binding of the drug to dihydrofolate reductase in the tissue. In this case, in vivo binding isotherms consist of a linear and a saturable term. Drug concentration in tissue is given by

$$C_t = R_t C_B + \frac{aC_B}{E + C_B} \qquad (9.45)$$

where a is the strong binding constant and E is the dissociation constant [22]. At high methotrexate concentrations the second term of (9.45) is negligible and binding is approximately linear. A similar approach has been suggested to handle nonlinear plasma protein binding [23].

MEMBRANE-LIMITED MODELS

Physiologic-pharmacokinetic studies with certain drugs, including methotrexate [22], tetraethylammonium ion [24], and actinomycin D [6], have revealed tissue uptake characteristics that are not consistent with a blood flow rate-limited distribution process. For example, the declining concentrations of actinomycin D in dog testes do not parallel the declining drug concentrations in plasma after a rapid intravenous injection (see Fig. 9.7). Figure 9.8 shows methotrexate concentrations determined simultaneously in plasma and bone marrow of the rat at several doses and clearly reveals that no unique relationship exists for the methotrexate tissue-to-blood ratios, unlike the situation described in Fig. 9.6. At a given methotrexate concentration in plasma, (e.g., 0.1 μg/ml), there are different concentrations in bone marrow, depending on the dose administered and the time the tissue sample was taken. These data indicate that the bone marrow is not a blood flow rate-limited equilibrium compartment and suggest a membrane-limited transport. Similar results have been found with respect to tumor uptake of methotrexate in spontaneous canine lymphosarcoma [25].

Figure 9.9 is a scheme for a body region where membrane-limited transport prevails. The model assumes that all concentrations represent free drug concentrations. Exchange across the capillary membrane is probably so rapid that the blood and interstitial fluid may be assumed to form one equilibrium compartment, termed the extracellular space. For the extracellular compartment the mass-balance rate equation is

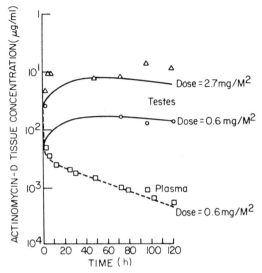

Fig. 9.7 Actinomycin-D concentrations in plasma and testes following a 0.6 mg/m^2 intravenous dose, and in testes following a 2.7 mg/m^2 intravenous dose, in the beagle dog. Drug concentrations in testes do not parallel the declining plasma curve. Simulations that assume cellular membrane resistance (solid lines) are in reasonable agreement with the tissue data. [From Ref. 6, © 1977 American Society for Pharmacology and Experimental Therapeutics, The Williams and Wilkins Company (agent).]

$$V_E \frac{dC_E'}{dt} = Q_i(C_B' - C_E') - \text{net flux} \qquad (9.46)$$

where V_E is the extracellular space (sum of capillary blood and inter-stitial fluid volume), C_E' is the free drug concentration in the extra-cellular space, Q_i is the blood flow rate to the region, and C_B' is free drug concentration in the blood pool. The mass-balance rate equation for the intracellular space is

$$V_I \frac{dC_I'}{dt} = \text{net flux} \qquad (9.47)$$

where V_I and C_I' are the volume and free drug concentration, re-spectively, of the intracellular fluid.

Net flux (transport) may be assumed preliminarily to be diffusive but in some cases must be handled as a saturable, facilitated process demonstrating Michaelis-Menten kinetics. In the case of diffusive transport, which appears to apply to actinomycin D uptake in dog testes [6], net flux is given by the equation

$$\text{net flux} = K_i(C_E' - C_I') \qquad (9.48)$$

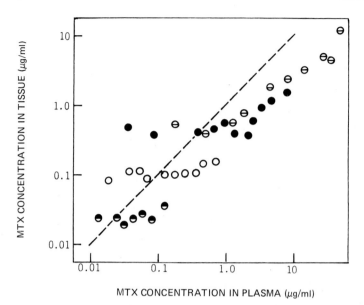

MTX CONCENTRATION IN PLASMA (μg/ml)

Fig. 9.8 Relative distribution of methotrexate (MTX) between plasma
and bone marrow in the rat following intravenous doses of 0.05 (◖),
0.25 (○), 2.5 (●), and 25 (⊖) mg/kg. Unlike the situation described
in Fig. 9.6, no unique thermodynamic relationship is seen between drug
in tissue and that in plasma. The dependence of drug concentration
in tissue on dose as well as on drug concentration in plasma suggests
a model that includes membrane resistance to transport. (From Ref.
22, reprinted with permission.)

where K_i is the effective membrane permeability coefficient. Membrane
resistance to drug transport is limiting only if the diffusion parameter
K_i is much smaller than the tissue perfusion rate per unit volume [6].
    Studies with methotrexate [22] and tetraethylammonium ion [24]
suggest that the assumption of simple diffusive transport is not sufficient to describe membrane-limited uptake of these drugs into certain
tissues. These uptake data have been rationalized by expressing net
flux as a concentration-dependent term:

$$\text{net flux} = \frac{V_m C'_E}{K'_m + C'_E} - \frac{V_m C'_I}{K'_m + C'_I} + K_i(C'_E - C'_I) \tag{9.49}$$

where V_m is the maximum facilitated transport rate and K'_m is the
Michaelis constant with respect to unbound drug. It is assumed that
the efflux and influx of the facilitated process are characterized by
the same parameters (i.e., membrane transport is symmetric). It is
of interest to note that for both drugs the passive permeability term
$K_i(C'_E - C'_I)$ was assumed to be negligible for the doses used. Mintum

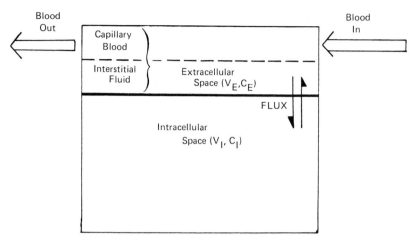

Fig. 9.9 Schematic representation of a tissue region in a physiological pharmacokinetic model which assumes membrane resistance. For most drugs the capillary membrane is very permeable, diffusion to the interstitial fluid is very fast, and the plasma and interstitial fluid can be combined into one equilibrium space termed the extracellular space. The volume of and drug concentration in this space are designated V_E and C_E, respectively. For some drugs the uptake rate (flux) by the cell is limited by the resistance of the membrane to drug transport. The volume of and drug concentration in the intracellular space are designated V_I and C_I, respectively.

et al. [24] have described the use of total rather than free drug concentrations for membrane-limited models.

The incorporation of *both* nonlinear binding and facilitated membrane-limited transport into a physiological pharmacokinetic model is a more formidable task but has been required and successfully accomplished in the case of methotrexate [22,26].

SPECIES SIMILARITY AND SCALE-UP

The development of a detailed physiological pharmacokinetic model for a drug in humans is a very difficult proposition. The almost insurmountable barrier is the vast amount and array of data needed to validate the model, particularly the need for tissue concentration data. Limited tissue-to-blood partition coefficient data for certain drugs in humans are available from studies conducted during surgery or on necropsy, but the reliability of these data as well as their applicability to general populations are suspect. Thus we must often rely substantially on in vitro or animal studies supplemented by clinical pharmacokinetic studies.

Table 9.2 Relationship Between Certain Physiological or Anatomical
Properties and Body Weight Among Mammals

Property	Exponent
Creatinine clearance	0.69
Inulin clearance	0.77
PAH clearance	0.80
Basal O_2 consumption	0.73
Endogenous N output	0.72
O_2 consumption by liver slices	0.77
Kidney weight	0.85
Heart weight	0.98
Liver weight	0.87
Stomach and intestines weight	0.94
Blood weight	0.99

Note: Data from different species were fitted to the following equation: property = (body weight)^{exponent}. (From Ref. 28.)

Dedrick and Bischoff [27] have noted: "There are many similar-
ities in the anatomy and physiology of mammalian species. A general
belief in this similarity has been the cornerstone of most biomedical
research. We share a remarkable geometric similarity. The same
blood flow diagram could be used for all mammals, and most organs
and tissues are similar fractions of the body weight. Major qualitative
differences, such as the absence of a gall bladder in some species, are
the exception." Adolph [28] observed that many anatomical and physiological variables can be correlated among mammals as exponential functions of body weight. Some examples are presented in Table 9.2. The
anatomical variables are more nearly proportional (as indicated by an
exponent of unity) to body weight than are the metabolic or physiological properties. Generally, physiologic function per unit of organ
weight or per unit of animal weight decreases as size increases.
Bischoff et al. [11] have presented scaling graphs for certain organ
blood flow rates (specifically, kidney, liver, and muscle) as a function
of body weight (see Fig. 9.10). Edwards [29] has found excellent
correlations for renal processes (including inulin clearance, PAH
clearance, renal blood flow, creatinine clearance, and daily urine output) among mammals as exponential functions of body weight (see Fig.
9.11). The values of the exponents were in the order of 0.7 to 0.8.
Edwards also suggests that renal blood flow is generally 26% of cardiac

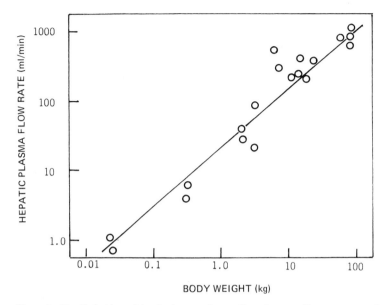

Fig. 9.10 Relationship between hepatic plasma flow rate and total body weight in several animal species. (Data from Ref. 11.)

output in mammals, independent of body weight. In this respect, renal blood flow differs from hepatic portal blood flow, which represents a relatively greater proportion of cardiac output in larger species [29].

If drug distribution involved purely physical interactions between xenobiotics and biological tissues or fluids, it might be expected to follow principles of thermodynamic partitioning with relatively minor interspecies variation. An equilibrium distribution ratio (R value) determined for a given tissue in a laboratory animal might then be useful for a model to be applied to humans. This seems to be a plausible idea for certain fat-soluble compounds, including dieldrin [30], thiopental [31], and kepone [32], but less encouraging results have been found for other compounds such as methotrexate [11] and digoxin [8,10]. At this time more work needs to be done to examine the merits of this hypothesis. It is reasonable to suggest that even a preliminary interest in this approach requires as a minimum that V_{ss} values for the drug be rather similar in the two or more species. This comparability is not sufficient but it is necessary. There has been some interest in using in vitro data to estimate in vivo binding parameters [31].

The most significant species differences that may confound pharmacokinetic predictability are in the pathways and kinetic characteristics of metabolism. Although humans usually metabolize drugs less rapidly then other animal species that are commonly used in drug development studies, and microsomal enzyme activities per kilogram of

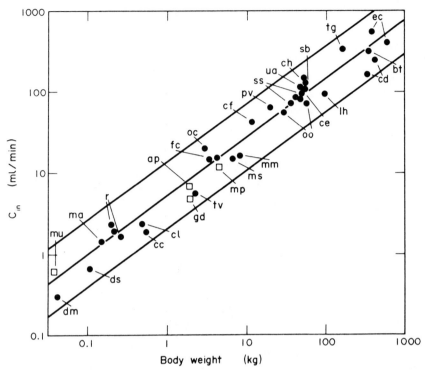

Fig. 9.11 Relationship between inulin clearance C_{in} and total body weight for mammals (●) and for four species of birds (□) C_{in} = $5.359 \, BW^{0.72}$. The key to species is provided in Ref. 29. (From Ref. 29.)

body weight tend to decrease as body weight increases, many exceptions exist. Quite different metabolic pathways may dominate in different species and toxicity may sometimes correlate with the concentration of a reactive intermediate that represents only a minor elimination pathway.

On the other hand, there is increasing evidence that metabolic information from in vitro systems may be used for quantitative parameter estimation in pharmacokinetic models. These in vitro systems have included both crude and purified enzyme preparations, other cell extracts such microsomes, cell suspensions, tissue slices, and isolated organs. Dedrick and Bischoff [27] propose that it should be possible to use metabolism data from properly designed in vitro systems in conjunction with pharmacokinetic models to provide a basis for predicting pharmacokinetic behavior of xenobiotics in any mammalian species, including humans. They have recently reviewed the evidence in support of this hypothesis. The most notable in vitro-

Table 9.3 Comparison of Extraction Ratios Predicted from In Vitro Estimates of V_m and K_m, and Observed in Isolated Perfused Rat Liver

Drug	V_m/K_m ml/ min (g liver)$^{-1}$	K_m (mM)	Extraction Ratio Predicted	Extraction Ratio Observed
Alprenolol	23.5	0.017	0.92	>0.90
Propranolol	10.0	0.005	0.83	>0.90
Lidocaine	8.2	0.058	0.80	>0.90
Phenytoin	2.0	0.031	0.50	0.53
Hexobarbital	1.6	0.105	0.44	0.33
Carbamazepine	0.11	0.73	0.05	0.04
Antipyrine	0.08	22.0	0.04	0.01

Source: From Ref. 19.

in vivo correlations have been observed by Rane et al. [19]. The results of their comparison of observed hepatic extraction ratios with those calculated from V_{max}/K_m ratios obtained from rat liver preparations are summarized in Table 9.3.

Probably the most fascinating approach to interspecies correlation of drug concentration data has been offered by Dedrick et al. [33] with methotrexate. This analysis is empirical and perhaps limited to a few compounds but is nevertheless interesting, informative, and exciting. Figure 9.12 shows methotrexate concentrations in plasma or serum after injection of various doses to different animal species, including the mouse, rat, monkey, dog, and humans. The range of variables is as follows: body weight, 22 to 70,000 g (ratio of 3000 to

Table 9.4 Equivalent Times for Several Species

Species	Average Body Weight (g)	Body Weight$^{1/4}$ (g$^{1/4}$)	Equivalent Time (min)
Mouse	22	2.16	0.13
Rat	160	3.56	0.22
Monkey	4,000	7.95	0.49
Dog	5,000	8.42	0.52
Humans	70.000	16.3	1.00

Source: From Ref. 33.

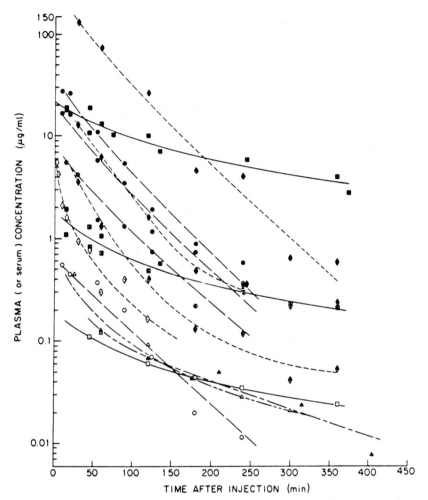

Fig. 9.12 Plasma (or serum) concentration of methotrexate after intravenous or intraperitoneal injection of different doses. The species
are indicated by diamonds (mice), circles (rats), closed triangles
(monkey), open triangles (beagle dog), and squares (humans). (Data
from Ref. 33.)

1); dose per unit body weight, 0.1 to 450 mg/kg (4500 to 1); and
methotrexate concentrations in plasma or serum, 0.0077 to 130 μg/ml
(17,000 to 1).

An attempt was made to represent all the data by a single curve.
Normalization of the ordinate in Fig. 9.12 was achieved by dividing
observed drug concentrations by the dose per unit body weight.
Such normalization implicitly assumes linear relationships among rele-

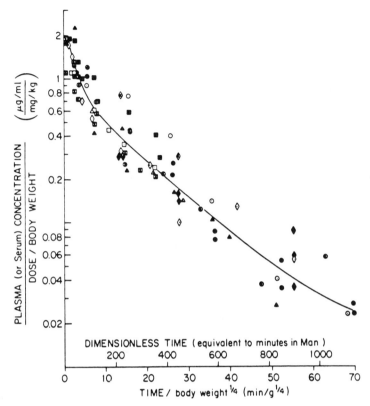

Fig. 9.13 Correlation of methotrexate concentration data in plasma
(or serum) in mouse, rat, monkey, dog, and humans. Symbols are as
indicated in Fig. 9.12. (From Ref. 33.)

vant thermodynamic phenomena such as equilibrium distribution in
major tissues. It would not be expected to apply to a drug that is
strongly and nonlinearly bound to proteins or other macromolecules.
These assumptions may be reasonably applied to methotrexate for
some time after injection (when concentrations are high), but are
inappropriate at later times.

Normalization of the abscissa in Fig. 9.12 requires introduction of
an interesting kinetic concept. It is evident that changes are taking
place more rapidly in the smaller animals than in the larger animals.
Dedrick et al. [33] developed the idea of *equivalent time* to account
for these kinetic differences. For example, since the decline of
methotrexate concentrations in plasma or serum occurs about an order
of magnitude faster in the mouse than in humans, an equivalent time
might be the mean residence time of the vascular system or the ratio
of blood volume to cardiac output. The latter has a value of about

1 min in humans and varies as a function of body weight to the 0.2 power. In the case of methotrexate concentrations, Dedrick and co-workers chose to use an empirical function of body weight (i.e., to normalize the abscissa by dividing time by body weight raised to the 0.25 power). Table 9.4 shows the correspondence between the fourth root of weight and an equivalent time based on unity for humans.

The correlation developed in this manner is shown in Fig. 9.13. All data from Fig. 9.12 have been included up to a time parameter of 70 $(min/g^{1/4})$. Accordingly, mouse data beyond 150 min and rat data beyond 250 min are not included. Agreement is very good and variations appear to be principally random. The application of this approach to other drugs that demonstrate linear pharmacokinetics and are essentially excreted unchanged is a distinct possibility; the success of this approach for drugs that are substantially metabolized is probably unlikely.

The development, validation, and application of physiologic pharmacokinetic models is a very exciting area of research. A great deal of credit must be accorded to Bischoff and Dedrick for their pioneering effort and prolific contributions. In all its ramifications, this pharmacokineric approach offers the possibility of unusual insight into complex biological systems.

REFERENCES

1. K. J. Himmelstein and R. J. Lutz. A review of the applications of physiologically based pharmacokinetic modeling. *J. Pharmacokinet. Biopharm.* *7*:127 (1979).
2. N. Benowitz, R. P. Forsyth, K. L. Melmon, and M. Rowland. Lidocaine disposition kinetics in monkey and man: II. Effects of hemmorrhage and sympathomimetic drug administration. *Clin. Pharmacol. Ther.* *16*:99 (1974).
3. R. L. Dedrick. Animal scale-up. *J. Pharmacokinet. Biopharm.* *1*:435 (1973).
4. K. B. Bischoff. Some fundamental considerations of the applications of pharmacokinetics to cancer chemotherapy. *Cancer Chemother. Rep.* *59*:777 (1975).
5. M. Rowland, L. Z. Benet, and G. G. Graham. Clearance concepts in pharmacokinetics. *J. Pharmacokinet. Biopharm.* *1*:123 (1973).
6. R. J. Lutz, W. M. Galbraith, R. L. Dedrick, R. Shrager, and L. B. Mellett. A model for the kinetics of distribution of actinomycin-D in the beagle dog. *J. Pharmacol. Exp. Ther.* *200*:469 (1977).
7. F. G. King and R. L. Dedrick. Pharmacokinetic model for 2-amino-1,3,4-thiadiazole in mouse, dog, and monkey. *Cancer Treat. Rep.* *63*:1939 (1979).

8. L. I. Harrison and M. Gibaldi. Physiologically based pharmaco-
    kinetic model for digoxin disposition in dogs and its preliminary
    application to humans. *J. Pharm. Sci.* *66*:1679 (1977).
9. A. Tsuji, E. Miyamoto, T. Terasaki, and T. Yamana. Physio-
    logical pharmacokinetics of β-lactam antibiotics: Penicillin V
    distribution and elimination after intravenous administration in
    rats. *J. Pharm. Pharmacol.* *31*:116 (1979).
10. L. I. Harrison and M. Gibaldi. Physiologically based pharma-
    cokinetic model for digoxin distribution and elimination in the
    rat. *J. Pharm. Sci.* *66*:1138 (1977).
11. K. B. Bischoff, R. L. Dedrick, D. S. Zaharko, and J. A.
    Longstreth. Methotrexate pharmacokinetics. *J. Pharm. Sci.*
    60:1128 (1971).
12. K. B. Bischoff, R. L. Dedrick, and D. S. Zaharko. Preliminary
    model for methotrexate pharmacokinetics. *J. Pharm. Sci.* *59*:149
    (1970).
13. N. Benowitz, R. P. Forsyth, K. L. Melmon, and M. Rowland.
    Lidocaine disposition kinetics in monkey and man: I. Prediction
    by perfusion model. *Clin. Pharmacol. Ther.* *16*:87 (1974).
14. H-S. G. Chen and J. F. Gross. Estimation of tissue-to-plasma
    partition coefficients used in physiological pharmacokinetic models.
    J. Pharmacokinet. Biopharm. *7*:117 (1979).
15. G. R. Wilkinson and D. G. Shand. A physiological approach to
    hepatic drug clearance. *Clin. Pharmacol. Ther.* *18*:377 (1975).
16. A. Yacobi and G. Levy. Comparative pharmacokinetics of cou-
    marin anticoagulants: XIV. Relationship between protein
    binding, distribution and elimination kinetics of warfarin in rats.
    J. Pharm. Sci. *64*:1660 (1975).
17. G. Levy, C.-M. Lai, and A. Yacobi. Comparative pharmaco-
    kinetics of coumarin anticoagulants: XXXII. Interindividual
    differences in binding of warfarin and dicumarol in rat liver
    and implications for physiological pharmacokinetic modeling.
    J. Pharm. Sci. *67*:229 (1978).
18. J. M. Collins, R. L. Dedrick, F. G. King, J. L. Speyer, and
    C. E. Myers. Nonlinear pharmacokinetic models for 5-fluorouracil
    in man: Intravenous and intraperitoneal routes. *Clin. Pharmacol.
    Ther.* *28*:235 (1980).
19. A. Rane, G. R. Wilkinson, and D. G. Shand. Prediction of
    hepatic extraction ratio from in vitro measurement of intrinsic
    clearance. *J. Pharmacol. Exp. Ther.* *200*:420 (1977).
20. R. L. Dedrick, D. D. Forrester, and D. H. W. Ho. In vitro-in
    vivo correlation of drug metabolism—deamination of 1-β-D-
    arabinofuranosylcytosine. *Biochem. Pharmacol.* *21*:1 (1972).
21. R. L. Dedrick and D. D. Forrester. Blood flow limitations in
    interpreting Michaelis constant for ethanol oxidation in vivo.
    Biochem. Pharmacol. *22*:1133 (1973).

22. R. L. Dedrick, D. S. Zaharko, and R. J. Lutz. Transport and
     binding of methotrexate in vivo. *J. Pharm. Sci. 62*:882 (1973).
23. D. S. Greene, R. Quintiliani, and C. H. Nightingale. Physio-
     logical perfusion model for cephalosporin antibiotics: I. Model
     selection based on blood concentrations. *J. Pharm. Sci. 67*:191
     (1978).
24. M. Mintum, K. J. Himmelstein, R. L. Schroder, M. Gibaldi, and
     D. D. Shen. Tissue distribution kinetics of tetraethylammonium
     ion in the rat. *J. Pharmacokinet. Biopharm. 8*:373 (1980).
25. R. J. Lutz, R. L. Dedrick, J. A. Straw, M. M. Hart, P. Klubes,
     and D. S. Zaharko. The kinetics of methotrexate distribution
     in spontaneous canine lymphosarcoma. *J. Pharmacokinet.
     Biopharm. 3*:77 (1975).
26. K. H. Yang, W. P. Fung, R. J. Lutz, R. L. Dedrick, and
     D. S. Zaharko. In vivo methotrexate transport in murine Lewis
     lung tumor. *J. Pharm. Sci. 68*:941 (1979).
27. R. L. Dedrick and K. B. Bischoff. Species similarity in phar-
     macokinetics. *Fed. Proc. 39*:54 (1980).
28. E. F. Adolph. Quantitative relations in the physiological con-
     stitutions of mammals. *Science 109*:579 (1949).
29. N. A. Edwards. Scaling of renal functions in mammals. *Comp.
     Biochem. Physiol.* [A] *52*:63 (1975).
30. C. G. Hunter, J. Robinson, and M. Roberts. Pharmacodynamics
     of dieldrin (HEOD): Ingestion by human subjects for 18 to 24
     months and post-exposure for eight months. *Arch. Environ.
     Health 18*:12 (1969).
31. K. B. Bischoff and R. L. Dedrick. Thiopental pharmacokinetics.
     J. Pharm. Sci. 57:1346 (1968).
32. P. M. Bungay, R. L. Dedrick, and H. B. Matthews. Pharma-
     cokinetics of halogenated hydrocarbons. *Ann. N.Y. Acad. Sci.
     320*:257 (1979).
33. R. L. Dedrick, K. B. Bischoff, and D. S. Zaharko. Inter-
     species correlation of plasma concentration history of metho-
     trexate. *Cancer Chemother. Rep. 54*:95 (1970).

10

Application of Pharmacokinetic Principles

Previous chapters have concerned basic pharmacokinetic principles, and have emphasized the development of pharmacokinetic theory. It is the purpose of this chapter to consider the application of these principles to drug utilization in the clinical setting. There will be little emphasis on the development of equations. Where appropriate, the practical utility of selected equations from previous chapters will be discussed.

MULTIPLE DOSING

The most common approach for the maintenance of therapeutic plasma concentrations is through the repetitive adminstration of oral doses at given time intervals. Although oral administration is the most frequently used route of administration, the basic principles of multiple dosing will apply regardless of the route of administration and the pharmacokinetic model used to describe the drug, as long as the kinetic behavior of the drug can be described by linear or first-order kinetics.

The general objective of drug treatment is to obtain quickly and to maintain drug plasma concentrations which fluctuate above some minimum effective concentration, and below those concentrations that have been associated with adverse effects (i.e., to maintain concentrations within the therapeutic range). The application of pharmacokinetic principles can have the greatest impact on therapy with drugs having a narrow therapeutic range. Frequently, a therapeutic range is perceived as being an absolute concentration range within which all patients will respond and no adverse effects will be observed. Unfortunately, this is not the case, and one must look at a therapeutic range as that concentration range within which there will be the greatest probability for a therapeutic response and the least probability for adverse effects. For example, 0.5 to 2 ng/ml is frequently

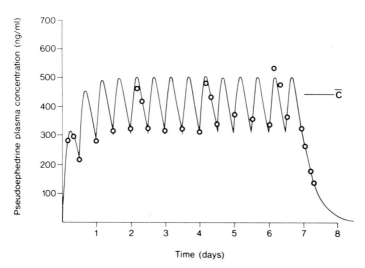

Fig. 10.1 Pseudoephedrine concentrations in plasma on twice-a-day oral administration of a slow-release product. The horizontal line, to the right of the curve, denotes the average steady-state drug concentration (see Ref. 1).

quoted as the therapeutic range for digoxin. However, there is about a 10% risk of seeing toxic symptoms at a concentration of 1.5 ng/ml. This risk increases with concentration and one sees about an 85% risk of adverse effects at concentrations greater than 2 ng/ml. Thus toxicity can be observed within a therapeutic range, and concentrations greater than the upper end of the therapeutic range may be found in patients demonstrating no adverse effects. Therefore, a therapeutic range can only be used as a guide to therapy.

When an oral multiple dosing regimen is initiated, plasma concentrations will increase, reach a maximum, and begin to decline (see Fig. 10.1). Generally, before all of the absorbed drug from the first dose is eliminated, a second dose will be administered. Consequently, plasma concentrations resulting from the second dose will be higher than those from the first dose. This increases in concentration with dose, or accumulation, will continue to occur until a steady state is reached. At steady state the rate of drug entry into the body will equal the rate of exit; hence the concentration at any time during a dosing interval should be the same from dose to dose. The extent to which a drug will accumulate relative to the first dose can be quantified by an accumulation factor R which is dependent on the relative magnitudes of the dosing interval τ and the half-life $t_{1/2}$ of a drug:

$$R = \frac{1}{1 - e^{-0.693\tau/t_{1/2}}} \qquad (10.1)$$

This relationship is depicted graphically in Fig. 10.2 and illustrates that the smaller the ratio $\tau/t_{1/2}$, the greater will be the extent of accumulation. Of interest is the fact that when the dosing interval equals the half-life of a drug, the average steady-state concentrations will be about twice the average concentration after the first dose.

Although the time to reach steady state will generally be a complex function of several pharmacokinetic parameters (see Chap. 3), it is usually found that regardless of the complexity of the pharmacokinetic

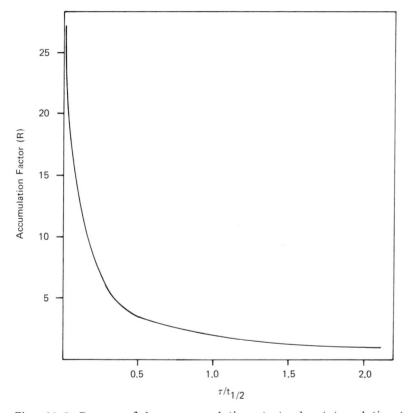

Fig. 10.2 Degree of drug accumulation at steady state relative to a single dose (expressed as an accumulation factor, R) as a function of the ratio of dosing interval to half-life of the drug, $\tau/t_{1/2}$. Administration of a fixed dose at a constant dosing interval equal to the half-life of the drug results in a twofold accumulation.

model, about 90% of steady state will be reached within approximately four half-lives. Whereas the time to reach steady state depends primarily on the half-life of a drug, the average drug concentration at steady state, $\bar{C}$, is a function of the maintenance dose X_0, the fraction of the dose absorbed F, the dosing interval, and the clearance Cl_s of the drug. This relationship is

$$\bar{C} = \frac{FX_0}{Cl_s \tau} \tag{10.2}$$

or

$$\bar{C} = \frac{1.44FX_0 t_{1/2}}{V\tau} = \frac{AUC}{\tau} \tag{10.3}$$

where V is the apparent volume of distribution of a drug, and AUC is the area under the plasma concentration versus time curve from time zero to infinity following a single maintenance dose. These equations, although very useful, give no insight into the degree of fluctuation in steady-state plasma concentrations. For example, administration of a drug with a half-life of 12 h according to the following regimens: 600 mg daily, 300 mg twice a day, and 200 mg three times a day, will produce identical values for $\bar{C}$. However, 600 mg daily will result in greater fluctuations in steady-state concentrations than will 300 mg twice a day, which will in turn produce greater fluctuations than 200 mg three times a day. Although absorption rate will influence the degree of fluctuation in steady-state concentrations, the relative magnitude of τ and $t_{1/2}$ will be a major factor governing these fluctuations. This is illustrated by Fig. 10.3, which assumes a one-compartment system with intravenous bolus administration. As can be seen, the greater the ratio of $\tau/t_{1/2}$, the larger will be the ratio of $C_{max}/\bar{C}$ at steady state, and the smaller will be the ratio of $C_{min}/\bar{C}$ at steady state.

Equations (10.2) and (10.3) illustrate how the absorption, distribution, and elimination characteristics of a drug affect steady-state drug concentrations. The influence of such factors as disease states, drug interactions, and age on steady-state concentrations can also be readily appreciated from these equations by knowing which process is influenced by these factors. One can also utilize these relationships as tools to gain insight into a patient's therapy and to determine whether a patient's regimen may produce subtherapeutic or toxic concentrations of a drug. Equations (10.2) and (10.3) can also be rearranged to yield the following expression for maintenance dose:

$$X_0 = \frac{\bar{C}Cl_s \tau}{F} = \frac{\bar{C}V\tau}{1.44Ft_{1/2}} \tag{10.4}$$

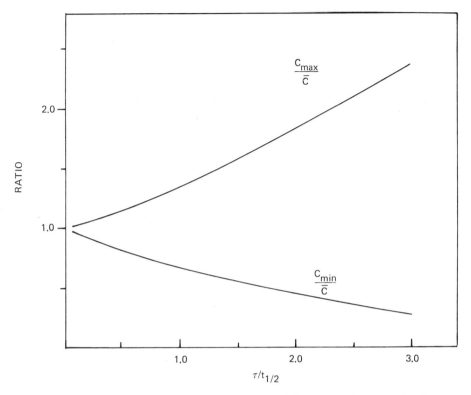

Fig. 10.3 Relationship between the ratio of C_{max} or C_{min} at steady state to the average drug concentration at steady state, $\bar{C}$ and the ratio of dosing interval to drug half-life, $\tau/t_{1/2}$. Assuming a fixed daily dose of drug, the larger the value of $\tau/_{1/2}$, the greater the fluctuations of drug concentration in plasma at steady state.

This equation can be used to predict an initial maintenance dose of a drug for a given patient. Knowledge of the therapeutic range will enable $\bar{C}$ and τ to be selected. It is generally appropriate to aim for a steady-state concentration which is safe (i.e., a concentration associated with a very low incidence of toxicity). A concentration midway between the limits of the therapeutic range or one just below this midpoint would generally be reasonable. Determination of τ requires information on a drug's half-life as well as its therapeutic range. If, for example, a drug has an optimum therapeutic range of 10 to 20 µg/ml, τ should probably be equal to or less than one half-life, since concentrations could fall from the upper to the lower end of the range in one half-life. If, however, the therapeutic range was between 2 and 20 µg/ml, it may be appropriate to use a dosing interval equal to approximately three half-lives. For reasons of compliance, it is often desirable to have a dosing interval as long as possible, but it probably should not exceed one day. In addition, patients should not be expected to take a dose more frequently than four times a day. If a drug has a narrow therapeutic range and a short half-life (e.g., procainamide), it may be necessary to dose more frequently than four times a day for optimum effects. Sustained-release dosage forms are very desirable for such drugs.

Once $\overline{C}$ and τ are selected, one must usually rely on literature data for values of F, the availability of the dosage form being used, and clearance. Generally, average parameters are used even though we know that there is considerable interpatient variability in these parameters. Interpatient variability is a particular problem with estimates of F for poorly absorbed drugs and Cl_s for drugs eliminated predominantly by metabolism. Another problem frequently encountered is the fact that most pharmacokinetic studies are performed in young, healthy male populations rather in the patient population in which the drug is to be used, although this information is becoming more available. Although the use of Eq. (10.4) does have some pitfalls due to the limitation of not having individual patient parameters available, it does provide a rational basis for the initiation of therapy.

Because of the problem of interpatient variability, it would be desirable to be able to determine a maintenance dose based on one or more measurable parameters in the individual patient. From a practical point of view this is generally not feasible. Recently, however, publications have appeared which indicate that a maintenance dose producing therapeutic plasma concentrations can be estimated based on a single plasma concentration at a specific time t* following the oral administration of a test dose X_0^* [2−4]. The plasma concentration C* following the test dose, assuming that it is in the postabsorptive-postdistributive phase of a plasma concentration versus time curve, can be given by the following equation:

$$C^* = FX_0^* Z e^{-0.693 t^*/t_{1/2}}$$

(10.5)

where Z is a constant dependent on the pharmacokinetic model and route of administration. Dividing Eq. (10.2) by (10.5) and solving for the reciprocal of the maintenance dose, $1/X_0$, yields

$$\frac{1}{X_0} = \frac{e^{0.693 t^*/t_{1/2}}}{\overline{C} Cl_s \tau Z X_0^*} C^*$$

(10.6)

Plots of $1/X_0$ versus C* have resulted in a linear relationship, as illustrated in Figs. 10.4 and 10.5. Once data have been generated

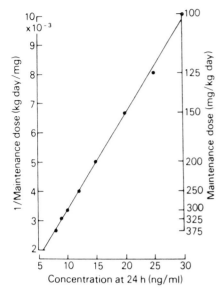

Fig. 10.4 Relationship between the reciprocal of the maintenance dose of imipramine needed to achieve a steady-state total tricyclics (imipramine and desipramine) concentration of 250 ng/ml and the concentration of total tricyclics 24 h after a single 50 mg oral test dose of imipramine (see Ref. 4).

such as those presented in Figs. 10.4 and 10.5, the administration of a test dose to a given patient followed by the measurement of C^* should permit the prediction of a maintenance dose that would yield the desired $\bar{C}$. This method can be applied to a patient population with a relatively wide range of half-lives [4]. However, different $1/X_0$ versus C^* data sets should be developed for the same drug in patient populations that have different ranges of half-lives. The optimum sampling time following the test dose equals the average half-life divided by 0.693 [5].

A more comprehensive single-point method has been described by Sheiner et al. [6]. This method requires a computer system with a large data base. In the case of digoxin, information concerning sex, age, height, weight, outpatient or inpatient status, presence or absence of moderate or severe heart failure, values of kidney function tests, as well as measured plasma concentration data must be available. The matching of patient characteristics and resulting plasma concentration(s) for a given patient to a typical member of a subgroup permits the forecasting of an individual's course of therapy based on known outcomes of this subgroup member. It has been

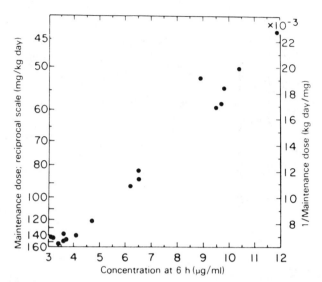

Fig. 10.5 Relationship between the reciprocal of the maintenance dose
of chloramphenicol needed to achieve a steady-state concentration of
15 μg/ml and the concentration of chloramphenicol 6 h after a single
25 mg/kg test dose (see Ref. 4).

demonstrated that information from one plasma concentration is more
valuable than all information on patient features, and if two plasma
concentrations are available, forecast accuracy and precision are as
good as theoretically possible.

The time required to reach steady-state concentrations and obtain
a maximum response from a given dosing regimen may be excessive
because of the half-life of a given drug. This problem can be overcome by the administration of a loading dose followed by administration of maintenance doses. As discussed in Chap. 3, a loading dose
X_0' can be estimated by multiplying the maintenance dose by the accumulation factor R, which is equal to $1/(1 - e^{-0.693\tau/t_{1/2}})$ [Eq.
(10.1)]. Therefore,

$$X_0' = X_0 \frac{1}{1 - e^{-0.693\tau/t_{1/2}}} \tag{10.7}$$

Equation (10.7) assumes that each does is administered in the postabsorptive-postdistributive phase of each previous dose. For certain
drugs it may be advisable not to administer the loading dose as a
single dose, but rather to spread it over the first dosing inverval
or even longer if necessary. For example, a 1 mg loading dose of
digoxin should probably be given as three divided doses of 0.5, 0.25,
and 0.25 mg at 4- to 8-h intervals.

Although consideration is given to the fluctuation in the steady-state plasma concentrations of a drug when the dosing interval τ is selected, more precise estimates may be obtained by utilizing Fig. 10.3. Once τ has been selected and $t_{1/2}$ has been estimated, the ratios $C_{max}/\bar{C}$ and $C_{min}/\bar{C}$ at steady state can be estimated from this figure using the $\tau/t_{1/2}$ ratio. Simply multiplying the chosen $\bar{C}$ by the $C_{max}/\bar{C}$ and $C_{min}/\bar{C}$ ratios will yield estimates of C_{max} and C_{min} at steady state. Since Fig. 10.3 is based on equations where instantaneous absorption is assumed, the measured C_{max} would be expected to be less than the predicted value, while the measured C_{min} should be greater than the predicted value.

DOSE ADJUSTMENTS IN RENAL FAILURE

There is generally a great deal of interpatient variability in the elimination rates of drugs which are predominantly eliminated by metabolism. Other than employing the method discussed above, which involves the administration of a test dose, there is no practical way to obtain a priori a measure of the ability of a given patient to eliminate such drugs. However, for drugs eliminated primarily by renal mechanisms, creatinine clearance and serum creatinine have been successfully employed to evaluate renal function in a given patient, thereby enabling estimates of the clearance or half-life of a drug. The use of serum creatinine measurements to determine renal function has been discussed by Bjornsson [7]. Creatinine is a useful marker of renal function since it is produced endogenously as an end product of muscle metabolism and is eliminated by the kidney at a rate that approximates glomerular filtration rate. It has been shown for a number of drugs that the elimination of creatinine directly reflects drug elimination.

The apparent first-order elimination rate constant of a drug, K, is equal to the sum of the rate constants for renal and nonrenal excretion, k_r and k_{nr}, respectively. That is,

$$K = k_r + k_{nr} \tag{10.8}$$

Assuming that renal elimination is directly related to creatinine clearance Cl_{cr} it follows that

$$K = aCl_{cr} + k_{nr} \tag{10.9}$$

where a is a proportionality constant. A plot of K versus Cl_{cr} will, therefore, be linear (see Fig. 10.6). Data relating K to creatinine clearance are available for many drugs, and summaries of such information appear in several publications [9–11]. Although the discussion above is concerned with adjusting an individual patient's K for changes in renal function, the same approach can be used to relate renal clearance or total body clearance of a drug to creatinine

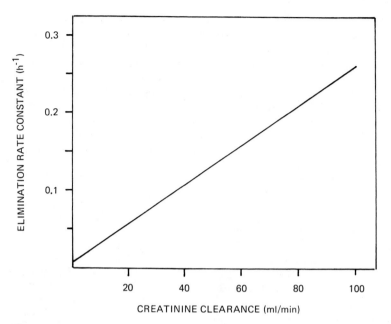

Fig. 10.6 Relationship between the elimination rate constants of 5-fluorocytosine and creatinine clearance, based on studies in patients with imparied renal function. The line intercepts the y axis at a value of 0.0067 h^{-1}. (Data from Ref. 8.)

clearance. Although these relationships have been established for digoxin [12], there are few data available for other drugs.

Because of the practical problem of obtaining a 24 h urine collection for the purpose of calculating creatinine clearance, serum creatinine is generally used as an index of renal function. Since serum creatinine C_c is inversely related to creatinine clearance by the relationship

$$C_c = \frac{PR}{Cl_{cr}} \tag{10.10}$$

where PR is endogenous production rate of creatinine, one would expect that a decrease in renal function would produce a corresponding increase in serum creatinine. Solving (10.10) for Cl_{cr} and substituting this value of creatinine clearance for Cl_{cr} in (10.9) yields

$$K = \frac{aPR}{C_c} + k_{nr} \tag{10.11}$$

which in terms of half-life $t_{1/2}$ is

$$\frac{1}{t_{1/2}} = \frac{aPR}{0.693} \frac{1}{C_c} + \frac{k_{nr}}{0.693} \qquad (10.12)$$

since $K = 0.693/t_{1/2}$ [Eq. (1.12)]. Therefore, a plot of K versus $1/C_c$, or $1/t_{1/2}$ versus $1/C_c$, will be linear (see Fig. 10.7).

Essential to the appropriate use of serum creatinine as an index of renal function and drug elimination is that the production rate of creatinine must be relatively constant. Since production rate depends on the muscle mass in a given individual, one would expect sex, age, and body weight to influence the relationship between serum creatinine and creatinine clearance. Because of this, serum creatinine may be a relatively poor index of renal function. One such example is illustrated in Table 10.1. Renal function decreases with increasing age, whereas serum creatinine remains relatively constant; the decrease in creatinine clearance is associated with a corresponding increase in kanamycin half-life. Therefore, serum creatinine alone may have limited utility as an index of renal function and drug elimination under certain conditions. Serum creatinine can, however, be employed in conjunction with the age, sex, and weight of an individual to predict

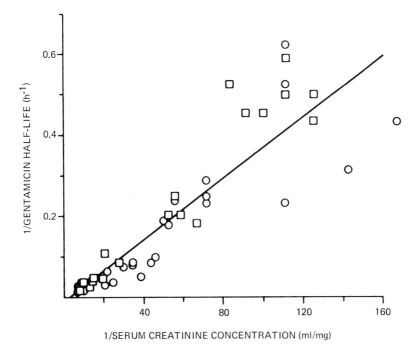

Fig. 10.7 Double reciprocal plot of gentamicin half-life versus serum creatinine concentration (see Ref. 13).

Table 10.1 Creatinine Clearance, Serum Creatinine, and Kanamycin Half-Life as a Function of Age in Healthy Humans

Age (yr)	n	Cl_{cr} (ml/min)	C_c (mg%)	$t_{1/2}$ (min)
20−50	13	94 ± 17[a]	0.97 ± 0.12	107 ± 27
50−70	21	75 ± 20	0.95 ± 0.23	149 ± 49
70−90	27	43 ± 12	0.98 ± 0.21	282 ± 99

[a]Mean ± SD.

Notes: The increase in kanamycin half-life $t_{1/2}$ with age is consistent with the decrease in creatinine clearance Cl_{cr}. Serum creatinine C_c appears to be independent of age. From Ref. 14.

a creatinine clearance. Although several approaches have been used for such a prediction [15,16], the following equation [17], based on the data of Kampmann et al. [18], is particularly useful:

$$Cl_{cr} = \frac{wt(144 - age)}{71C_c} \qquad (10.13)$$

where age is in years, C_c is in mg%, Cl_{cr} is in ml/min, and wt is in kg. Since creatinine is an end product of muscle metabolism, total body weight should not be used in (10.13) for obese individuals. Rather, some weight between total and ideal body weight is appropriate [19]. Equation (10.13) is intended for use with males. For females the value obtained from (10.13) should be multiplied by 0.85 to correct for the average difference in creatinine production between males and females. As mentioned previously, (10.13) is only one of several approaches that has been used to predict creatinine clearance. A study correlating predictions using Eq. (10.13) to measure clearance has found a correlation coefficient of 0.84 [15], which is as high as any method to which it was compared.

Once a creatinine clearance has been either determined directly or predicted from a serum creatinine value using (10.13), an estimate of the elimination rate constant or clearance can be obtained for the patient from data such as those presented in Fig. 10.6. Once this elimination parameter has been determined, it can be used in Eqs. (10.4) and (10.7) to calculate a maintenance dose and a loading dose, respectively. The adjustment of doses of renally excreted drugs is most critical for those drugs that have a narrow therapeutic range, examples of which are digoxin and the aminoglycoside antibiotics. Drugs such as the penicillins and cephalosporins, which are also eliminated primarily by the kidneys, probably require dose adjust-

ments only when renal function is significantly compromised (i.e.,
a creatinine clearance less than 20 ml/min), since they have a much
wider therapeutic range.

HEMODIALYSIS

Additional dose adjustments may be necessary in severe renal failure
patients who require routine dialysis. Hemodialysis, peritoneal dialysis, or hemoperfusion may result in drug removal from the body
and require replacement of this amount to maintain therapeutic concentrations. Hemodialysis is the most common method of removing
endogenous waste material in chronic renal failure patients, although
chronic ambulatory peritoneal dialysis is becoming more popular.
Hemoperfusion appears to be used primarily to remove drugs from the
body in cases of drug overdose.

A number of factors may influence the hemodialyzability of a drug
[20−23]. Since hemodialysis membranes have discrete pores through
which drug must diffuse to be dialyzed, one might expect that the
larger the molecular size, the more poorly a drug will be dialyzed.
However, the clinical significance of molecular weight has not been
clearly established. Blood flow, dialysate flow, and aqueous solubility
are also factors that will influence dialyzability. A decrease in each
of these factors will tend to decrease the extent to which a drug is
dialyzed, with the relative effect of each being governed by their
influence on the concentration gradient between blood and dialysate.

The pharmacokinetic characteristics of a drug will also have a
significant impact on the ability of a drug to be dialyzed. Those
drugs that have a large volume of distribution and/or are highly
plasma protein bound tend to be poorly dialyzed. When the ratio of
percent unbound/volume of distribution (in liters/kg) is less than 20,
a small and probably insignificant amount (i.e., less than 10%) of
drug will be removed from the body by a 6 h dialysis, while a value
greater than 80 suggests that between 20 and 50% of the amount of
drug in the body will be removed by dialysis (see Fig. 10.8).

The use of binding and distribution data will give one a general
appreciation of the dialyzability of a given drug, but more precise
estimates of the amount removed may be desirable for the purpose of
dose adjustments. One approach involves the use of the half-lives
of drug during dialysis, $(t_{1/2})_d$, and when dialysis is not being performed, $t_{1/2}$. The fraction of drug in the body removed by dialysis,
f, can be given by [24]

$$f = \frac{t_{1/2} - (t_{1/2})_d}{t_{1/2}} (1 - e^{-0.693t/(t_{1/2})_d}) \qquad (10.14)$$

where t is the duration of dialysis. The half-lives $t_{1/2}$ and $(t_{1/2})_d$
can be obtained from the literature for a number of drugs, some of

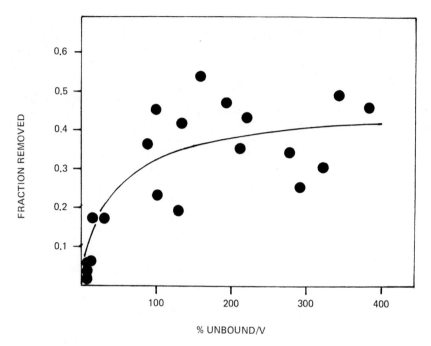

Fig. 10.8 Plot of the fraction of drug in the body removed by a 6 h hemodialysis treatment versus the ratio of the percentage of drug in the plasma unbound to plasma proteins to the apparent volume of distribution V of the drug expressed in liters/kg. (From Ref. 24.)

which have been tabulated [24]. A predialysis concentration C and the volume of distribution V of the drug must also be known. This information then enables the amount of drug that will be removed from the body by dialysis, X_d, to be estimated. The relationship is

$$X_d = fCV \qquad (10.15)$$

This amount of drug can then be administered at the end of the dialysis.

Another approach for estimating the amount of drug removed during dialysis involves the use of dialysis clearance. The rate of appearance of drug in the dialysate, dX_d/dt, is given by

$$\frac{dX_d}{dt} = k_d X \qquad (10.16)$$

where k_d is the first-order rate constant for appearance of drug in the dialysate, and X is the amount of drug in the body. Over a finite period of time (e.g., dialysis time), dX_d/dt can be replaced by $\Delta X_d/\Delta t$. The amount of drug in the body is equal to the product of the plasma concentration C_p and volume of distribution V. Since dX_d/dt is replaced by $\Delta X_d/\Delta t$, plasma concentration must be measured at the midpoint (i.e., C_{pm}). Equation (10.16) can therefore be written as

$$\frac{\Delta X_d}{\Delta t} = k_d V C_{pm} \tag{10.17}$$

The product $k_d V$ will equal dialysis clearance Cl_d; therefore,

$$\frac{\Delta X_d}{\Delta t} = Cl_d C_{pm} \tag{10.18}$$

Equation (10.18) can be solved for the amount of drug appearing in the dialysate, ΔX_d or X_d, during a given dialysis time Δt or t:

$$\Delta X_d = Cl_d \Delta t C_{pm} \tag{10.19}$$

or

$$X_d = Cl_d t C_{pm} \tag{10.20}$$

To determine the amount of drug in the dialysate, one must know the duration of dialysis, the plasma concentration at the midpoint of the dialysis interval, and dialysis clearance. A value for dialysis clearance must be obtained from the literature and should have been determined based on plasma concentration-time rather than blood concentration-time data.

Dialysis clearance measured in terms of plasma $(Cl_d)_p$ is given by

$$(Cl_d)_p = Q_p \frac{C_{ap} - C_{vp}}{C_{ap}} \tag{10.21}$$

and

$$(Cl_d)_p = Q_d \frac{C_{do}}{C_{vp}} \tag{10.22}$$

where Q_p is plasma flow through the dialyzer, Q_d is dialysate flow, C_{ap} and C_{vp} are arterial and venous plasma concentrations of drug (i.e., the plasma concentrations entering and leaving the dialyzer), and C_{do} is the dialysate concentration leaving the dialyzer. Equation (10.22) can be readily applied if dialysate concentrations can be measured. This may be a problem because of the low concentrations frequently encountered and the inconvenience of collecting the large volume of dialysate.

The use of (10.21) requires an estimate of plasma flow through the dialyzer. This can be calculated from blood flow, which is quite readily measured. Blood concentration C_{vb} is related to plasma concentration C_{vp} by the relationship

$$C_b = C_p \left(1 - H + \frac{C_{vrbc}}{C_{vp}} H \right) \tag{10.23}$$

where H is hematocrit and C_{vrbc} is the drug concentration in the red blood cells. Since drug removal rates will be equal no matter whether clearance is expressed in terms of blood or plasma, it follows that [25]

$$(Cl_d)_b C_{vb} = (Cl_d)_p C_{vp} \tag{10.24}$$

where $(Cl_d)_b$ is dialysis clearance based on blood concentrations. Solving Eqs. (10.23) and (10.24) for the ratio of blood to plasma concentrations and setting the right sides of the resulting equations equal to each other yields

$$\frac{(Cl_d)_p}{(Cl_d)_b} = 1 - H + \frac{C_{vrbc}}{C_{vp}} H \tag{10.25}$$

An equation analogous to (10.21) can be written in terms of blood concentrations C_{ab} and C_{vb}, flow Q_b, and clearance $(Cl_d)_b$:

$$(Cl_d)_b = Q_b \frac{C_{ab} - C_{vb}}{C_{ab}} \tag{10.26}$$

The extraction ratios $(C_{ap} - C_{vp})/C_{ap}$ and $(C_{ab} - C_{vb})/C_{ab}$ in (10.21) and (10.26) are equal if the red blood cell-to-plasma concentration ratio is constant on both sides of the dialyzer. Therefore, the ratio of (10.21) to (10.26) is given by

$$\frac{(Cl_d)_p}{(Cl_d)_b} = \frac{Q_p}{Q_b} \tag{10.27}$$

Substituting for $(Cl_d)_p/(Cl_d)_b$ according to (10.25) and solving for Q_p yields

$$Q_p = Q_b \left(1 - H + \frac{C_{vrbc}}{C_{vp}} H \right) \tag{10.28}$$

Therefore, to calculate dialysis clearance based on (10.21), plasma flow should be calculated using (10.28). As can be seen, red blood cell concentration and hematocrit in addition to plasma concentration must be measured to permit this calculation.

The plasma flow calculated by (10.28) is actually an apparent plasma flow and will only equal real plasma flow as given by

$$Q_p = Q_b(1 - H) \qquad (10.29)$$

if no drug distributes into the red blood cells. The use of (10.29) instead of (10.28) will result in an underestimate of the true dialysis clearance if the drug partitions to any significant degree into red blood cells. It is also readily apparent from (10.28) that plasma flow equals blood flow if the concentrations of drug in the red blood cells and plasma are equal.

Utilizing a correctly determined dialysis clearance [i.e., one calculated using (10.21) or (10.22)] will permit an estimate of the amount of drug removed during dialysis. This amount can then be replaced at the end of the dialysis to permit the maintenance of therapeutic plasma concentrations.

In general, the same principles apply to the dialyzability of a drug by peritoneal dialysis as were mentioned for hemodialysis, the primary difference being the properties of the membrane to be traversed by the drug, the peritoneal membrane versus the synthetic membrane in hemodialysis. It has been suggested that the peritoneal membrane appears more permeable to larger molecules (e.g., molecular weights of 5000 or more) than does a hemodialysis membrane [26]. Also, the characteristics of the peritoneal membrane would require that to be dialyzable a drug must have a certain degree of lipid solubility. Overall peritoneal dialysis tends to be much less efficient than hemodialysis in removing drugs. Although there is much less quantitative information available on peritoneal dialysis, it would seem reasonable that the amount of drug removed from the body due to peritoneal dialysis, and hence the amount of additional drug necessary to maintain therapeutic plasma concentrations, could be determined using either (10.14), or (10.20) and (10.22).

METHODS FOR DETERMINATION OF INDIVIDUAL PATIENT PARAMETERS

Most individualized drug dosing and/or dose adjustment methods have relied on population data and individual patient characteristics. A more precise approach would be to assess the pharmacokinetics of a drug directly in the patient receiving the drug. The single-point method [2–5] described earlier in this chapter is one such approach to estimate clearance in individuals within a defined population. The method described by Sheiner et al. [6] is a more general approach. Other methods which require several blood samples after administration of test doses have been applied to gentamicin [27,28] and phenytoin [29,30]. These methods may be used for drugs with similar pharmacokinetic properties.

If the half-life $t_{1/2}$ or elimination rate constant K and volume of distribution V can be determined in a patient for a drug that obeys first-order kinetics and essentially confers on the body the pharmacokinetic characteristics of a one-compartment model, a total dosing regimen can be designed. This has been demonstrated with gentamicin [27,28]. Following a 1 h intravenous infusion of gentamicin the maximum plasma concentration of gentamicin, C_{max}, is given by (see Chap. 1)

$$C_{max} = \frac{k_0}{VK} (1 - e^{-KT}) + C_0 e^{-KT} \qquad (10.30)$$

where k_0 is the zero-order infusion rate, T the infusion time, and C_0 the preinfusion drug concentration, which will be zero if the patient has not recently received drug prior to this dose. Collection of blood samples prior to the infusion and at 1, 2, and 4 h after the start of the infusion will yield a value for C_{max} (i.e., the 1 h concentration), C_0, and K. The rate constant is obtained by applying linear regression to the logarithms of the 1, 2, and 4 h concentrations plotted against time.

Solving (10.30) for volume of distribution yields

$$V = \frac{k_0 (1 - e^{-KT})}{K(C_{max} - C_0 e^{-KT})} \qquad (10.31)$$

Since all of the terms are known, V can be readily calculated. The estimated values of V and K can then be used to calculate the amount of gentamicin to be infused over 1 h to provide the desired maximum or minimum steady-state concentrations, $(C_{ss})_{max}$ and $(C_{ss})_{min}$. $(C_{ss})_{max}$ is given by [27]

$$(C_{ss})_{max} = \frac{k_0 (1 - e^{-KT})}{VK(1 - e^{-K\tau})} \qquad (10.32)$$

where τ is the dosing interval. Equation (10.32) can be solved for the infusion rate required to obtain the desired maximum steady-state concentration, that is

$$k_0 = \frac{VK(C_{ss})_{max}(1 - e^{-K\tau})}{1 - e^{-KT}} \qquad (10.33)$$

The predicted minimum steady-state concentration will be given by the following equation:

$$(C_{ss})_{min} = (C_{ss})_{max} e^{-K(\tau - T)} \qquad (10.34)$$

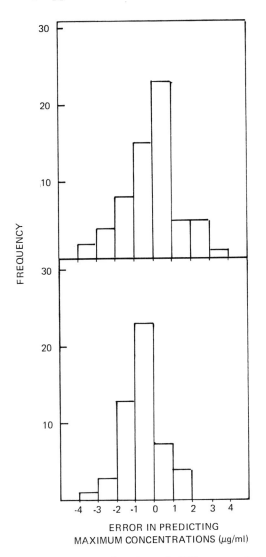

Fig. 10.9 Distribution of differences between predicted and observed peak (upper panel) and nadir (lower panel) concentrations of gentamicin in serum at steady state. (From Ref. 28.)

This method was evaluated in 63 patients for whom it was desirable to produce maximum and minimum gentamicin concentrations ranging from 6 to 10 μg/ml and 0.5 to 2 μg/ml, respectively [28]. The results are presented in Fig. 10.9. Sixty percent of the maximum values and 56% of the minimum values were within 1 μg/ml of those predicted.

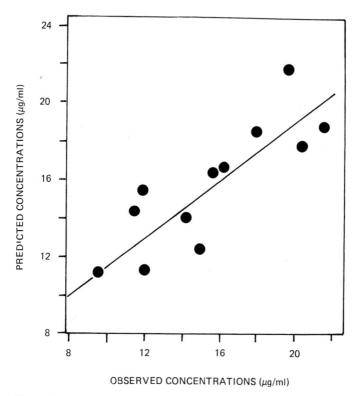

Fig. 10.10 Correlation of predicted and observed concentrations of phenytoin in serum. (From Ref. 29.)

Other methods have been recommended for the dosing of the anticonvulsant phenytoin based on its pharmacokinetic parameters in the patient receiving the drug. Since phenytoin is eliminated by a nonlinear process, the assessment of the necessary parameters becomes somewhat demanding. The elimination rate dX_e/dt of phenytoin can be adequately described by the equation (see Chap. 7)

$$\frac{dX_e}{dt} = \frac{V_m C}{K_m + C} \qquad (10.35)$$

where C is plasma concentration, V_m the maximum rate of elimination, and K_m the concentration at which dX_e/dt equals one-half V_m. At steady state the rate of drug administration RA in mg/day equals the rate of elimination, and concentration will then be the steady-state concentration. Therefore,

$$RA = \frac{V_m C_{ss}}{K_m + C_{ss}} \qquad (10.36)$$

This relationship can be rearranged to yield

$$RA = -K_m \frac{RA}{C_{ss}} + V_m \qquad (10.37)$$

Therefore, a plot of dose rate versus dose rate divided by steady-state concentration (i.e., RA versus RA/C_{ss}) will yield a straight line with a slope of $-K_m$ and an intercept of V_m. Thus this method requires that the phenytoin be dosed to at least two steady states. Once estimates of these parameters are obtained, the daily dose required to produce a desired steady-state concentration can be calculated from (10.36). The predictive ability of this approach is illustrated in Fig. 10.10.

Although this method is sufficiently accurate for clinical purposes, it is simply too time consuming to be of much value in routine practice. Simpler methods have been described [30,31] but are probably less accurate. Thus far, no widely accepted method has been proposed for individualized dosing with drugs having nonlinear pharmacokinetics.

In conclusion, we wish to reiterate that this chapter does nothing more than provide a few examples of the potential usefulness of pharmacokinetics in the clinical setting. There is general agreement that such applications have permitted us to use certain drugs more safely and more sensibly.

REFERENCES

1. J. Dickerson, D. Perrier, M. Mayersohn, and R. Bressler. Dose tolerance and pharmacokinetic studies of L(+)pseudoephedrine capsules in man. *Eur. J. Clin. Pharmacol. 14*:253 (1978).
2. J. R. Koup, C. M. Sack, A. L. Smith, and M. Gibaldi. Hypothesis for the individualization of drug dosage. *Clin. Pharmacokinet. 4*:460 (1979).
3. J. T. Slattery. A pharmacokinetic model-independent approach for estimating dose required to give desired steady-state trough concentrations of drug in plasma. *J. Pharmacokinet. Biopharm. 8*:105 (1980).
4. J. T. Slattery, M. Gibaldi, and J. R. Koup. Prediction of maintenance dose required to attain a desired drug concentration at steady-state from a single determination of concentration after an initial dose. *Clin. Pharmacokinet. 5*:377 (1980).
5. J. T. Slattery. Single-point maintenance dose prediction: role of interindividual differences in clearance and volume of distribution in choice of sampling time. *J. Pharm. Sci. 70*:1174 (1981).

6. L. B. Sheiner, S. Beal, B. Rosenberg, and V. V. Marathe. Forecasting individual pharmacokinetics. *Clin. Pharmacol. Ther.* 26:294 (1979).

7. T. D. Bjornsson. Use of serum creatinine concentrations to determine renal function. *Clin. Pharmacokinet.* 4:200 (1979).

8. J. Schonebeck, A. Polak, M. Fernex, and H. J. Scholer. Pharmacokinetic studies on the oral antimycotic agent 5-fluorocytosine in individuals with normal and impaired kidney function. *Chemotherapy* 18:321 (1973).

9. L. Dettli, P. Spring, and S. Ryter. Multiple dose kinetics and drug dosage in patients with kidney disease. *Acta Pharmacol. Toxicol.* 29(Suppl. 3):211 (1971).

10. L. Dettli. Drug dosage in patients with renal disease. *Clin. Pharmacol. Ther.* 16:274 (1974).

11. L. Dettli. Individualization of drug dosage in patients with renal disease. *Med. Clin. North Am.* 58:977 (1974).

12. J. R. Koup, W. J. Jusko, C. M. Elwood, and R. K. Kohli. Digoxin pharmacokinetics: Role of renal failure in dosage regimen design. *Clin. Pharmacol. Ther.* 18:9 (1975).

13. D. Perrier and M. Gibaldi. Estimation of drug elimination in renal failure. *J. Clin. Pharmacol.* 13:458 (1973).

14. M. Kristensen, J. M. Hansen, J. Kampmann, B. Lumholtze, and K. Siersbaek-Nielsen. Drug elimination and renal function. *J. Clin. Pharmacol.* 14:307 (1974).

15. D. W. Cockcroft and M. H. Gault. Prediction of creatinine clearance from serum creatinine. *Nephron* 16:31 (1976).

16. J. H. Hull, L. J. Hak, G. G. Koch, W. A. Wargin, S. L. Chi, and A. M. Mattocks. Influence of range of renal function and liver disease on predictability of creatinine clearance. *Clin. Pharmacol. Ther.* 29:516 (1981).

17. W. N. Jones and D. Perrier. Prediction of creatinine clearance, *Am. J. Hosp. Pharm.* 35:1183 (1978).

18. J. Kampmann, K. Siersbaek-Nielsen, M. Kristensen, and J. M. Hansen. Rapid evaluation of creatinine clearance. *Acta Med. Scand.* 196:517 (1974).

19. R. E. Dionne, L. A. Bauer, G. A. Gibson, W. O. Griffen, and R. A. Blouin. Estimation of creatinine clearance in the morbidly obese. *Am. J. Hosp. Pharm.* 38:841 (1981).

20. A. L. Babb, R. P. Popovich, T. G. Christopher, and B. H. Scribner. The genesis of the square meter-hour hypothesis. *Trans. Am. Soc. Artif. Intern. Organs* 17:81 (1971).

21. P. M. Galletti. Theoretical considerations about artificial kidneys. *Proc. 3rd Int. Congr. Nephrol.* 3:237 (1967).

22. T. P. Gibson and H. A. Nelson. Drug kinetics and artificial kidneys. *Clin. Pharmacokinet.* 2:403 (1977).

23. T. G. Christopher, A. D. Blair, A. W. Forrey, and R. E. Cutler. Hemodialyzer clearances of gentamicin, kanamycin, tobramycin, amikacin, ethambutol, procainamide and flucytosine, with a technique for planning therapy. *J. Pharmacokinet. Biopharm.* *4*:427 (1976).

24. P. R. Gwilt and D. Perrier. Plasma protein binding and distribution characteristics of drugs as indices of their hemodialyzability. *Clin. Pharmacol. Ther.* *24*:154 (1978).

25. C. S. Lee, T. C. Marburg, and L. Z. Benet. Clearance calculations in hemodialysis: Application to blood, plasma, and dialysate measurements for ethambutol. *J. Pharmacokinet. Biopharm.* *8*:69 (1980).

26. T. P. Gibson. Influence of renal diseases on pharmacokinetics, In *Applied Pharmacokinetics*, W. E. Evans, J. J. Schentag, and W. J. Jusko (Eds.). Applied Therapeutics, Inc., San Francisco, 1980, pp. 32–56.

27. R. J. Sawchuck and D. F. Zaske. Pharmacokinetics of dosing regimens which utilize multiple intravenous infusions: Gentamicin in burn patients. *J. Pharmacokinet. Biopharm.* *4*:183 (1976).

28. R. J. Sawchuck, D. E. Zaske, R. J. Cipolle, W. A. Wargin, and R. G. Strate. Kinetic model for gentamicin dosing with the use of individual patient parameters. *Clin. Pharmacol. Ther.* *21*:362 (1977).

29. T. M. Ludden, J. P. Allen, J. P. Valutsky, A. V. Vicuna, J. M. Nappi, S. F. Hoffman, J. E. Wallace, D. Lalka, and J. L. McNay. Individualization of phenytoin dosage regimens. *Clin. Pharmacol. Ther.* *21*:287 (1977).

30. E. Martin, T. N. Tozer, L. B. Sheiner, and S. Riegelman. The clinical pharmacokinetics of phenytoin. *J. Pharmacokinet. Biopharm.* *5*:579 (1977).

31. B. Rambeck, H. E. Boenigk, A. Dunlop, P. W. Mullen, J. Wadsworth, and A. Richens. Predicting phenytoin dose—a revised nomogram. *Ther. Drug Monit.* *1*:325 (1979).

11

Noncompartmental Analysis Based on Statistical Moment Theory

Throughout this text we have used noncompartmental methods for the estimation of certain pharmacokinetic parameters without specifically referring to them as such. These methods are usually based on the estimation of the area under a plot of drug concentration versus time. Noncompartmental methods have been used to estimate bioavailability, clearance, apparent volume of distribution, and the fraction of a dose of a drug that is converted to a specific metabolite, based on data following single doses of drug and metabolite. These methods have also been used to predict the average steady-state concentration of a drug or its metabolites, based on data following a single dose of the drug, and the time required to reach a given fraction of the steady-state concentration when a fixed dose of a drug is given at regular intervals.

Noncompartmental methods do not require the assumption of a specific compartmental model for either drug or metabolite. In fact, these methods can be applied to virtually any compartmental model, provided that we can assume linear pharmacokinetics. Noncompartmental methods are hardly new. However, the idea that noncompartmental methods provide a general approach for pharmacokinetic analysis is both new and important. During the preparation of this edition of *Pharmacokinetics*, there has been a distinct shift away from computer-based curve-fitting of experimental data and elaboration of compartmental models and toward noncompartmental methods of analysis. In the final stages of preparation of the text, this shift was so evident, that the authors concluded that a separate section dealing with the subject matter was required. Therefore, this chpater has been added in proof. The scope of this chapter is by necessity limited: we shall briefly introduce the basis for noncompartmental analysis, summarize the various noncompartmental methods that have been presented in different sections of the text, modestly extend the applications of noncompartmental analysis, and, perhaps, provide some direction for future developments.

STATISTICAL MOMENTS

Statistical moments have been used extensively for data analysis in chemical engineering [1]. One of the earliest applications to biological systems was provided by Perl and Samuel [2] in a report concerned with the kinetics of body cholesterol. In 1975 Oppenheimer et al. [3] applied statistical moments to the analysis of iodothyronine metabolism and distribution in man. The application of statistical moments to pharmacokinetics was reported in 1979 by Yamaoka et al. [4] and Cutler [5]. In 1980, Riegelman and Collier [6] applied statistical moment theory to the evaluation of drug absorption.

The time course of drug concentration in plasma can usually be regarded as a statistical distribution curve [1]. Irrespective of the route of administration, the first three (zero to second) moments are defined as follows:

$$AUC = \int_0^\infty C \, dt \tag{11.1}$$

$$MRT = \frac{\int_0^\infty tC \, dt}{\int_0^\infty C \, dt} = \frac{AUMC}{AUC} \tag{11.2}$$

$$VRT = \frac{\int_0^\infty t^2 C \, dt}{\int_0^\infty C \, dt} = \frac{\int_0^\infty (t - MRT)^2 \, C \, dt}{AUC} \tag{11.3}$$

where MRT is the mean residence time and VRT is the variance of the mean residence time of a drug in the body. AUC, MRT, and VRT are termed the zero, first, and second moment, respectively, of the drug concentration-time curve. The area under the curve of a plot of the product of concentration and time versus time from zero time to infinity is often referred to as the area under the (first) moment curve, AUMC [7]. The moments defined above can be calculated by numerical integration using the trapezoidal rule (see App. D) from concentration-time data following drug administration. Only the zero and first moments have been used in pharmacokinetic analysis because the higher moments are prone to an unacceptable level of computational error.

In the usual single-dose pharmacokinetic study, blood sampling is stopped at some time t^* when drug concentration, C^*, is measurable. Hence, estimation of the area under the blood level-time curve from zero time to infinity, AUC, must be carried out in two steps. The area under the curve from zero time to t^* is calculated by means of the trapezoidal rule. To this partial area we must add the area under the curve from t^* to infinity, which is usually estimated as follows:

$$\int_{t*}^{\infty} C \, dt = \frac{C*}{\lambda_n} \tag{11.4}$$

where λ_n is 2.303 times the slope of the terminal exponential phase of a plot of log drug concentration versus time. The sum of the two partial areas is AUC.

The same approach must be used to estimate total AUMC. The area under the first moment curve from t* to infinity is estimated as follows [7]:

$$\int_{t*}^{\infty} tC \, dt = \frac{t*C*}{\lambda_n} + \frac{C*}{\lambda_n^2} \tag{11.5}$$

BIOAVAILABILITY

Bioavailability often refers to the fraction (F) of an oral dose that actually reaches the systemic circulation. Since the availability of an intravenous dose is usually unity, we can estimate F as follows:

$$F = \frac{D_{i.v.} AUC_{oral}}{D_{oral} AUC_{i.v.}} \tag{11.6}$$

Hence, F is simply the ratio of the zero moments after oral and intravenous (i.v.) administration, respectively, adjusted for differences in the size of the dose. Equation (11.6) assumes equal clearances in the oral and intravenous studies. The fraction of the oral dose available relative to a standard other than an intravenous injection (F_r) may be estimated by means of a similar equation.

CLEARANCE

Increasingly, clearance is viewed as the single most important parameter to describe the pharmacokinetics of a drug. One can define clearance as the reciprocal of the zero moment of a blood level-time curve normalized for dose. In other words,

$$Cl = \frac{D_{i.v.}}{AUC} \tag{11.7}$$

Clearance is usually calculated after an intravenous dose ($D_{i.v.}$) of a drug, but may sometimes be calculated after intramuscular administration. Clearance cannot be estimated after oral administration of a drug unless it can be assured that the total dose reaches the systemic circulation.

For drugs that are completely absorbed from the gastrointestinal tract and that are eliminated only by metabolism in the liver, the ratio of oral dose to AUC is equal to the hepatic intrinsic clearance of the drug. Under certain conditions intrinsic clearance may be related to the V_{max} and K_m of the drug-metabolizing enzyme process.

HALF-LIFE

The first moment of the blood level-time curve, mean residence time, is the statistical moment analogy to half-life ($t_{1/2}$). In effect, the MRT represents the time for 63.2% of the administered dose to be eliminated. Therefore, the MRT of a drug that can be described by a one-compartment model after intravenous administration is given by the following equation [3]:

$$MRT_{i.v.} = \frac{1}{K}$$ (11.8)

where K is the first-order elimination rate constant. It follows that

$$t_{1/2} = 0.693 \cdot MRT_{i.v.}$$ (11.9)

The MRT of a drug that distributes slowly and requires multi-compartment characterization is a function of the model rate constants for distribution and elimination. However, in noncompartmental terms the following relationship is useful [7].

$$MRT_{i.v.} = \frac{1}{\overline{K}}$$ (11.10)

where $\overline{K}$ is a first-order rate constant equal to the ratio of clearance to apparent volume of distribution at steady state (V_{ss}). For drugs requiring multicompartment characterization, $\lambda_1 < \overline{K} < \lambda_n$. It may be appropriate in most instances to consider the product of 0.693 and $MRT_{i.v.}$ as the *effective* half-life of a drug requiring a multicompartment model.

Irrespective of the distribution characteristics of drug, MRT represents the time for 63.2% of a intravenous bolus dose to be eliminated. As such, it may be possible to estimate MRT from urinary excretion data alone by determining the time required to excrete 63.2% of that amount of the dose which is ultimately excreted in the urine.

Mean residence time is a function of how a drug is administered. MRT values for noninstantaneous administrations will always be greater than the MRT following intravenous bolus administration. However, $MRT_{i.v.}$ may sometimes be estimated following other modes of drug administration. For example, following a short-term constant-rate intravenous infusion, the first moment of the blood level-time curve is given by

$$MRT_{inf} = MRT_{i.v.} + \frac{T}{2} \qquad (11.11)$$

where T is the infusion time. Therefore, MRT_{inf} can be calculated from the data according to Eq. (11.2), and $MRT_{i.v.}$ may be estimated by rearranging Eq. (11.11).

ABSORPTION KINETICS

Statistical moment methods for estimating rates of absorption after oral or intramuscular administration of a drug are based on differences in mean residence times after different modes of administration [5]. In general,

$$MAT = MRT_{ni} - MRT_{i.v.} \qquad (11.12)$$

where MAT is the mean absorption time, MRT_{ni} is the mean residence time after administration of the drug in a noninstantaneous manner, and $MRT_{i.v.}$ is the mean residence time after intravenous bolus administration.

When drug absorption can be described by a single first-order process,

$$MAT = \frac{1}{k_a} \qquad (11.13)$$

where k_a is the apparent first-order absorption rate constant. Under these conditions the absorption half-life is given by

$$Absorption\ t_{1/2} = 0.693 \cdot MAT \qquad (11.14)$$

When drug absorption is a zero-order process,

$$MAT = \frac{T}{2} \qquad (11.15)$$

where T is the time over which absorption takes place.

Deconvolution, described in Chap. 4, is another example of the application of statistical moment theory for the estimation of absorption kinetics. Riegelman and Collier [6] have applied statistical moment theory to the gastrointestinal absorption of a drug after oral administration of a solid dosage form. Their analysis permits the estimation of a mean dissolution time of a drug from its dosage form.

APPARENT VOLUME OF DISTRIBUTION

Of the many parameters used to describe drug distribution, the most useful is the apparent volume of distribution at steady state, V_{ss}.

According to statistical moment theory [3,7], V_{ss} is simply the product of clearance and mean residence time, after a single intravenous bolus dose of a drug. Therefore,

$$V_{ss} = Cl \cdot MRT = \frac{D_{i.v.} \cdot AUMC}{AUC^2} \tag{11.16}$$

Although Eq. (11.16) applies only to intravenous bolus administration, the relationship can be modified easily to accommodata other modes of drug administration [8]. If a drug is given by a short-term constant rate intravenous infusion [9], then

$$V_{ss} = \frac{infused\ dose \cdot AUMC}{AUC^2} - \frac{infused\ dose \cdot T}{2 \cdot AUC} \tag{11.17}$$

where T is the infusion time. Since the infused dose is equal to the product of the zero-order infusion rate, k_0, and T, we can also express Eq. (11.17) as follows:

$$V_{ss} = \frac{k_0T \cdot AUMC}{AUC^2} - \frac{k_0T^2}{2 \cdot AUC} \tag{11.18}$$

FRACTION METABOLIZED

It is sometimes useful to know the fraction of a dose of a drug that is converted to a certain metabolite. An unambiguous estimation requires that a single dose of both drug and metabolite be admimistered [10]. Although statistical moment theory does not reduce the experimental difficulties in making this estimation, it does facilitate the analysis.

It can be shown that the fraction metabolized, F_m, to a specific metabolite is simply equal to the ratio of the zero moment of the metabolite level-time curve after administering the drug to the zero moment of the metabolite level-time curve after administering an equimolar dose of the metabolite [10]:

$$F_m = \frac{AUC'_x}{AUC'} \tag{11.19}$$

where AUC'_x is the area under the curve of metabolite concentration in plasma versus time from zero time to infinity after an intravenous dose of the drug, and AUC' is the total area under the metabolite concentration-time curve after an equimolar intravenous dose of the metabolite.

PREDICTING STATE-STATE CONCENTRATIONS

When a dose of a drug is repetitively given at regular intervals, the area under the drug concentration-time curve during a dosing interval at steady state is equal to the total area under the curve after a single dose. Therefore, we can demonstrate that the average drug concentration at steady state, which is equal to the area under the drug level-time curve during a single dosing interval at steady state divided by the duration of the dosing interval, can be estimated after a single dose of the drug according to the following equation:

$$\overline{C} = \frac{AUC}{\tau} \qquad (11.20)$$

where AUC is the total area under the curve after a single dose and τ is the dosing interval.

The ratio of metabolite to drug concentration at steady state can also be predicted after a single dose of the drug [11,12]. This requires determination of the zero moment of both the metabolite level- and drug level-time curves after administering the drug (see Chap. 8).

PREDICTING TIME TO STEADY STATE

To carry out a pharmacokinetic analysis at steady state, or to determine whether a patient is stabilized after continuous administration of a drug, we must be able to estimate the time required for the drug concentrations in plasma to reach some substantial fraction (e.g., 90-99%) of the steady-state concentration. For drugs that distribute rapidly and can be described by a one-compartment model, the time to reach a certain fraction of steady state is a relatively simple function of the half-life of a drug. The situation is more complicated for drugs that require multicompartment characterization. Statistical moment theory provides a unique solution to this problem. Chiou [13] has recently shown that by means of area analysis one can predict the time to reach a given fraction of steady state from a single dose administered in the same way that will be used for repetitive dosing. In essence, the time required, after giving a single dose, for the partial area under the curve, AUC_0^t, to be equal to a certain fraction of the total area under the curve, AUC, is the same as the time required to reach the same fraction of steady-state on repetitive dosing of the drug [14]. This relationship is expressed in the following equation:

$$f_{ss} = \frac{AUC_0^t}{AUC} \qquad (11.21)$$

where f_{ss} is the fraction of the steady-state reached at time t on repetitive dosing, and the area terms refer to a single dose.

CONCLUSIONS

This overview of noncompartmental methods based on statistical moment theory, albeit circumscribed, is sufficient in our view to demonstrate the power of the approach. It is evident that statistical moment theory permits a wide range of analyses that, in most instances, will be adequate to characterize the pharmacokinetics of a drug.

There are, of course, certain problems that are not addressed by this theory. Nonlinear events are not adequately treated at this time by statistical moment theory. Statistical moments provide only limited information regarding the time course of drug concentrations; for the most part, we deal with averages. However, we point out that other types of noncompartmental methods such as superposition (see App. E) can be used to augment statistical moment theory in this case.

We strongly suspect that future developments will remove many of the limitations that now exist. We predict that these trends in pharmacokinetic analysis, coupled with the impressive developments in microcomputer technology, will remove the reliance on main frame computers and may make compartmental analysis a matter of historical interest.

REFERENCES

1. D. M. Himmelblau and K. B. Bischoff. Process analysis and simulation. In *Deterministic Systems,* Wiley, New York, 1968.
2. W. Perl and P. Samuel. Input-ouput analysis for total input rate and total traced mass of body cholesterol in man. *Cir. Res.* 25:191 (1969).
3. J. H. Oppenheimer, H. L. Schwartz, and M. I. Surks. Determination of common parameters of iodothyronine metabolism and distribution in man by noncompartmental analysis. *J. Clin. Endocrinol. Metab.* 41:319 (1975).
4. K. Yamaoka, T. Nakagawa, and T. Uno. Statistical moments in pharmacokinetics. *J. Pharmacokin. Biopharm.* 6:547 (1978).
5. D. J. Cutler. Theory of the mean absorption time, an adjunct to conventional bioavailability studies. *J. Pharm. Pharmacol.* 30:476 (1978).
6. S. Riegelman and P. Collier. The application of statistical moment theory to the evaluation of in vivo dissolution time and absorption time. *J. Pharmacokin. Biopharm.* 8:509 (1980).
7. L. Z. Benet and R. L. Galeazzi. Noncompartmental determination of the steady-state volume of distribution. *J. Pharm. Sci.* 68:1071 (1979).
8. D. Perrier and M. Mayersohn. Noncompartmental determination of the steady-state volume of distribution for any mode of administration. *J. Pharm. Sci.* 71:372 (1982).

9. C. S. Lee, D. C. Brater, J. G. Gambertoglio, and L. Z. Benet. Disposition kinetics of ethambutol in man. *J. Pharmacokin. Biopharm.* *8*:335 (1980).

10. S. A. Kaplan, M. L. Jack, S. Cotler, and K. Alexander. Utilization of area under the curve to elucidate the disposition of an extensively biotransformed drug. *J. Pharmacokin. Biopharm.* *1*:201 (1973).

11. E. A. Lane and R. Levy. Prediction of steady-state behavior of metabolite from dosing of parent drug. *J. Pharm. Sci.* *69*:610 (1980).

12. E. A. Lane and R. Levy. Metabolite to parent drug concentration ratio as a function of parent drug extraction ratio: Cases of nonportal route of administration. *J. Pharmacokin. Biopharm.* *9*:489 (1981).

13. W. L. Chiou. Rapid compartment- and model-independent estimation of times required to attain various fractions of steady-state plasma level during multiple dosing of drugs obeying superposition principle and having various absorption or infusion kinetics *J. Pharm. Sci.* *68*:1546 (1979).

14. D. Perrier and M. Gibaldi. General derivation of the equation for the time to reach a certain fraction of steady-state. *J. Pharm. Sci.* *71*:474 (1982).

Appendix A
Method of Laplace Transforms

Rate equations that describe apparent zero-order or first-order processes are termed linear equations. The Laplace transform is used for solving linear differential equations and hence is applicable to the solution of many equations used for pharmacokinetic analysis. A rigorous mathematical development of the Laplace transform method will not be provided herein. However, the basic idea of the method and its application in solving relatively simple differential equations in pharmacokinetics will be examined. For a more detailed treatment, the reader is referred to several books [1–3] and particularly to a programmed text [4] that should prove useful.

Essentially what the Laplace transform does is replace the time domain of a rate expression by the complex domain of the Laplace operator s. This is achieved by eliminating the independent variable (in pharmacokinetics this variable is always time) and replacing it with the Laplace operator. The Laplace transform enables complex rate expressions to be manipulated easily by conventional algebraic techniques once the time variable has been replaced by the Laplace operator s. Since most problems fall into certain patterns, the transformed expression may be rearranged into a form that can generally be found in a table of Laplace transforms. Values for initial conditions may be included in the transformed expression. Consequently, upon transformation back into the time domain, the complete solution to the differential equation is obtained.

The means by which a time-dependent expression is transformed into the s domain is given by the Laplace integral $Lf(t)$, which is defined by

$$Lf(t) = \int_0^\infty e^{-st} f(t)\, dt \tag{A.1}$$

where $f(t)$ is the time-dependent function. Thus the function is multiplied by e^{-st}, and this product is evaluated by integration from time zero to time infinity.

The Laplace transform of several expressions will be derived using the Laplace integral simply to illustrate how the transforms are obtained. However, once certain transformed functions that are used repeatedly in pharmacokinetics are established, the use of the integral may be dispensed with for future transformations simply by constructing an appropriate table of transforms and referring to this table for the transform of the desired time-dependent expression. For example, to obtain the transform of a constant A, the Laplace integral can be applied:

$$L(A) = \int_0^\infty e^{-st} A \, dt \tag{A.2}$$

which when integrated becomes

$$L(A) = A\left(-\frac{1}{s}\right) e^{-st} \Big|_0^\infty \tag{A.3}$$

Evaluation of this equation between the limits of time zero and infinity yields

$$L(A) = \frac{A}{s} \tag{A.4}$$

Thus the transform of any constant will take the form given in Eq. (A.4). The transform of the constant k_0, for example, will simply be k_0/s. Initially, derivation of the transform of a function requires some knowledge of integral calculus. However, once these transforms are known, no integration is required.

The transformation of an exponential function is also readily accomplished. Proceeding as before, the Laplace integral may be applied to the function e^{-at}:

$$L(e^{-at}) = \int_0^\infty e^{-st}(e^{-at}) \, dt = \int_0^\infty e^{-(s+a)t} \, dt \tag{A.5}$$

which when integrated yields

$$L(e^{-at}) = -\frac{1}{s+a} e^{-(s+a)t} \Big|_0^\infty = \frac{1}{s+a} \tag{A.6}$$

If this exponential is multiplied by a constant, for example Ae^{-at}, the resulting transform is found to be $A/(s+a)$.

A function that is used quite often is the derivative expression $df(t)/dt$. The Laplace integral is

$$L \frac{df(t)}{dt} = \int_0^\infty e^{-st} \frac{df(t)}{dt} \, dt \tag{A.7}$$

Solving this integral by integration by parts yields

$$\int_0^\infty e^{-st} \frac{df(t)}{dt} \, dt = e^{-st} f(t) \Big|_0^\infty - \int_0^\infty - se^{-st} f(t) \, dt \tag{A.8}$$

since

$$\int_a^b h(x) \frac{dg(x)}{dx} dx = h(x)g(x) \Big|_a^b - \int_a^b \frac{dh(x)}{dx} g(x) \, dx \tag{A.9}$$

and

$$\frac{de^{-st}}{dt} = -se^{-st} \tag{A.10}$$

Equation (A.8) may be simplified to

$$\int_0^\infty e^{-st} \frac{df(t)}{dt} \, dt = -f(0) + \int_0^\infty e^{-st} f(t) \, dt \tag{A.11}$$

In this equation $\int_0^\infty e^{-st} f(t) \, dt$ equals $Lf(t)$ [see (A.1)]. Therefore,

$$\int_0^\infty e^{-st} \frac{df(t)}{dt} \, dt = -f(0) + sLf(t) \tag{A.12}$$

Hence the Laplace transform of $df(t)/dt$ is given by

$$L \frac{df(t)}{dt} = sLf(t) - f(0) \tag{A.13}$$

where $f(t)$ is the time-dependent function we are interested in finding, $df(t)/dt$ is the derivative of this function (as in a rate expression, for example dC/dt), and $f(0)$ is the value of the function at time zero (initial condition).

The approach outlined above has been used in determining the Laplace transforms of many functions. Some of the most useful of these are presented in Table A.1. On the left side of the table are the time-domain functions that are commonly encountered in rate expressions. The corresponding, s-domain, Laplace transforms are shown on the right side of Table A.1, opposite their time functions.

There are examples throughout Chap. 1 illustrating the use of the method of Laplace transforms for solving linear differential equations. The derivation of the expression describing the time course of the amount of drug in the body during zero-order intravenous infusion will be presented here to illustrate the steps that should be followed in solving such equations. Initially, the rate expression for the species of interest should be written. In this example the rate expression is

$$\frac{dX}{dt} = k_0 - KX \tag{A.14}$$

Table A.1 Laplace Transforms of Some Common Functions

Function, $F(t)$	Laplace Transform, $f(s)$
1	$\dfrac{1}{s}$
A	$\dfrac{A}{s}$
t	$\dfrac{1}{s^2}$
t^m	$\dfrac{m!}{s^{m+1}}$
Ae^{-at}	$\dfrac{A}{s+a}$
Ate^{-at}	$\dfrac{A}{(s+a)^2}$
$\dfrac{A}{a}(1 - e^{-at})$	$\dfrac{A}{s(s+a)}$
$\dfrac{A}{a}e^{-(b/a)t}$	$\dfrac{A}{as+b}$
$\dfrac{(B - Aa)e^{-at} - (B - Ab)e^{-bt}}{b-a} \quad (b \neq a)$	$\dfrac{As+B}{(s+a)(s+b)}$
$\dfrac{A}{b-a}(e^{-at} - e^{-bt})$	$\dfrac{A}{(s+a)(s+b)}$
$e^{-at}[A + (B - Aa)t]$	$\dfrac{As+B}{(s+a)^2}$
$-\dfrac{1}{PQR}[P(Aa^2 - Ba + C)e^{-at}$ $+ Q(Ab^2 - Bb + C)e^{-bt} + R(Ac^2 - Bc + C)e^{-ct}]$ $(P = b - c,\ Q = c - a,\ R = a - b)$	$\dfrac{As^2 + Bs + C}{(s+a)(s+b)(s+c)}$
$A\left[\dfrac{1}{ab} + \dfrac{1}{a(a-B)}e^{-at} - \dfrac{1}{b(a-b)}e^{-bt}\right]$	$\dfrac{A}{s(s+a)(s+b)}$
$\dfrac{A}{a}t - \dfrac{A}{a^2}(1 - e^{-at})$	$\dfrac{A}{s^2(s+a)}$
$\dfrac{B}{ab} - \dfrac{Aa - B}{a(a-b)}e^{-at} + \dfrac{Ab - B}{b(a-b)}e^{-bt}$	$\dfrac{As+B}{s(s+a)(s+b)}$
$\dfrac{B}{ab} - \dfrac{a^2 - Aa + B}{a(b-a)}e^{-at} + \dfrac{b^2 - Ab + B}{b(b-a)}e^{-bt}$	$\dfrac{s^2 + As + B}{s(s+a)(s+b)}$

From Ref. 5.

where X is the amount of drug in the body, k_0 the zero-order infusion rate, and K the apparent first-order rate constant for elimination of drug from the body. Taking the Laplace transform of each term yields

$$sLf(X) - X(0) = \frac{k_0}{s} - KLf(X) \tag{A.15}$$

For simplicity in writing such transformed expressions, the following convention will be employed. A bar will be placed over the dependent variable that is being transformed. Thus

$$s\overline{X} - X(0) = \frac{k_0}{s} - K\overline{X} \tag{A.16}$$

This greatly facilitates representation of transformed expressions.

The symbol X_0 or D (dose) rather than $X(0)$ is generally employed for the initial amount of X present at time zero. In the present example X_0 equals zero since there is no drug in the body at time zero. Setting $X(0)$ equal to zero in (A.16) and solving for $\overline{X}$ yields

$$\overline{X} = \frac{k_0}{s(s + K)} \tag{A.17}$$

which is the transform of the desired quantity X. An expression identical in form to the right-hand side of (A.17) may be found under the column for Laplace transforms in Table A.1. This expression is $A/s(s + a)$.

The time-dependent function $F(t)$ for this transform is $A(1 - e^{-at})/a$ (see Table A.1). Since k_0 is A and K is a, the expression for the amount of drug in the body X as a function of time following intravenous infusion may be readily written

$$X = \frac{k_0}{K} (1 - e^{-Kt}) \tag{A.18}$$

This equation is the complete solution to the differential equation given in (A.14).

REFERENCES

1. N. F. Nixon. *Handbook of Laplace Transformation: Fundamentals, Application, Tables, and Examples,* 2nd ed. Prentice-Hall, Englewood Cliffs, N.J., 1965.
2. N. F. Nixon. *Handbook of Laplace Transformation: Fundamentals, Applications, Tables, and Examples—Workbook* (with answers), 2nd ed. Prentice-Hall, Englewood Cliffs, N.J., 1965.

3.   H. S. Bear, Jr. *Differential Equations.* Addison-Wesley,
     Reading, Mass., 1962.
4.   R. D. Strum and J. R. Ward. *Laplace Transformation Solutions
     of Differential Equations: A Programmed Text.* Prentice-Hall,
     Englewood Cliffs, N.J., 1968.
5.   A. Rescigno and G. Segre. *Drug and Tracer Kinetics,* Blaisdell,
     Waltham, Mass., 1966, p. 204.

Appendix B
Method for Solving Linear Mammillary Models

A method is available which permits, by means of some very simple general treatments, the derivation of equations for any linear mammillary compartment model with any first- or zero-order, or bolus (instantaneous) input process. This is accomplished by the use of (1) general input and disposition functions, (2) a method for solving partial fractions to obtain solutions to Laplace transforms, and (3) a multiple-dosing function. The input function and the disposition function are defined such that the product of these two functions yields the Laplace transform of the equation describing the time course of a drug in a model compartment. A disposition function defines the model necessary to describe drug levels in the body or a compartment thereof. Disposition describes everything that happens to a drug (i.e., distribution and elimination through all possible routes) when input into the system occurs instantaneously. Input functions describe the processes necessary to get the drug into the body. They may either describe an intravenous bolus injection, an intravenous infusion, or first- or zero-order absorption from a site such as the gastrointestinal tract or a muscle.

The following general equation has been empirically derived to describe the Laplace transform for the disposition function of the central compartment in a linear N-compartment mammillary model where elimination of drug from any compartment is allowed:

$$d_{s,c} = \frac{\displaystyle\prod_{i=2}^{N} (s + E_i)}{\displaystyle\prod_{i=1}^{N} (s + E_i) - \sum_{j=2}^{N} \left[k_{1j} k_{j1} \prod_{\substack{m=2 \\ m \neq j}}^{N} (s + E_m) \right]} \qquad (B.1)$$

In this equation:

$d_{s,c}$ = disposition function for compartment 1, the central compartment; it is a function of s, the Laplace operator (see Appendix A)

Π = continued product where any term is defined as equal to 1 when the index takes a forbidden value; that is, i = 1 in the numerator or m = j in the denominator

Σ = continued summation where any term is defined as equal to zero when the index takes a forbidden value

k_{1j}, k_{j1} = first-order intercompartmental transfer rate constants

E_i, E_m = sum of the exit rate constants out of compartments i or m

N = number of driving force compartments in the disposition model (i.e., compartments having exit rate constants)

This equation has been employed in the text for the determination of disposition functions for several multicompartment models.

The following input functions describe the usual ways drugs get to the systemic circulation: intravenous bolus, in_s = dose; first-order absorption, $in_s = k_a \, dose/(s + k_a)$, where k_a is the first-order absorption rate constant. The input function for absorption may describe absorption from any site but will usually be used for either oral or intramuscular dosing. The term "dose" in this input function refers to the amount of drug that actually gets into the system as such. Frequently, an F may appear in equations describing oral dosing, where F is the systemic availability of the drug. For intravenous infusion or zero-order absorption, $in_s = k_0(e^{-t_0 s} - e^{-Ts})_s$, where k_0 is the zero-order infusion rate in units of amount per time and t_0 and T are the times when infusion begins and ends, respectively. In most cases, the intravenous infusion begins at time zero (t_0 = 0) and, therefore, the input function for intravenous infusion is generally $in_s = k_0(1 - e^{-Ts})/s$. This input function may be used to define zero-order input from the gastrointestinal tract as well as constant rate intravenous infusion. Input functions may also be combined if a drug is given by more than one route of administration. For example, it is common to given an intravenous bolus injection of a drug to produce therapeutic blood levels quickly followed by a zero-order infusion so that these blood levels may be maintained. In this case, the input function in_s would equal dose + $k_0(1 - e^{-Ts})/s$ if the infusion began at the same time that the bolus injection was administered.

The product of the input and disposition functions yields the Laplace transform for the amount of drug in the central compartment, $a_{s,c}$:

$$a_{s,c} = in_s d_{s,c} \tag{B.2}$$

The anti-Laplace of the resulting transform may be found in an extensive table of Laplace transforms. However, the method of partial fractions is generally easier to apply. The use of a general partial fraction theorem for obtaining inverse Laplace transforms, denoted L^{-1}, has been described [1]. If the quotient of two polynomials $P(s)/Q(s)$ is such that $Q(s)$ has a higher degree and contains the factor $s - \Lambda_i$, which is not repeated, then

$$L^{-1} \frac{P(s)}{Q(s)} = \sum_{i=1}^{N} \frac{P(\Lambda_i)}{Q_i(\Lambda_i)} e^{\Lambda_i t} \tag{B.3}$$

where Λ_i's are the roots of the polynomial $Q(s)$. $Q_i(\Lambda_i)$ is the value of the denominator when Λ_i is substituted for all s terms except for the term originally containing Λ_i, this term being omitted. The $P(\Lambda_i)$ terms are obtained by substitution of the appropriate root for every value of s in the numerator. If a repeating function appears in the denominator, an alternative approach discussed in Ref. 2 must be used. The complex symbolism of Eq. (B.3) will be clarified in the following illustration.

To illustrate the application of this approach for solving linear differential equations, a two-compartment model with zero-order input will be employed. This model is represented by the following scheme:

where k_0 is the zero-order infusion rate constant, k_{12} and k_{21} are apparent first-order intercompartmental rate constants, and k_{10} is the apparent first-order elimination rate constant from the central compartment. The disposition function for the central compartment can readily be written by setting N equal to 2, in Eq. (B.1), since there are two driving force compartments in a two-compartment model. Hence

$$d_{s,c} = \frac{s + E_2}{(s + E_1)(s + E_2) - k_{12}k_{21}} \tag{B.4}$$

where E_1 and E_2 are the sum of the exit rate constants from the central and peripheral compartments, respectively, that is, $E_1 = k_{10} + k_{12}$ and $E_2 = k_{21}$.

A term with s to the second power appears in the denominator of Eq. (B.4), since there are two driving force compartments in the model. As a result, the equation describing the disposition function for the central compartment is biexponential. Therefore, Eq. (B.4) may be rewritten

$$d_{s,c} = \frac{s + E_2}{(s + \lambda_1)(s + \lambda_2)} \tag{B.5}$$

The constants λ_1 and λ_2 may be expressed in terms of the individual rate constants when the denominators of (B.4) and (B.5) are expanded in terms of the coefficients of the powers of s.

Multiplication of this disposition function by the input function for an intravenous infusion beginning at time zero [i.e., $in_s = k_0(1 - e^{-Ts})/s$] yields the following Laplace transform for the amount of drug in the central compartment:

$$a_{s,c} = \frac{k_0(s + E_2)(1 - e^{-Ts})}{s(s + \lambda_1)(s + \lambda_2)} \tag{B.6}$$

The two polynomials in this equation fulfill the requirements for the use of (B.3). Hence the solution for the amount of drug in the central compartment X_c as a function of time may be readily written

$$X_c = \frac{k_0(E_2 - \lambda_1)(1 - e^{\lambda_1 T})}{-\lambda_1(\lambda_2 - \lambda_1)} e^{-\lambda_1 t} + \frac{k_0(E_2 - \lambda_2)(1 - e^{\lambda_2 T})}{-\lambda_2(\lambda_1 - \lambda_2)} e^{-\lambda_2 t} \tag{B.7}$$

Note that even though there are three roots $(0, -\lambda_1, \text{ and } -\lambda_2)$ in the denominator of (B.6), there are only two terms in (B.7). This is because the numerator of (B.6) becomes zero when the root zero is substituted for every value of s. It should also be noted that (B.7), a single equation, describes the amount of drug in the central compartment as a function of time while infusion is being carried out and after infusion stops. While infusion is continuing, T = t and varies with time. However, when infusion ceases, T becomes a constant corresponding to the time infusion was stopped.

Haborak et al. [3] have pointed out that although the constant rate infusion input function leads to a correct equation for the time course of drug in the central compartment [Eq. (B.7)], the approach is technically incorrect because the presence of the term $1 - e^{-Ts}$ in the numerator of (B.6) destroys the polynomial character of the numerator. Benet [4] acknowledges this discrepancy but suggests that apparently the restriction concerning the polynomial character of the numerator may be relaxed when exponential functions appear in the numerator due to the inclusion of a zero-order input function. The approach outlined above gives the correct equations for the usual multicompartment pharmacokinetic models with zero-order input into the central or peripheral compartments.

A mammillary model may also be solved for compartments other than the central compartment. For example, to obtain an equation that would describe the time course of drug in the peripheral compartment of a two-compartment model following intravenous infusion, the following approach can be employed. The differential equation describing the peripheral compartment is

$$\frac{dX_p}{dt} = k_{12}X_c - k_{21}X_p \qquad (B.8)$$

where X_p is the amount of drug in the peripheral compartment and k_{12}, k_{21}, and X_c are as defined previously. Taking the Laplace transform of (B.8) yields

$$s(a_{s,p}) = k_{12}a_{s,c} - k_{21}a_{s,p} \qquad (B.9)$$

where $a_{s,p}$ is the Laplace transform for the amount of drug in the peripheral compartment. Solving this equation for $a_{s,p}$ and substituting the value of $a_{s,c}$ as given in (B.6) into the resulting equation yields the following expression for $a_{s,p}$:

$$a_{s,p} = \frac{k_{12}k_0(s + E_2)(1 - e^{-Ts})}{s(s + k_{21})(s + \lambda_1)(s + \lambda_2)} \qquad (B.10)$$

Since E_2 equals, k_{21}, Eq. (B.10) reduces to

$$a_{s,p} = \frac{k_{12}k_0(1 - e^{-Ts})}{s(s + \lambda_1)(s + \lambda_2)} \qquad (B.11)$$

This equation can be readily solved for the amount of drug in the peripheral compartment employing the method of partial fractions [i.e., Eq. (B.3)]. Hence

$$X_p = \frac{k_{12}k_0(1 - e^{\lambda_1 T})}{-\lambda_1(\lambda_2 - \lambda_1)} e^{-\lambda_1 t} + \frac{k_{12}k_0(1 - e^{\lambda_2 T})}{-\lambda_2(\lambda_1 - \lambda_2)} e^{-\lambda_2 t} \qquad (B.12)$$

It has been shown [5] that any equation describing the time course of drug in a driving force compartment after a single dose may be changed into a multiple-dose equation by multiplying each exponential term containing t (time), $e^{-k_i t}$, by the function

$$\frac{e^{(n-1)k_i\tau} - e^{-k_i\tau}}{1 - e^{-k_i\tau}}$$

where τ is the constant dosing interval, k_i is the apparent first-order rate constant in each exponential term, and n equals the number of doses. It can be demonstrated that

$$\frac{e^{(n-1)k_i\tau} - e^{-k_i\tau}}{1 - e^{-k_i\tau}}e^{-k_i t} = \frac{1 - e^{-nk_i\tau}}{1 - e^{-k_i\tau}}e^{-k_i[t-(n-1)\tau]}$$

$$= \frac{1 - e^{-nk_i\tau}}{1 - e^{-k_i\tau}}e^{-k_i t'} \qquad\qquad (B.13)$$

where $t' = t - (n - 1)\tau$, the time since the last dose was given (i.e., the time during a dosing interval where $0 \leq t' \leq \tau$). The application of the function

$$\frac{1 - e^{-nk_i\tau}}{1 - e^{-k_i\tau}}$$

for converting single-dose equations to multiple-dose equations is discussed in Chap. 3.

In addition to the material covered in this appendix, a situation where one mammillary model serves as an input function into a second mammillary model has also been considered [2].

A model that has appeared in the pharmacokinetic literature and may not be solved employing the techniques presented in this appendix is depicted in the following scheme:

In this model k_{12}, k_{21}, k_{13}, and k_{31} are apparent first-order inter-compartmental rate constants, k_a is an apparent first-order absorption rate constant, and k_{20} is the apparent first-order elimination rate constant of drug from the hepatoportal system. This particular model has been employed to describe the disposition of a drug subject to first-pass metabolism following oral drug administration. Since drug enters the body via the hepatoportal compartment, this model behaves mathematically like a catenary rather than a mammillary system. The method of Laplace transforms (Appendix A) can be used to obtain a solution. A general treatment of simultaneous input into and elimination from a peripheral compartment has been described by Vaughan and Trainor [6].

REFERENCES

1. L. Z. Benet and J. S. Turi. Use of a general partial fraction theorem for obtaining inverse Laplace transforms in pharmacokinetic analysis. *J. Pharm. Sci.* *60*:1593 (1971).
2. L. Z. Benet. General treatment of linear mammillary models with elimination from any compartment as used in pharmacokinetics. *J. Pharm. Sci.* *61*:536 (1972).
3. G. E. Haborak, J. D. Bennaman, and J. W. Warren, Jr. Mathematical treatment of linear mammillary models using inverse Laplace transforms. *J. Pharm. Sci.* *68*:932 (1979).
4. L. Z. Benet. Mathematical treatment of linear mammillary models using inverse Laplace transforms: A reply. *J. Pharm. Sci.* *68*:933 (1979).
5. F. H. Dost. *Der Blutspiegel.* Georg Thieme, Leipzig, East Germany, 1953, pp. 252--255.
6. D. P. Vaughan and A. Trainor. Derivation of general equations for linear mammillary models when the drug is administered by different routes. *J. Pharmacokin. Biopharm.* *3*:203 (1975).

Appendix C
Method of Residuals

The method of residuals is a commonly used technique in pharmacokinetics for resolving a curve into its various exponential components.
The terms feathering, peeling, and stripping are also used to describe
this technique. Application of the method of residuals is probably
most clearly illustrated by employing specific numerical examples.
Hence four examples have been selected to demonstrate the application of this technique.

The first example is the case where a drug administered orally
is absorbed by apparent first-order kinetics and confers the characteristics of a one-compartment model on the body. The following
equation has been employed to describe the time course of such a
drug in the body:

$$C = \frac{k_a F X_0}{V(k_a - k)} (e^{-Kt} - e^{-k_a t})$$

(C.1)

where C is the plasma concentration of drug at any time t following
the administration of dose X_0, V is the apparent volume of distribution, F is the fraction of the orally administered dose which is absorbed, and k_a and K are the apparent first-order absorption and
elimination rate constants, respectively. Assuming that $k_a > K$, the
term $e^{-k_a t}$ in (C.1) will approach zero, whereas the term e^{-Kt} retains
a finite value. At some time (C.1) will reduce to

$$C = \frac{k_a F X_0}{V(k_a - K)} e^{-Kt}$$

(C.2)

which can be written in terms of common logarithms as follows:

$$\log C = \log \frac{k_a F X_0}{V(k_a - K)} - \frac{Kt}{2.303}$$

(C.3)

433

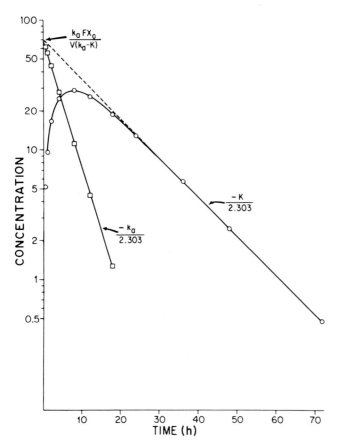

Fig. C.1 Drug concentration in plasma (O) after oral administration of a drug (see Table C.1). Residual values are denoted by (□). See Eqs. (C.1) to (C.5).

Based on these relationships, a plot of the logarithm of plasma drug concentration versus time following oral administration will be biexponential with a terminal linear phase having a slope of $-K/2.303$ (see Fig. C.1, which is a plot of the concentration-time data presented in Table C.1). Since the terminal linear phase is described by (C.3), extrapolation of this straight line to time zero will yield an intercept equal to log $[k_aFX_0/V(k_a - K)]$.

Subtraction of the true plasma drug concentration-time values in the absorptive phase from the corresponding concentration-time values on the extrapolated line yields a series of residual concentration values (see Table C.1). These residual values are described by the following equation, which is obtained by subtracting (C.1) from (C.2):

Table C.1 Application of the Method of Residuals to Data Obtained
After Oral Administration of a Drug

Time (h)	Plasma Concentration (μg/ml)	Extrapolated Concentration (μg/ml)	Residual Concentration (μg/ml)
0.5	5.36	69.0	63.64
1.0	9.95	66.5	56.55
2.0	17.18	62.5	45.32
4.0	25.78	54.0	28.22
8.0	29.78	41.2	11.42
12.0	26.63	31.2	4.57
18.0	19.40	20.7	1.30
24.0	13.26		
36.0	5.88		
48.0	2.56		
72.0	0.49		

Notes: First-order absorption and a one-compartment model are
assumed. $K = 0.0693 \text{ h}^{-1}$, $k_a = 0.231 \text{ h}^{-1}$, $V = 10$ liters, $X_0 = 500$
mg, $F = 1$.

$$C_r = \frac{k_a FX_0}{V(k_a - K)} e^{-k_a t} \qquad (C.4)$$

where C_r is the residual plasma concentration. In terms of common
logarithms Eq. (C.4) becomes

$$\log C_r = \log \frac{k_a FX_0}{V(k_a - K)} - \frac{k_a t}{2.303} \qquad (C.5)$$

Hence a plot of the logarithm of the residual concentrations versus
time will yield a straight line with a slope of $-k_a/2.303$ and a zero-
time intercept equal to $\log [k_a FX_0/V(k_a - K)]$. Application of the
method of residuals has enabled resolution of the plasma level-time
curve in Fig. C.1 into its two exponential components.

A second example is the resolution of a plasma concentration-time
curve obtained following intravenous administration of a drug that
confers multicompartment characteristics on the body. To illustrate
this type of curve, a two-compartment model is employed. The resulting curve can be described by the following biexponential equation:

$$C = Ae^{-\alpha t} + Be^{-\beta t} \qquad (C.6)$$

where α and β are the apparent first-order fast and slow disposition rate constants, respectively, and A and B are the corresponding zero-time intercepts. Since α is larger than β, by definition, the term $Ae^{-\alpha t}$ will approach zero more rapidly than will the term $Be^{-\beta t}$, and Eq. (C.6) will then reduce to

$$C = Be^{-\beta t} \qquad (C.7)$$

which in terms of common logarithms is

$$\log C = \log B - \frac{\beta t}{2.303} \qquad (C.8)$$

This equation describes the terminal linear phase of the curve resulting from a plot of the logarithm of plasma concentration versus time. This terminal linear phase has a slope of $-\beta/2.303$, and when extrapolated to zero yields an intercept of log B (see Fig. C.2).

By subtracting the concentration-time values on the extrapolated line from the corresponding true plasma concentration-time values, a series of residual concentration-time values will be obtained (see Table C.2). These residual concentrations C_r are described by

Table C.2 Application of the Method of Residuals to Data Obtained After Intravenous Administration of a Drug

Time (h)	Plasma Concentration ($\mu g/ml$)	Extrapolated Concentration ($\mu g/ml$)	Residual Concentration ($\mu g/ml$)
0.165	65.03	4.65	60.38
0.5	28.69	4.26	24.43
1.0	10.04	3.73	6.31
1.5	4.93	3.30	1.63
3.0	2.29		
5.0	1.36		
7.5	0.71		
10.0	0.38		

Notes: An instantaneous intravenous bolus dose and a two-compartment open model are assumed. A = 95 $\mu g/ml$, B = 4.85 $\mu g/ml$, $\alpha = 2.718$ h^{-1}, $\beta = 0.254$ h^{-1}, $X_0 = 1$ g.

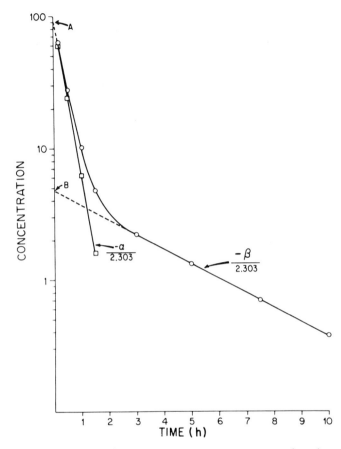

Fig. C.2 Drug concentration in plasma (O) after intravenous administration of a drug (see Table C.2). Residual values are denoted by
(□). See Eqs. (C.6) to (C.10).

$$C_r = Ae^{-\alpha t} \qquad\qquad (C.9)$$

which is arrived at by subtracting (C.7) from (C.6). When expressed
as common logarithms, Eq. (C.9) becomes

$$\log C_r = \log A - \frac{\alpha t}{2.303} \qquad\qquad (C.10)$$

Therefore, a plot of the logarithm of the residual concentration values
versus time will yield a straight line with a slope of $-\alpha/2.303$ and a
zero-time intercept of log A (see Fig. C.2). Resolution of the biexponential curve thereby enables the determination of all parameters
in Eq. (C.6), which will in turn permit the estimation of the two-

compartment model parameters k_{12}, k_{21}, k_{10}, and V_c (see Chap. 2).
The method of residuals can also be employed to resolve plasma-level
curves which require more than two exponentials for their description.

Urinary excretion data can also be resolved employing the method
of residuals. For example, following the oral administration of a drug
that confers the characteristics of a one-compartment model on the
body, the urinary excretion of unchanged drug can be evaluated employing the sigma-minus method according to the equation

$$X_u^\infty - X_u = \frac{X_u^\infty}{k_a - K}(k_a e^{-Kt} - Ke^{-k_a t}) \tag{C.11}$$

In this equation X_u^∞ and X_u are the cumulative amounts of unchanged
drug excreted in the urine to time infinity (i.e., at least seven half-
lives) and time t, respectively. The constants k_a and K are as defined previously in this appendix.

Absorption is generally assumed to occur at a faster rate than
elimination. Therefore, the term $Ke^{-k_a t}$ will approach zero while the
term $k_a e^{-Kt}$ has a finite value resulting in Eq. (C.11) reducing to

$$X_u^\infty - X_u = \frac{X_u^\infty k_a}{k_a - K} e^{-Kt} \tag{C.12}$$

Writing this equation in common logarithms yields

$$\log (X_u^\infty - X_u) = \log \frac{X_u^\infty k_a}{k_a - K} - \frac{Kt}{2.303} \tag{C.13}$$

Based on these relationships, if urine samples were collected at sufficiently frequent intervals immediately following oral administration,
a plot of $\log (X_u^\infty - X_u)$ versus time should result in a biexponential
curve with a terminal linear phase having a slope of $-K/2.303$. Extrapolation of this terminal phase to time zero will yield an intercept
of $\log [X_u^\infty k_a/(k_a - K)]$ (see Fig. C.3, which is a plot of the data
presented in Table C.3).

Subtracting the true $X_u^\infty - X_u$ values from the values on the extrapolated line at the same time period [i.e., (C.12) minus (C.13)]
yields a series of residual $X_u^\infty - X_u$ values (Table C.3) which can be
described by the equation

$$(X_u^\infty - X_u)_r = \frac{X_u^\infty K}{k_a - K} e^{-k_a t} \tag{C.14}$$

In this equation $(X_u^\infty - X_u)_r$ is the residual sigma-minus value. Writing
Eq. (C.14) in terms of common logarithms yields

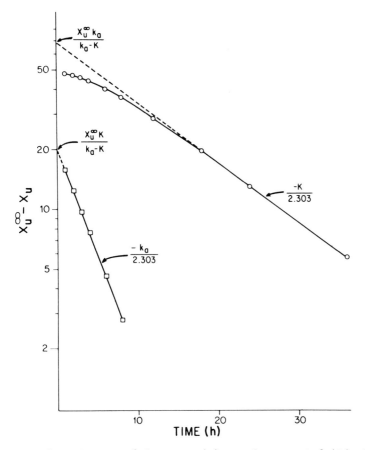

Fig. C.3 Amount of drug remaining to be excreted (O) after oral administration (see Table C.3). Residual values are denoted by (□). See Eqs. (C.11) to (C.15).

$$\log (X_u^\infty - X_u)_r = \log \frac{X_u^\infty K}{k_a - K} - \frac{k_a t}{2.303} \tag{C.15}$$

Therefore, by plotting the logarithm of the residual $X_u^\infty - X_u$ values [log $(X_u^\infty - X_u)_r$] versus time, a straight line with a slope of $-k_a/2.303$ and an intercept of log $[X_u^\infty K/(k_a - K)]$ would result (see Fig. C.3). The method of residuals, therefore, permits the resolution of a sigma-minus plot into its exponential components.

A final example illustrating the application of the method of residuals is the resolution of the plasma concentration-time curve of a

Table C.3 Application of the Method of Residuals to Urinary Excretion Data Obtained After Oral Administration of a Drug

Time (h)	X_u^a (mg)	$X_u^\infty - X_u$ (mg)	Extrapolated $X_u^\infty - X_u$ (mg)	Residual $X_u^\infty - X_u$ (mg)
1.0	0.36	49.64	65.8	16.16
2.0	1.32	48.68	61.5	12.82
3.0	3.70	47.30	57.3	10.0
4.0	4.37	45.63	53.5	7.87
6.0	8.23	41.77	46.5	4.73
8.0	12.35	37.65	40.5	2.85
12.0	20.24	29.76		
18.0	29.82	20.18		
24.0	36.55	13.45		
36.0	44.11	5.90		
∞	50.00			

^{a}Cumulative amount of drug in the urine.

Notes: The data are analyzed using the sigma-minus method. First-order absorption and a one-compartment model are assumed. $K = 0.0693$ h^{-1}, $k_a = 0.231\ h^{-1}$, $V = 10$ liters, $X_0 = 500$ mg, $F = 1$.

drug which when administered orally confers the pharmacokinetic characteristics of a two-compartment model on the body. The equation describing such a curve is

$$C = Ne^{-k_a t} + Le^{-\alpha t} + Me^{-\beta t} \qquad (C.16)$$

where k_a, α, and β are as defined previously in this appendix and L, M, and N are coefficients.

Since α is by definition larger than β, and since k_a is generally assumed to be larger than β, the terms $Ne^{-k_a t}$ and $Le^{-\alpha t}$ will approach zero while the term $Me^{-\beta t}$ will retain some finite value. Equation (C.16) will then reduce to

$$C = Me^{-\beta t} \qquad (C.17)$$

This equation can be written in terms of common logarithms as follows:

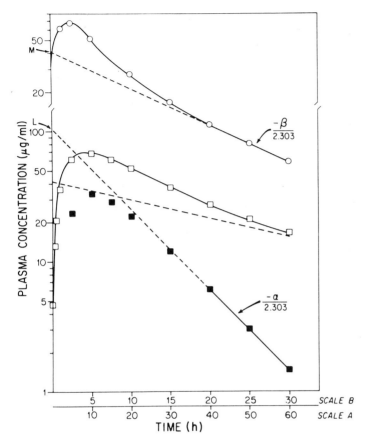

Fig. C.4 Drug concentration in plasma (O, time scale A; □, time
scale B) after oral administration of a drug (see Table C.4). First
residual values are denoted by (■) and are plotted on time scale B.
See Eqs. (C.16) to (C.21).

$$\log C = \log M - \frac{\beta t}{2.303} \qquad \text{(C.18)}$$

which describes the terminal lines phase of the curve resulting from a
plot of the logarithm of the plasma concentration versus time. The slope
of this terminal linear phase is $-\beta/2.303$, and when extrapolated to time
zero yields an intercept of $\log M$ (see Fig. C.4).

Subtraction of the concentration-time values on the extrapolated
line from the corresponding true plasma concentration-time values
produces a series of residual concentration-time values (see Table
C.4). The equation describing the time course of these residual concentrations C_{r1} is obtained by subtracting (C.17) from (C.16):

Table C.4 Application of the Method of Residuals to Data Obtained After Oral Administration of a Drug

Time (h)	Plasma Concentration, C (μg/ml)	$Me^{-\beta t}$ (μg/ml)	C_{r1} (μg/ml)	$Le^{-\alpha t}$ (μg/ml)	C_{r2} (μg/ml)
0.1	4.7	41.2	−36.5	104.0	140.5
0.3	13.2	40.9	−27.7	101.0	128.7
0.5	20.8	40.6	−19.8	98.2	118.0
1	36.3	40.0	−3.7	91.5	95.2
2.5	61.4	38.0	23.4	74.0	50.6
5	68.1	35.0	33.1	51.9	18.8
7.5	61.1	32.2	28.9	36.5	7.6
10	52.1	29.7	22.4	25.6	3.2
15	37.3	25.2	12.1		
20	27.5	21.3	6.2		
25	21.1	18.1	3.0		
30	16.9	15.4	1.5		
40	11.4				
50	8.2				
60	5.9				

Notes: First-order absorption and a two-compartment open model are assumed. It is assumed further that $k_a > \alpha > \beta$. See Eqs. (C.16) to (C.23). L = 105.0 μg/ml, M = 41.3 μg/ml, N = −146.3 μg/ml, α = 0.141 h^{-1}, β = 0.033 h^{-1}, k_a = 0.40 h^{-1}, X_0 = 1 g, V_c = 10 liters, F = 1.

$$C_{r1} = Ne^{-k_a t} + Le^{-\alpha t} \qquad (C.19)$$

A plot of the positive residual concentration values versus time will yield a biexponential curve (see Fig. C.4). Assuming that k_a is greater than α, the term $Ne^{-k_a t}$ will approach zero while the term $Le^{-\alpha t}$ still has a finite value, and (C.19) will then reduce to

$$C_{r1} = Le^{-\alpha t} \qquad (C.20)$$

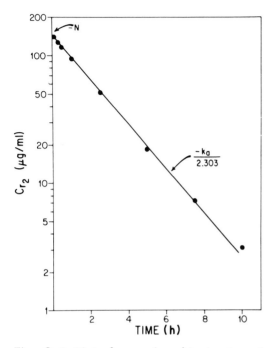

Fig. C.5 Plot of second residual values (see Table C.4) to estimate the apparent first-order absorption rate constant. See Eqs. (C.22) and (C.23).

which in terms of common logarithms is

$$\log C_{r1} = \log L - \frac{\alpha t}{2.303} \tag{C.21}$$

This equation describes the terminal linear phase of the residual curve resulting from a plot of $\log C_{r1}$ versus time. The slope of the resulting straight line will be $-\alpha/2.303$, and when extrapolated to time zero will yield an intercept of $\log L$ (see Fig. C.4).

This residual curve can be resolved further. Subtracting the residual concentration values C_{r1} from the corresponding concentration-time values on the extrapolated residual line yields a second series of residual concentration-time values (see Table C.4). These residual concentrations C_{r2} are described by the following equation, which is obtained by subtracting (C.19) from (C.20):

$$C_{r2} = -Ne^{-k_a t} \tag{C.22}$$

which when transformed to common logarithms becomes

$$\log C_{r2} = \log (-N) - \frac{k_a t}{2.303} \qquad\qquad (C.23)$$

Hence a plot of the logarithm of C_{r2} versus time will yield a straight line with a slope of $-k_a/2.303$ and a zero-time intercept of $\log (-N)$ (see Fig. C.5). Application of the method of residuals thus permits the resolution of Eq. (C.16) into its three exponential components, and hence estimation of the parameters k_a, α, β, N, L, and M.

The method of residuals is a useful technique for resolving essentially any multiexponential curve encountered in pharmacokinetic analysis into the individual exponential components.

Appendix D
Estimation of Areas

The estimation of areas under blood level-time curves is often re-quired for pharmacokinetic analysis. These areas are usually estimated by employing an approximate integration formula. The trapezoidal rule is one such formula. This particular method involves the descrip-tion of a given plasma concentration-time curve by a function that de-picts the curve as a series of straight lines, thereby enabling the area under the curve to be divided into a number of trapezoids (see Fig. D.1). The area of each trapezoid is easily calculated, and the sum of all the areas of all the trapezoids yields an estimate of the true area under the curve.

We will let $f(t)$ be a function that describes a given plasma con-centration-time curve and $\phi(t)$ be a second function that coincides with $f(t)$ but is linear between two consecutive blood level-time points (see Fig. D.1). Consequently, the area under the curve described by the function $\phi(t)$ [i.e., $\int_{t_0}^{t_n} \phi(t)\ dt$] will only be an approximation of the true area under the curve, $\int_{t_0}^{t_n} f(t)\ dt$.

The integral $\int_{t_0}^{t_n} \phi(t)\ dt$ can be expressed as the sum of n inte-grals, where n equals the number of trapezoids into which the curve is divided. Hence

$$\int_{t_0}^{t_n} \phi(t)\ dt = \int_{t_0}^{t_1} \phi(t)\ dt + \int_{t_1}^{t_2} \phi(t)\ dt + \cdots + \int_{t_{n-1}}^{t_n} \phi(t)\ dt$$

(D.1)

Since each integral on the right side of this equation is the area of a trapezoid, it follows that

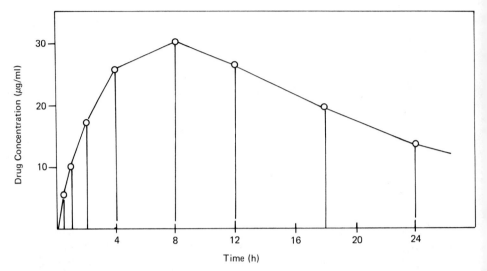

Fig. D.1 Representation of drug concentration in plasma-time profile after oral administration for the application of linear trapezoidal method to estimate areas. See Table D.1.

$$\int_{t_0}^{t_1} \phi(t)\ dt = \frac{t_1 - t_0}{2}\ (C_0 + C_1) \qquad\qquad (D.2)$$

where C_0 and C_1 are the plasma concentrations at times t_0 and t_1, respectively. After a single oral dose of a drug, C_0 is usually zero. C_0 has a positive value following a single intravenous dose of drug and during a dosing interval of a multiple-dose regimen. By the same token,

$$\int_{t_1}^{t_2} \phi(t)\ dt = \frac{t_2 - t_1}{2}\ (C_1 + C_2) \qquad\qquad (D.3)$$

and

$$\int_{t_{n-1}}^{t_n} \phi(t)\ dt = \frac{t_n - t_{n-1}}{2}\ (C_{n-1} + C_n) \qquad\qquad (D.4)$$

Therefore, Eq. (D.1) can be rewritten

$$\int_{t_0}^{t_n} \phi(t) \, dt = \frac{t_1 - t_0}{2} (C_0 + C_1) + \frac{t_2 - t_1}{2} (C_1 + C_2) + \cdots$$

$$+ \frac{t_n - t_{n-1}}{2} (C_{n-1} + C_n) \qquad (D.5)$$

If the time intervals between sampling of the plasma were the same,

$$\int_{t_0}^{t_n} \phi(t) \, dt = \frac{\Delta t}{2} (C_0 + 2C_1 + 2C_2 + \cdots + 2C_{n-1} + C_n) \qquad (D.6)$$

where Δt is the sampling time interval. However, sampling intervals are often different and a more general expression such as Eq. (D.5) must usually be employed. This equation can be written more consisely as follows:

$$\int_{t_0}^{t_n} \phi(t) \, dt = \sum_{i=0}^{n-1} \frac{t_{i+1} - t_i}{2} (C_i + C_{i+1}) \qquad (D.7)$$

The use of the trapezoidal rule as a method for approximating the area under a plasma concentration-time curve is probably best illustrated by employing a numerical example. The data from which the plasma concentration versus time curve in Fig. D.1 was constructed will be used. These data were generated by assuming first-order absorption and a one-compartment model (see Table D.1). In this particular example, 11 plasma samples were obtained after drug administration for the characterization of the curve; hence n equals 11. The approximate area under the curve can be estimated by determining the area under the 11 trapezoids and then summing these areas. The total area under the curve from zero to 72 h [$\int_0^{72} \phi(t) \, dt$] was found to be 724 μg-h/ml, which is in reasonable agreement with the true area under the curve [$\int_0^{72} f(t) \, dt$], 714 μg-h/ml.

The accuracy to which this method approximates the true area under a curve depends on the number of plasma concentration-time points within the time interval t_0 to t_n. The larger the number of samples within a given time interval, the more closely will $\int_{t_0}^{t_n} \phi(t) \, dt$ estimate $\int_{t_0}^{t_n} f(t) \, dt$, since the straight-line function $\phi(t)$ will be a more exact representation of the true function, $f(t)$. For example, if plasma samples had been taken only at times 1, 4, 12, 24, 48, and 72 h, the estimated area would be 734 μg-h/ml, which is a poorer approximation of the true area than when the plasma was sampled more frequently.

As we have noted in the text, the *total* area under the drug concentration in blood or plasma versus time curve from t = 0 to t = ∞

Table D.1 Drug Concentration in Plasma Following Oral Administration of a Fully Absorbed 500 mg Dose, and Areas Under the Curve During Successive Time Intervals Calculated According to the Linear Trapezoidal Method

i	Time (h)	Concentration (μg/ml)	Area Under[a] Trapezoid (μg-h/ml)
0	0	0	
1	0.5	5.4	1.3
2	1.0	10.0	3.9
3	2.0	17.2	13.6
4	4.0	25.8	43.0
5	8.0	29.8	111.1
6	12.0	26.6	112.8
7	18.0	19.4	138.1
8	24.0	13.3	98.0
9	36.0	5.9	114.8
10	48.0	2.6	50.6
11	72.0	0.5	36.6

$$\int_{t_0}^{t_n} \phi(t)\,dt = 723.8$$

[a]Determined employing Eq. (D.7).

Note: Data generated by assuming first-order absorption ($k_a = 0.231$ h^{-1}) and a one-compartment model ($V = 10$ liters) with first-order elimination ($K = 0.0693$ h^{-1}).

following a single dose is calculated by combining the area to t_n, estimated by the trapezoidal rule, to the area from t_n to ∞, estimated by assuming log-linear decline. Under these conditions, this residual area is given by C_n/K or C_n/λ_n.

Yeh and Kwan [1] have noted that the linear interpolation between data points that is required to apply the trapezoidal rule tends to overestimate or underestimate the area, depending on the concavity of the curve. In cases where changes in curvature between data points are pronounced or there are long intervals between data points, large errors are known to occur. In some instances, area estimates can be obtained by linear interpolation of logarithmically transformed data. In the log trapezoidal method the area is given by [1]

$$\text{AUC} \Big|_{t_1}^{t_2} = \frac{(C_1 - C_2)(t_2 - t_1)}{\ln C_1 - \ln C_2} \tag{D.8}$$

Equation (D.8) is most appropriate when applied to data that appear to decline exponentially. However, the method may produce large errors when used in an ascending curve, near a peak, or in a steeply descending polyexponential curve. Furthermore, the method cannot be used if either concentration is zero or if the two values are equal. Despite these limitations, the log trapezoidal method can be used advantageously in combination with a second method, such as the linear trapezoidal rule, to yield optimal estimates.

Two alternative algorithms based on known interpolating functions have been devised for area calculation. In the Lagrange method, the linear interpolations are replaced by cubic polynomial interpolations. In the spline method, the cubic functions are modified so that the fitted curves are smooth. The advantages and disadvantages of the Lagrange and spline methods relative to the trapezoidal or log trapezoidal method are discussed by Yeh and Kwan [1].

REFERENCE

1. K. C. Yeh and K. C. Kwan. A comparison of numerical integrating algorithms by trapezoidal, Lagrange, and spline approximations. *J. Pharmacokinet. Biopharm.* 6:79 (1978).

Appendix E

Prediction of Drug Concentrations on Mutliple Dosing Using the Principle of Superposition

Assuming that a drug may be characterized by linear pharmacokinetics, concentrations in blood or plasma on multiple dosing can be predicted from the corresponding concentrations after a single dose. The usual approach requires computer fitting of the data to a particular compart-

Table E.1 Predicting Drug Concentrations During Multiple Dosing Using the Principle of Superposition

Dose Number	Time (h)	Dose 1	Dose 2	Dose 3	Dose 4	Drug Concentration
1	0	0				0
	1	59				59
	2	70				70
	4	58				58
2	6	42	0			42
	7	35	59			94
	8	30	70			100
	10	21	58			79
3	12	15	42	0		57
	13	13	35	59		107
	14	10	30	70		110
	16	7	21	58		86
4	18	5	15	42	0	62
	19	4	13	35	59	111
	20	4	10	30	70	114
	22	3	7	21	58	89
	24	2	5	15	42	64

Note: It is assumed that a constant dose is given every 6 h.
From Ref. 2.

Table E.2 Predicting Drug Concentrations During Multiple Dosing
Using the Principle of Superposition

Dose Number	Time (h)	Dose 1	Dose 2	Dose 3	Dose 4	Drug Concentration
1	0	0				0
	1	59				59
	2	70				70
2	4	58	0			58
	5	50	59			109
	6	42	70			112
3	8	30	58	0		88
	9	25	50	59		134
	10	21	42	70		133
4	12	15	30	58	0	103
	13	13	25	50	59	147
	14	10	21	42	70	143
	16	7	15	30	58	110
	17	6	13	25	50	94
	18	5	10	21	42	78
	20	4	7	15	30	56
	21	3	6	13	25	47
	22	3	5	10	21	39
	24	2	4	7	15	28

Note: It is assumed that the same dose of drug is given four times
a day (i.e., at 9 a.m., 1 p.m., 5 p.m., and 9 p.m.).

mental model and some necessarily simplistic assumption concerning
the absorption kinetics of the drug. An alternative approach that requires no assumptions regarding a pharmacokinetic model or absorption kinetics is based on the principle of superposition and employs
an overlay technique [1,2]. This method merely requires the assumptions that each dose of drug, in essence, acts independently of every
other dose, that the rate and extent of absorption and average systemic clearance are the same for each dosing interval, and that linear
pharmacokinetics apply so that a change in dose during the multiple
dosing regimen can be accommodated. The overlay technique also requires a rather complete characterization of the concentration-time
profile after a single dose.

    In the example shown in Table E.1, it is assumed that one wishes
to predict the drug concentrations in blood on multiple dosing when the
same dose is taken every 6 h. The concentration data in the column

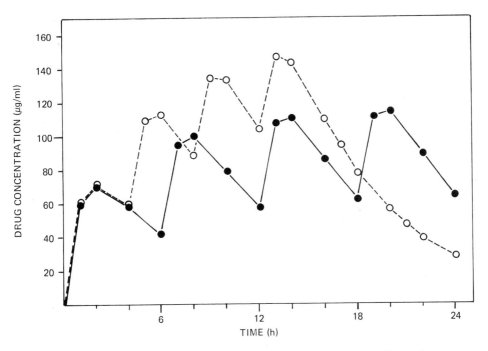

Fig. E.1 Drug concentrations in blood during multiple dosing of a constant dose given every 6 h (●) or four times a day (○). Data from Tables E.1 and E.2.

labeled "Dose 1" was either determined after a single dose, or interpolated or extrapolated from such data. The values are repeated under each "dose" column at the appropriate time. The drug concentration at any time during multiple dosing is predicted by simply adding all the concentration values in a given row. The drug concentration 2 h after the fourth dose is equal to the sum of the drug concentration 2 h after a single dose and all residual concentrations resulting from doses preceding the fourth dose.

A particular advantage of this overlay technique is that it permits one to almost as easily predict drug concentrations during multiple dosing using unequal dosing intervals, unequal doses, or both. In the example shown in Table E.2, it is assumed that one wishes to predict drug concentrations during multiple dosing when the same dose of drug is given four times a day (i.e., at 9 a.m., 1 p.m., 5 p.m., and 9 p.m.) rather than every 6 h. The example in Table E.3 is similar to that shown in Table E.1 except that a loading dose that is twice the usual dose is given. Note that drug concentrations after dose 1 are doubled to account for the dosing change.

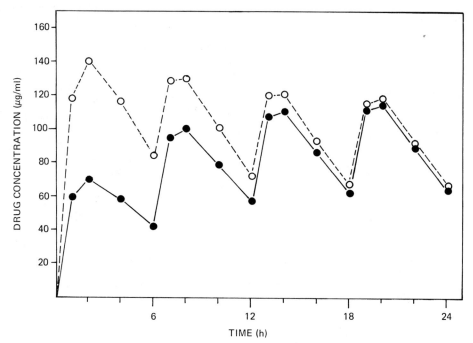

Fig. E.2 Drug concentrations in blood during multiple dosing of a constant dose given every 6 h with (O) or without (●) a loading dose. Data from Tables E.1 and E.3.

Figure E.1 compares the data from Tables E.1 and E.2. It is evident that dosing a drug four times a day results in a different drug concentration profile than that produced by dosing the drug every 6 h. Assuming a therapeutic concentration range of 60 to 140 µg/ml, it is evident that dosing the drug every 6 h results in therapeutic concentrations shortly after the second dose which are maintained throughout the course of therapy. On the other hand, dosing the drug four times a day results in rather high concentrations following the last dose of each day and subtherapeutic concentrations for several hours preceding the first dose of each day of therapy.

Figure E.2 compares the data from Tables E.1 and E.3. As we have noted in the text, an appropriate loading dose can safely allow more rapid attainment of therapeutic concentrations.

In those cases where the same dose of drug is given at constant dosing intervals and where the dosing interval is sufficiently large so that drug concentrations reflect the postabsorptive and postdistributive phase of the concentration-time profile, it is possible to describe the overlay technique by simple equations that are readily solved by means of a calculator.

Table E.3 Predicting Drug Concentrations During Multiple Dosing
Using the Principle of Superposition

Dose Number	Time (h)	Dose 1	Dose 2	Dose 3	Dose 4	Drug Concentration
1	0	0				0
	1	118				118
	2	140				140
	4	116				116
2	6	84	0			84
	7	70	59			129
	8	60	70			130
	10	42	58			100
3	12	30	42	0		72
	13	26	35	59		120
	14	20	30	70		120
	16	14	21	58		93
4	18	10	15	42	0	67
	19	8	13	35	59	115
	20	8	10	30	70	118
	22	6	7	21	58	92
	24	4	5	15	42	66

Note: It is assumed that the same dose is given every 6 h but that
the first dose is a loading dose (i.e., twice the usual dose).

To predict the drug concentration at time t (where $0 < t < \tau$)
during the nth dosing interval [i.e., $C_n(t)$] under these conditions,
the following approach can be used. Drug concentration at time t
following the first dose is defined as $C_1(t)$. At t hours after the
second dose, drug concentration is given by

$$C_2(t) = C_1(t) + Be^{-\lambda_n(t+\tau)} \tag{E.1}$$

where B and λ_n are as defined in Fig. E.3. Similarly, drug concentration at t hours after the third dose is given by

$$C_3(t) = C_1(t) + Be^{-\lambda_n(t+\tau)} + Be^{-\lambda_n(t+2\tau)} \tag{E.2}$$

The first term on the right-hand side of Eq. (E.2) is contributed by
the third dose, the second term by the second dose, and the third
term by the first dose.

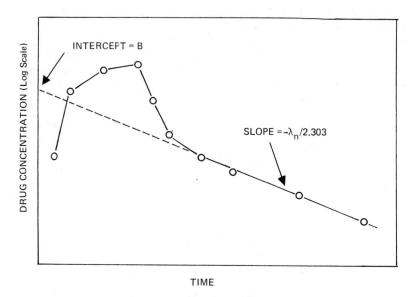

Fig. E.3 Drug concentration-time profile on semilogarithmic coordinates following a single oral dose.

It follows that drug concentration after the nth dose is given by

$$C_n(t) = C_1(t) + Be^{-\lambda_n(t+\tau)} + Be^{-\lambda_n(t+2\tau)} + \cdots$$
$$+ Be^{-\lambda_n[t+(n-1)\tau]}$$

$$(E.3)$$

which can be simplified to

$$C_n(t) = C_1(t) + Be^{-\lambda_n\tau}[1 + e^{-\lambda_n\tau} + e^{-2\lambda_n\tau} + \cdots$$
$$+ e^{-(n-2)\lambda_n\tau}]e^{-\lambda_n t}$$

$$(E.4)$$

The term in brackets can be shown to be equal to

$$\frac{1 - e^{-(n-1)\lambda_n\tau}}{1 - e^{-\lambda_n\tau}}$$

Therefore, Eq. (E.4) can be written as follows:

$$C_n(t) = C_1(t) + \frac{Be^{-\lambda_n \tau}[1 - e^{-(n-1)\lambda_n \tau}]e^{-\lambda_n t}}{1 - e^{-\lambda_n \tau}}$$ (E.5)

At steady-state the term in brackets approaches one and Eq. (E.5) may be simplified to

$$C_{ss}(t) = C_1(t) + \frac{(Be^{-\lambda_n \tau})(e^{-\lambda_n t})}{1 - e^{-\lambda_n \tau}}$$ (E.6)

where $C_{ss}(t)$ is the drug concentration at any time t during a dosing interval at steady state.

REFERENCES

1. W. J. Westlake. Problems associated with analysis of pharma-
    cokinetic models. *J. Pharm. Sci.* *60*:82 (1971).
2. J. G. Wagner. Relevant pharmacokinetics of antimicrobial drugs.
    Med. Clin. North Am. *58*:479 (1974).

Appendix F

Estimation of Rates

It is not possible experimentally to determine instantaneous rates of change of drug or metabolite concentrations in any body compartment. Hence it becomes necessary to approximate instantaneous rates by estimating average rates over finite periods of time. Possible limitations of employing average rates have been discussed [1]. We will illustrate this method by employing the equations for the excretion of unchanged drug in the urine following the intravenous administration of a drug, assuming a one-compartment model with first-order elimination.

The expression for the instantaneous rate of appearance of unchanged drug in the urine, dX_u/dt, is given as follows:

$$\frac{dX_u}{dt} = k_e X \tag{F.1}$$

where k_e is the apparent first-order excretion rate constant, X_u the cumulative amount of unchanged drug eliminated in the urine to time t, and X the amount of drug in the body at time t. Since the time course of drug in the body following intravenous administration in a one-compartment model is given by the equation

$$X = X_0 e^{-Kt} \tag{F.2}$$

the following expression for dX_u/dt can be written by substituting this value of X into Eq. (F.1):

$$\frac{dX_u}{dt} = k_e X_0 e^{-Kt} \tag{F.3}$$

which in terms of common logarithms is

$$\log \frac{dX_u}{dt} = \log k_e X_0 - \frac{Kt}{2.303} \tag{F.4}$$

459

In this equation K is the apparent first-order elimination rate constant for the drug and X_0 is the intravenous dose. Integration of Eq. (F.3) yields the following expression for the cumulative amount of unchanged drug in the urine as a function of time:

$$X_u = \frac{k_e X_0}{K} (1 - e^{-Kt}) \tag{F.5}$$

Hence the cumulative amount of drug in the urine at two consecutive sampling times t_1 and t_2 is given by

$$(X_u)_{t_1} = \frac{k_e X_0}{K} (1 - e^{-Kt_1}) \tag{F.6}$$

and

$$(X_u)_{t_2} = \frac{k_e X_0}{K} (1 - e^{-Kt_2}) \tag{F.7}$$

respectively. If Δt equals t_2 minus t_1 and t^* is the time at the mid-point of t_2 and t_1 [i.e., $t^* = (t_2 + t_1)/2$], then

$$t_1 = t^* - \Delta t/2 \tag{F.8}$$

and

$$t_2 = t^* + \Delta t/2 \tag{F.9}$$

Substitution of these values of t_1 and t_2 into Eqs. (F.6) and (F.7), respectively, yields

$$(X_u)_{t_1} = \frac{k_e X_0}{K} [1 - e^{-K(t^*-\Delta t/2)}] \tag{F.10}$$

and

$$(X_u)_{t_2} = \frac{k_e X_0}{K} [1 - e^{-K(t^*+\Delta t/2)}] \tag{F.11}$$

The amount of unchanged drug eliminated in the urine during the time interval Δt (i.e., ΔX_u) would be equal to $(X_u)_{t_2}$ minus $(X_u)_{t_1}$. Hence ΔX_u is given by the difference between Eqs. (F.11) and (F.10):

$$\Delta X_u = \frac{k_e X_0}{K} [e^{-K(t^*-\Delta t/2)} - e^{-K(t^*+\Delta t/2)}] \tag{F.12}$$

which can be simplified to

$$\Delta X_u = \frac{k_e X_0}{K} e^{-Kt^*} (e^{K\Delta t/2} - e^{-K\Delta t/2}) \qquad (F.13)$$

Since the amount of drug in the body X at time t^* equals $X_0 e^{-Kt^*}$, according to Eq. (F.2), substitution of X for $X_0 e^{-Kt^*}$ in Eq. (F.13) yields

$$\Delta X_u = \frac{k_e X}{K} (e^{K\Delta t/2} - e^{-K\Delta t/2}) \qquad (F.14)$$

Dividing both sides of Eq. (F.14) by Δt gives the average rate of appearance of unchanged drug in the urine over a finite period of time, $\Delta X_u / \Delta t$, which is an approximation of the instantaneous rate dX_u / dt:

$$\frac{\Delta X_u}{\Delta t} = \frac{k_e X}{K \Delta t} (e^{K\Delta t/2} - e^{-K\Delta t/2}) \qquad (F.15)$$

To account for any difference between $\Delta X_u / \Delta t$ and the instantaneous rate, the factor λ will be introduced such that

$$\frac{\Delta X_u}{\Delta t} = \lambda \frac{dX_u}{dt} \qquad (F.16)$$

Solving this equation for λ yields

$$\lambda = \frac{\Delta X_u / \Delta t}{dX_u / dt} \qquad (F.17)$$

Substituting for $\Delta X_u / \Delta t$ and dX_u / dt according to Eqs. (F.15) and (F.1), respectively, and canceling common terms results in the following expression for λ:

$$\lambda = \frac{e^{K\Delta t/2} - e^{-K\Delta t/2}}{K \Delta t} \qquad (F.18)$$

Therefore, λ is a constant that depends on the values of K and Δt. A plot of the logarithm of $\Delta X_u / \Delta t$ versus t^* would be linear and parallel to a plot of the logarithm of dX_u / dt versus t provided that Δt is the same for each point plotted. Consequently, no error will arise in the calculation of the elimination rate constant K from the slope (i.e., slope $= -K/2.303$) of a log ($\Delta X_u / \Delta t$) versus t^* plot if the sampling intervals are the same.

By expressing Δt in terms of the biologic half-life $t_{1/2}$ of a drug such that

$$\Delta t = \theta t_{1/2} \qquad (F.19)$$

and since

Table F.1 Relationship Between Average Excretion Rates Calculated over Varying Time Intervals and Instantaneous Excretion Rates

Δt [a]	$\dfrac{\Delta X_u/\Delta t}{dX_u/dt}$ [b]
0.25	1.001
0.5	1.005
1.0	1.020
2.0	1.082
3.0	1.190

[a] Expressed as a multiple of the elimination half-life of the drug, that is, values of θ, where $\theta = \Delta t/t_{1/2}$.
[b] The value of λ, that is, the extent of departure of $\Delta X_u/\Delta t$ from dX_u/dt.

$$t_{1/2} = \frac{\ln 2}{K} \tag{F.20}$$

then

$$\Delta t = \frac{\theta \ln 2}{K} \tag{F.21}$$

Substituting this value for Δt in Eq. (F.18) and canceling common terms yields

$$\lambda = \frac{e^{\theta(\ln 2)/2} - e^{-\theta(\ln 2)/2}}{\theta \ln 2} = \frac{2^{\theta/2} - 2^{-\theta/2}}{\theta \ln 2} \tag{F.22}$$

Based on this equation, the extent to which a semilogarithmic plot of $\Delta X_u/\Delta t$ versus the midpoint in time (i.e., t*) deviates from an instantaneous rate plot can be readily calculated. The larger the value of Δt, relative to the half-life, the greater will be the displacement of the log ($\Delta X_u/\Delta t$) plot above the log (dX_u/dt) plot (see Table F.1). If urine is collected, however, at intervals that are not larger than one half-life of the drug, there is only a 2% shift upward (i.e., $\lambda = 1.020$), which is insignificant.

Usually, urinary excretion rate plots are not based on constant time intervals. As can be seen from Table F.1, the error caused by employing unequal time intervals does not become significant until one of these intervals is at least twice the half-life of a drug. A problem may arise with drugs having very short half-lifes where urine collection intervals equal to or less than one half-life may be difficult to attain. With this type of drug the use of equal time intervals is suggested.

REFERENCE

1. B. K. Martin. Drug urinary excretion data—some aspects concerning the interpretation. *Br. J. Pharmacol. Chemother.* *29*:181 (1967).

Appendix G

Selective Derivations

MICHAELIS-MENTEN EQUATION

Based on the scheme

$$E + C \xrightleftharpoons[k_1]{k_{-1}} EC \xrightarrow{k_2} E + M$$

the differential equation for EC is

$$\frac{dEC}{dt} = k_1(E)(C) - (k_{-1} + k_2)EC \qquad (G.1)$$

where E, C, EC, and M are the concentrations of enzyme, drug, enzyme-drug complex, and metabolite, respectively. The constants k_{-1} and k_2 are first-order rate constants and k_1 is a second-order rate constant. Assuming that $dEC/dt = 0$ (steady-state assumption), the right-hand side of (G.1) can be rearranged to yield

$$\frac{k_{-1} + k_2}{k_1} = \frac{(E)(C)}{EC} \qquad (G.2)$$

since

$$k_1(E)(C) - (k_{-1} + k_2)\, EC = 0 \qquad (G.3)$$

The ratio $(E)(C)/EC$ is denoted as K_m, the Michaelis constant.
The following differential equation can be written for C:

$$-\frac{dC}{dt} = k_1(E)(C) - k_{-1}(EC) \qquad (G.4)$$

Expansion of Eq. (G.3) and rearrangement yields

$$k_1(E)(C) - k_{-1}(EC) = k_2(EC) \qquad (G.5)$$

465

Substitution of $k_2(EC)$ for $k_1(E)(C) - k_{-1}(EC)$ in (G.4) produces the following expression for $-dC/dt$:

$$- \frac{dC}{dt} = k_2(EC) \tag{G.6}$$

The total concentration of enzyme in the system, E_T, equals the sum of the concentrations of free and bound enzyme, E and EC, respectively. Therefore,

$$E_T = E + EC \tag{G.7}$$

Since there is only a finite amount of enzyme present in the system, all of the enzyme will exist as EC complex at a sufficiently high drug concentration. At this point the enzyme will be completely saturated with drug, and the rate of change in C will occur at a maximum rate. This maximum rate V_m will equal k_2ET. Therefore, at high drug concentrations

$$- \frac{dC}{dt} = k_2(EC) = k_2E_T = V_m \tag{G.8}$$

Taking the ratio of $V_m/(-dC/dt)$, where V_m equals k_2E_T and $-dC/dt$ is given by Eq. (G.6) yields

$$\frac{V_m}{-dC/dt} = \frac{k_2E_T}{k_2(EC)} = \frac{E_T}{EC} \tag{G.9}$$

As stated previously,

$$K_m = \frac{(E)(C)}{EC} \tag{G.10}$$

Substitution of $(E_T - EC)$ for E [according to a rearrangement of (G.7)] in (G.10) results in the relationship

$$K_m = \frac{(E_T - EC)(C)}{EC} \tag{G.11}$$

Dividing both sides of this equation by C and solving for the ratio E_T/EC gives

$$\frac{E_T}{EC} = \frac{K_m}{C} + 1 = \frac{K_m + C}{C} \tag{G.12}$$

Substituting the value of E_T/EC in (G.12) for E_T/EC in (G.9) and solving for $-dC/dt$ produces the Michaelis-Menten equation

$$- \frac{dC}{dt} = \frac{V_m C}{K_m + C} \tag{G.13}$$

TIME TO REACH A FRACTION OF STEADY STATE FOR A DRUG ELIMINATED BY PARALLEL FIRST-ORDER AND CAPACITY-LIMITED PROCESSES

Assuming a one-compartment model, consider the following situation: drug is administered by a constant rate (k_0) intravenous infusion and eliminated by parallel first-order and Michaelis-processes. The rate of change of drug concentration during infusion is given by

$$\frac{dC}{dt} = \frac{k_0}{V} - K'C - \frac{V_m C}{K_m + C} \tag{G.14}$$

where K' is the sum of the rate constants for the first-order elimination processes. Expansion and rearrangement of (G.14) yields

$$\frac{K_m}{-K'C^2 + [(k_0/V) - K'K_m - V_m]C + k_0 K_m/V} \, dC$$

$$+ \frac{C}{-K'C^2 + [(k_0/V) - K'K_m - V_m]C + K_0 K_m/V} \, dC = dt \tag{G.15}$$

This equation is of the form

$$\frac{g}{fx^2 + bx + a} \, dx + \frac{x}{fx^2 + bx + a} \, dx = dt \tag{G.16}$$

where

$$a = \frac{k_0 K_m}{V} \tag{G.17}$$

$$b = \frac{k_0}{V} - K'K_m - V_m \tag{G.18}$$

$$f = -K' \tag{G.19}$$

$$g = K_m \tag{G.20}$$

The integral of (G.16) is [1]

$$\frac{g}{\sqrt{-q}} \ln \frac{2fx + b - \sqrt{-q}}{2fx + b + \sqrt{-q}} + \frac{1}{2f} \ln (a + bx + fx^2)$$

$$- \frac{b}{2f} \frac{1}{\sqrt{-q}} \ln \frac{2fx + b - \sqrt{-q}}{2fx + b + \sqrt{-q}} = t + i \tag{G.21}$$

where

$$-q = b^2 - 4af = b^2 + 4aK' \tag{G.22}$$

Equation (G.21) can be simplified to

$$\frac{1}{2f} \ln (a + bx + fx^2) + \left(\frac{g}{\sqrt{-q}} - \frac{b}{2f \sqrt{-q}} \right) \ln \frac{2 fx + b - \sqrt{-q}}{2 fx + b + \sqrt{-q}} = t + i \tag{G.23}$$

At $t = 0$, $x = 0$ and therefore

$$i = \frac{1}{2f} \ln a + \left(\frac{g}{\sqrt{-q}} - \frac{b}{2f \sqrt{-q}} \right) \ln \frac{b - \sqrt{-q}}{b + \sqrt{-q}} \tag{G.24}$$

Substitution of the value of i in (G.24) into (G.21), setting x equal to C (i.e., drug concentration), substitution of $-K'$ for f and K_m for g according to (G.19) and (G.20), respectively, followed by rearrangement yields

$$t = \frac{1}{\sqrt{-q}} \left(K_m + \frac{b}{2K'} \right) \ln \left(\frac{-2K'C + b - \sqrt{-q}}{-2K'C + b + \sqrt{-q}} \right) \left(\frac{b + \sqrt{-q}}{b - \sqrt{-q}} \right)$$

$$- \frac{1}{2K'} \ln \frac{a + bC - K'C^2}{a} \tag{G.25}$$

The steady-state concentration of a drug eliminated by parallel first-order and saturable pathways is given by

$$C_{ss} = \frac{k_0}{Cl_s} = \frac{k_0}{[VV_m/(K_m + C_{ss})] + K'V} \tag{G.26}$$

where Cl_s at steady state is given by (7.53). Rearranging (G.26) produces the following quadratic equation:

$$-K'C_{ss}^2 + \left(\frac{k_0}{V} - VK'K_m - V_m \right) C_{ss} + \frac{k_0 K_m}{V} = 0 \tag{G.27}$$

or in terms of a and b where these values are given by (G.17) and (G.18), respectively.

$$-K'C_{ss}^2 + bC_{ss} + a = 0 \tag{G.28}$$

The solution for C_{ss} is

$$C_{ss} = \frac{b \pm \sqrt{b^2 + 4aK'}}{2K'} \tag{G.29}$$

The term $\sqrt{b^2 + 4aK'}$ will always be greater than b; therefore, the sign between these two terms must always be positive since C_{ss} must be positive. Consequently,

$$C_{ss} = \frac{b + \sqrt{b^2 + 4aK'}}{2K'} = \frac{b + \sqrt{-q}}{2K'} \tag{G.30}$$

Substitution of $2K'C_{ss}$ for $b + \sqrt{-q}$ in (G.25) yields

$$t = \frac{1}{\sqrt{-q}}\left(K_m + \frac{b}{2K'}\right)\ln \frac{-2K'C + b - \sqrt{-q}}{-2K'C + 2K'C_{ss}} \quad \frac{2K'C_{ss}}{b - \sqrt{-q}}$$

$$- \frac{1}{2K'}\ln \frac{a + bC - K'C^2}{a} \tag{G.31}$$

or

$$t = \frac{1}{\sqrt{-q}}\left(K_m + \frac{b}{2K'}\right)\ln \frac{-2K'C + b - \sqrt{-q}}{b - \sqrt{-q}} \quad \frac{1}{1 - C/C_{ss}}$$

$$- \frac{1}{2K'}\ln \frac{a + bC - K'C^2}{a} \tag{G.32}$$

The fraction of a given steady-state concentration, f_{ss}, equals C/C_{ss}. Therefore, substitution of f_{ss} for C/C_{ss} and rearrangement gives

$$t = \frac{1}{\sqrt{-q}}\left(K_m + \frac{b}{2K'}\right)\ln\left(\frac{-2K'C}{b - \sqrt{-q}} + 1\right)\frac{1}{1 - f_{ss}}$$

$$- \frac{1}{2K'}\ln\left(1 + \frac{bC - K'C^2}{a}\right) \tag{G.33}$$

Two limiting cases of Eq. (G.33) can be considered: the time to reach a certain fraction of steady state when there is a very high or a very low rate of drug administration. When the rate of drug administration is very low (i.e., $k_0 \underset{\sim}{} 0$) and hence $C \underset{\sim}{} 0$, Eqs. (G.18) and (G.22) can be approximated by

$$b \underset{\sim}{} - K'K_m - V_m \tag{G.34}$$

and

$$-q \underset{\sim}{} b^2 \underset{\sim}{} (K'K_m + V_m)^2 \tag{G.35}$$

respectively. Substitution of these values of b and $-q$ and the value of a as given by (G.17) into (G.33) yields

$$t = \frac{1}{K'K_m + V_m}\left(K_m - \frac{K'K_m + V_m}{2K'}\right)\ln\left(\frac{-2K'C}{b - \sqrt{-q}} + 1\right)\frac{1}{1 - f_{ss}}$$

$$- \frac{1}{2K'}\ln\left(1 - \frac{(K'K_m + V_m)VC + K'VC^2}{k_0 K_m}\right) \tag{G.36}$$

Recognizing that $-2K'C \approx 0$ and $(K'K_m + V_m)VC \gg K'VC^2$, and factoring out $1/2K'$ produces the following expression for t:

$$t = \frac{1}{2K'}\left(\frac{2K'K_m - K'K_m - V_m}{K'K_m + V_m}\ln\frac{1}{1 - f_{ss}}\right.$$

$$\left. - \ln\left\{1 - \frac{[K' + (V_m/K_m)]VC}{k_0}\right\}\right) \tag{G.37}$$

At a low rate of administration Eq. (G.26) reduces to

$$C_{ss} = \frac{k_0}{[K' + (V_m/K_m)]V} \tag{G.38}$$

since $K_m \gg C_{ss}$.

Substitution of $1/C_{ss}$ for $[K' + (V_m/K_m)]V/k_0$ in (G.37), and recognizing that $C/C_{ss} = f_{ss}$, yields

$$t = \frac{-1}{2K'}\left[\frac{K'K_m - V_m}{K'K_m + V_m}\ln(1 - f_{ss}) + \ln(1 - f_{ss})\right] \tag{G.39}$$

which, when $\ln(1 - f_{ss})$ is factored out, becomes

$$t = -\frac{1}{2K'}\left(\frac{K'K_m - V_m}{K'K_m + V_m} + 1\right)\ln(1 - f_{ss}) \tag{G.40}$$

Equation (G.27) can be further simplified to give

$$t = -\frac{1}{K' + (V_m/K_m)}\ln(1 - f_{ss}) \tag{G.41}$$

When the rate of drug administration is very high and the resulting value of C approaches infinity, Eqs. (G.18) and (G.22) can be approximated by

$$b \approx \frac{k_0}{V} \tag{G.42}$$

and

$$-q \underset{\sim}{\sim} b^2 \underset{\sim}{\sim} \left(\frac{k_0}{V}\right)^2 \tag{G.43}$$

respectively. Substitution of these values of b and $-q$ and the value of a as given by (G.17) into (G.33) yields

$$t = \frac{1}{k_0/V}\left(K_m + \frac{k_0/V}{2K'}\right)\ln\left(\frac{-2K'C}{b - \sqrt{-q}} + 1\right)\frac{1}{1 - f_{ss}}$$

$$- \frac{1}{2K'}\ln\left[1 + \frac{(k_0/V)C - K'C^2}{k_0 K_m/V}\right] \tag{G.44}$$

Since $(k_0/V)/2K' \gg K_m$, $-2K'C/(b - \sqrt{-q}) \gg 1$, and $[(k_0/V)C - K'C^2]/(k_0 K_m/V) \gg 1$, Eq. (G.44) can be simplified to

$$t = \frac{1}{2K'}\ln\frac{-2K'C}{b - \sqrt{-q}}\frac{1}{1 - f_{ss}} - \frac{1}{2K'}\ln\frac{k_0 C - K'VC^2}{k_0 K_m} \tag{G.45}$$

Factoring out $1/2K'$ and simplifying the resulting expression gives

$$t = \frac{1}{2K'}\ln\frac{1}{1 - f_{ss}}\frac{-2K'k_0 K_m}{(b - \sqrt{-q})(k_0 - K'VC)} \tag{G.46}$$

Further simplification requires that the term $b - \sqrt{-q}$ be evaluated. Substitution of the values of a and b as given by Eqs. (G.17) and (G.18), respectively, into Eq. (G.22) yields

$$-q = \left(\frac{k_0}{V} - K'K_m - V_m\right)^2 + \frac{4k_0 K_m K'}{V} \tag{G.47}$$

Expansion, collection of common terms, and further simplification results in the following relationship:

$$-q = \left(\frac{k_0}{V}\right)^2 + 2\frac{k_0}{V}(K'K - V_m) - (K'K_m + V_m)^2 \tag{G.48}$$

Factoring out $(k_0/V)^2$ produces

$$-q = \left(\frac{k_0}{V}\right)^2\left[1 + 2\frac{V}{k_0}(K'K_m - V_m) - \left(\frac{V}{k_0}\right)^2(K'K_m + V_m)^2\right] \tag{G.49}$$

the square root of which is given by

$$\sqrt{-q} = \frac{k_0}{V} \left[1 + 2 \frac{V}{k_0} (K'K_m - V_m) - \left(\frac{V}{k_0} \right)^2 (K'K_m + V_m)^2 \right]^{1/2}$$

(G.50)

This is of the form

$$\sqrt{-q} = \frac{k_0}{V} (1 + x)^n$$

(G.51)

where $n = 1/2$, and therefore

$$(1 + x)^{1/2} = \left[1 + 2 \frac{V}{k_0} (K'K_m - V_m) - \left(\frac{V}{k_0} \right)^2 (K'K_m + V_m)^2 \right]^{1/2}$$

(G.52)

The binomial expansion [1] of $(1 + x)^{1/2}$ is

$$(1 + x)^{1/2} = 1 + 1/2x - \frac{1}{8} x^2 + \frac{1}{16} x^3 + \cdots$$

(G.53)

or

$$(1 + x)^{1/2} = 1 + \left[\frac{V}{k_0} (K'K_m - V_m) - 1/2 \left(\frac{V}{k_0} \right)^2 (K'K_m + V_m)^2 \right]$$

$$- \frac{1}{8} \left[2 \frac{V}{k_0} (K'K_m - V_m) - \left(\frac{V}{k_0} \right)^2 (K'K_m + V_m)^2 \right]^2 + \frac{1}{16} \cdots$$

(G.54)

Since k_0 is very large, an approximation of $(1 + x)^{1/2}$ is

$$(1 + x)^{1/2} \simeq 1 + \frac{V}{k_0} (K'K_m - V_m)$$

(G.55)

Substitution of this value of $(1 + x)^n$ into (G.51) and simplification yields

$$\sqrt{-q} = \frac{k_0}{V} + K'K_m - V_m$$

(G.56)

The resulting expression for $b - \sqrt{-q}$, where b and $\sqrt{-q}$ are given by (G.18) and (G.56), respectively, is

$$b - \sqrt{-q} = \frac{k_0}{V} - K'K_m - V_m - \left(\frac{k_0}{V} + K'K_m - V_m \right)$$

(G.57)

which can be further reduced to give

$$b - \sqrt{-q} = -2K'K_m \tag{G.58}$$

The following relationship for t results when this value of $b - \sqrt{-q}$ is substituted into (G.46) and common terms are canceled:

$$t = \frac{1}{2K'} \ln \frac{1}{1 - f_{ss}} \frac{k_0}{k_0 - K'VC} \tag{G.59}$$

At a high rate of drug administration steady-state concentration is given by

$$C_{ss} \sim \frac{k_0}{K'V} \tag{G.60}$$

since under this condition K'V in (G.26) becomes $\gg VV_m/(K_m + C_{ss})$. Substituting k_0/C_{ss} for K'V in (G.59), canceling common terms, and recognizing that C/C_{ss} is f_{ss} produces

$$t = \frac{1}{2K'} \ln \left(\frac{1}{1 - f_{ss}} \right)^2 \tag{G.61}$$

or

$$t = -\frac{1}{K'} \ln(1 - f_{ss}) \tag{G.62}$$

REFERENCE

1. W. H. Beyer (Ed). *CRC Standard Mathematical Tables.* CRC Press, West Palm Beach, Fla., 1978.

Appendix H

Computer Programs

The corresponding appendix in the first edition of this book emphasized simulation programs and nonlinear least-squares regression
programs for use in large computers. In the intervening period,
pharmacokinetic analysis has undergone a distinct change and the ad-
vances in computer technology have been nothing short of revolu-
tionary.

The principal purpose of a pharmacokinetic analysis today is to
gain information regarding the clearance, renal clearance, volume of
distribution, metabolic disposition, accumulation characteristics on
multiple dosing, and absorption of a drug. As we have indicated
throughout this text, model-independent methods are now available
to attain these ends. There is very much less interest in characterizing the pharmacokinetics of a drug in terms of model-dependent constants. Thus there is far less need for nonlinear least-squares regression analysis. This type of analysis remains useful to estimate
the slope of the terminal exponential phase of a polyexponential curve
and the half-life of the drug, but such estimates can usually be
carried out with sufficient accuracy by logarithmic conversion of the
data and the application of linear regression. Moreover, a relatively
simple method termed direct linear plotting has recently been described
[1] which may be more robust than nonlinear least-squares regression
(weighted or unweighted), particularly when the assumption of equal
variance for all experimental data points is incorrect. This method can
be implemented using a programmable calculator or microcomputer [2].

Pharmacokinetic analysis based on curve-fitting is still best carried
out by means of nonlinear estimation programs such as BMDP [3],
NONLIN [4], and SAAM [5], which are designed for use with large
computers. These and similar programs have been discussed by
Metzler [6]. Although relatively little has been written concerning nonlinear least-squares regression programs for microcomputers, considerable development may take place over the next decade. Peck and
Barrett [7] have surveyed the available nonlinear regression programs

and found several written in BASIC, of which at least two [8,9] have
been successfully run on microcomputers with BASIC capability and
8K bytes of random access memory (RAM). These programs have been
found under certain conditions to perform at least as well as NONLIN
and BMDP but have several serious limitations, including limited accuracy and insufficient documentation [7]. More recently, Muir [10]
has described two programs for programmable calculators allowing
nonlinear least-squares fits to data conforming to the one-compartment oral (first-order absorption) and the two-compartment intravenous pharmacokinetic models.

Mathematical description of polyexponential curves by exponential
stripping [11] is easily implemented using a microcomputer or programmable calculator. Several programs have been described, including ESTRIP [12] and STRIPACT [13]. This method, however, is
widely acknowledged to provide an insufficiently definitive analysis.
The value of such programs is viewed in terms of improvement in
accuracy of final parameter estimates (e.g., avoiding unreasonable
final estimates arising from bad initial estimates) when used in conjunction with a nonlinear regression program. Koup [2] has recently
described an exponential stripping program for a microcomputer which
is based on the method of direct linear plotting. This approach may
prove to be more robust than previously described stripping methods.

Although the need for curve-fitting has decreased considerably,
the importance of simulation techniques in pharmacokinetics remains
high. However, these techniques may now be implemented with microcomputers. Koup and Benjamin [14] have described BASIC programs
for use with the Apple II Plus microcomputer which generate graphic
and hard copy simulations of various linear and Michaelis-Menten
pharmacokinetic models. The programs numerically integrate sets of
differential equations for appropriate models. Multiple oral, intramuscular, intravenous bolus, or intravenous infusion doses may be
simulated in any combination. Doses as well as pharmacokinetic
parameters may be changed at the end of each simulated dosing
interval.

It requires no great prescience to suggest that the computational
aspects of pharmacokinetic analysis will be substantially further
simplified in the years ahead.

REFERENCES

1. L. Endrenyi and H.-Y. Tang. Robust parameter estimation for a
    simple kinetic model. *Comput. Biomed. Res.* *13*:430 (1980).
2. J. Koup. Direct linear plotting method for estimation of phar-
    macokinetic parameters. *J. Pharm. Sci.* *70*:1093 (1981).
3. J. Garcia-Pena and S. P. Azen. A user's experience with a
    standard non-linear regression program (BMDP3R). *Comput.
    Programs Biomed.* *10*:185 (1979).

4. C. M. Metzler, G. L. Elfring, and A. J. McEwen. *A User's Manual for NONLIN and Associated Programs*. The Upjohn Co., Kalamazoo, Mich., 1974.

5. M. Berman and M. F. Weiss. *User's Manual for SAAM*. National Institutes of Health, Bethesda, Md., 1974.

6. C. M. Metzler. Factors affecting pharmacokinetic modeling. In *Drug Absorption and Disposition: Statistical Considerations*, K. S. Albert (Ed.). Academy of Pharmaceutical Science, American Pharmaceutical Association, Washington, D.C., 1980, pp. 15–30.

7. C. C. Peck and B. B. Barrett. Nonlinear least-squares regression programs for microcomputers. *J. Pharmacokinet. Biopharm.* 7:537 (1979).

8. E. Patlak and K. Pettigrew. Theoretical and Mathematics Branch, National Institutes of Mental Health, N.I.H., Bethesda, Md., personal communication to C. C. Peck and B. B. Barrett (see Ref. 7), 1976.

9. D. L. Horowitz and L. D. Homer. *Analysis of Biomedical Data by Time-Sharing Computers: I. Non-linear Regression Analysis*. Project No. MR 005:20-2087, Report No. 25, Naval Medical Research Institute, National Naval Medical Center, Bethesda, Md., 1970.

10. K. T. Muir. Nonlinear least-squares regression analysis in pharmacokinetics: Application of a programmable calculator in model parameter estimation. *Comput. Biomed. Res.* 13:307 (1980).

11. A. J. Sedman and J. G. Wagner. CSTRIP, a Fortran IV computer program for obtaining initial polyexponential parameter estimates. *J. Pharm. Sci.* 65:1006 (1976).

12. R. D. Brown and J. E. Manno. ESTRIP, a BASIC computer program for obtaining initial polyexponential parameter estimates. *J. Pharm. Sci.* 67:1687 (1978).

13. J. G. Leferink and R. A. A. Maes. STRIPACT, an interactive curve fit program for pharmacokinetic analysis. *Arzneim. Forsch.* 29:1894 (1979).

14. J. R. Koup and D. R. Benjamin. Numerical integration simulation programs for the microcomputer. *Ther. Drug Monit.* 2:243 (1980).

Author Index

Subject Index